Auto-Inflammatory Syndromes

Petros Efthimiou
Editor

Auto-Inflammatory Syndromes

Pathophysiology, Diagnosis, and Management

Springer

Editor
Petros Efthimiou
New York University School of Medicine
New York, NY
USA

ISBN 978-3-319-96928-2 ISBN 978-3-319-96929-9 (eBook)
https://doi.org/10.1007/978-3-319-96929-9

Library of Congress Control Number: 2018961006

This Springer imprint is published by the registered company Springer Nature Switzerland AG
The registered company address is: Gewerbestrasse 11, 6330 Cham, Switzerland

To my dear wife Olga and my parents, Vasilios and Angeliki, whose patience and unwavering faith and support made this publication possible.

Foreword

The concept of precision medicine came to the fore in early 2015 when President Barack Obama proposed a new Precision Medicine Initiative in his State of the Union Address, which was soon followed by a more detailed exposition from NIH Director Francis Collins and NCI Director Harold Varmus in the *New England Journal of Medicine.* Simply put, the concept of precision medicine entails "prevention and treatment strategies that take individual variability into account," and is based upon the availability of high-dimensional tools for analyzing human biology that have been developed over the last three decades. Of course, the best established of these tools is genomics, which created a human reference sequence through the Human Genome Project, and now includes databases of DNA sequences from literally hundreds of thousands of individuals and a rich set of bioinformatics tools to analyze those data. The functional consequences of genomic variability have been dramatically magnified through the lenses of cell biology, proteomics, and metabolomics. Precision medicine refers not only to a new NIH initiative, but, in a broader sense, to a systematic approach to biomedical science that began to emerge in the 1990s, entailing both an understanding of the genomic basis of human illness and a detailed accounting of how that inherited variability translates into disease phenotypes.

The concept of autoinflammation is a creature of this era, originally invoked almost exactly twenty years ago to describe two inherited diseases characterized by seemingly unprovoked inflammation, but without the high-titer autoantibodies or antigen-specific T cells seen in autoimmune diseases. Over time the concept has evolved to denote a much larger group of diseases, most of which were unknown twenty years ago, in which the innate immune system plays a primary role in disease pathogenesis. The refinement of the idea of autoinflammation, and the rapid expansion of its range, is a case study in how the tools of precision medicine have transformed our understanding of human disease and our approach to patients. Genomic analyses of patients, families, or cohorts have provided key insights into the underlying biology, which have, in turn, had profound implications for new diagnoses and targeted therapies. In the 1990s, genomic studies relied upon linkage analysis in families and the laborious process of positional cloning, but more recently the field has exploded with the advent of next-generation sequencing technologies and whole-exome sequencing (WES) or even whole-genome sequencing (WGS) that enable breakthrough discoveries based on small numbers of patients. Through these advances, clinical medicine and basic science have informed one another in a virtuous feedback loop to give rise to our current understanding of autoinflammatory disease.

Throughout this process, monogenic disease gene discovery has highlighted the importance of some of the newly discovered building blocks of the innate immune system, leading to predictions regarding targeted therapeutic trials that have vindicated emerging biologic concepts. For example, the discovery of gain-of-function *NLRP3* mutations in the three cryopyrin-associated periodic syndromes (CAPS; familial cold autoinflammatory syndrome [FCAS], Muckle-Wells syndrome [MWS], and neonatal-onset multisystem inflammatory disease [NOMID]) in 2001 and 2002 suggested the clinical relevance of Jürg Tschopp's concept of the NLRP3 inflammasome, and led directly to the targeted trials of anakinra, an IL-1 receptor antagonist, in all three conditions. The dramatic success of IL-1 inhibition in these disorders vindicated the concept of the NLRP3 inflammasome as an important driver of IL-1 production and provided the first well-documented example of an *inflammasomopathy*. More recently, the discovery of the intracellular double-stranded DNA sensor STING (stimulator of interferon genes) and shortly thereafter the description of SAVI, a devastating autoinflammatory disorder caused by gain-of-function mutations in STING, highlighted the importance of this molecule in human biology and has led to therapies targeting the JAK-STAT pathway downstream of type I interferons. Both the CAPS/NLRP3 and the SAVI/STING stories are excellent examples of the bedside to bench to bedside feedback loop made possible in the current era of precision medicine.

Identification of patients with mutations in new monogenic disease genes has also led to the discovery that some individuals with similar clinical phenotypes do not have mutations in that newly discovered gene, leading to the eventual identification of a second gene mutated in the patients without mutations in the first. For example, after the positional cloning of *MEFV*, the gene mutated in familial Mediterranean fever (FMF), it became clear that some recurrent fever patients do not have mutations in *MEFV*, even though they had been regarded as having an "FMF-like" illness. A subset manifesting prolonged attacks unresponsive to colchicine were found to have dominantly inherited mutations in *TNFRSF1A,* thus defining an entirely new autoinflammatory disorder, the TNF receptor-associated periodic syndrome (TRAPS). Similarly, the discovery of mutations in *IL1RN*, encoding the IL-1 receptor antagonist, led to the recognition of the deficiency of the IL-1 receptor antagonist (DIRA) in *NLRP3* mutation-negative patients initially thought to have NOMID. Moreover, some of the first patients described with the deficiency of adenosine deaminase 2 (DADA2) were also first thought to have NOMID before they were found to be *NLRP3* mutation-negative. In all of these examples, new diseases are defined through the progression from bedside to bench to bedside catalyzed by the tools of precision medicine.

The field of autoinflammation has also advanced through molecular discoveries that sometimes led to the lumping of seemingly disparate clinical syndromes into common monogenic disorders, rather than the splitting of similar cases into distinct illnesses. One of the earliest examples was the recognition that FCAS, MWS, and NOMID represent a spectrum of phenotypes all caused by mutations in *NLRP3*. This discovery not only simplified the understanding of these diseases, but (correctly) suggested that there might be patients manifesting illness on the continuum between FCAS and MWS or between MWS and NOMID and hastened clinical trials of IL-1 inhibitors across the disease spectrum. Later, the application of targeted deep resequencing of *NLRP3* in leukocyte subpopulations extended the CAPS spectrum to individuals with somatic mutations in *NLRP3* perhaps occurring even in adulthood, thus providing a scientific rationale for the successful use of IL-1 inhibitors in these patients. In another recent example, the discovery of mutations in *ADA2* (formerly *CECR1*) both in children with fevers and recurrent strokes and in an inherited form of polyarteritis nodosa led to the recognition that both are mechanistically related and part of the same spectrum of disease (DADA2). Molecular genetic testing has further extended the spectrum of DADA2 to include patients presenting with pure red cell aplasia, immunodeficiency, and bone marrow failure. Molecular genetics has dramatically accelerated the understanding that these patients are causally related long before the potential observation of individuals with disparate clinical manifestations in the same family.

While the tools of precision medicine have had the most obvious impact on our understanding of monogenic autoinflammatory diseases, they are now beginning to elucidate genetically complex disorders. The difference in pace is largely owing to the fact that the monogenic disorders, although rare, are caused by high-penetrance mutations with relatively easily discernible biologic effects, while the genetically complex disorders are often caused by combinations of common susceptibility variants each with relatively subtle biologic effects, combined with environmental stimuli that are often difficult to document. Although the genetically complex diseases are more common, their analysis requires many more subjects to analyze, primarily through genome-wide association studies (GWAS).

Among the genetically complex autoinflammatory diseases, Adamantiades-Behçet's disease (A-BD) stands out as a case in which the patient collections are sufficient to at least begin to scratch the surface of understanding pathophysiology. There are three major findings worth highlighting. The first is that GWAS performed in both Turkish and Japanese patient collections suggests a complex interaction between the microbiome and the host response in determining disease susceptibility. This includes host structural variants in the major histocompatibility complex and antigen-processing molecules, as well as additional variants controlling mucosal barrier function and the host inflammatory response. Taken individually, these genetic polymorphisms do not predict A-BD susceptibility, but, taken together, they begin to provide testable hypotheses regarding disease pathogenesis. The second major finding is that, at least to the current level of understanding, A-BD is not a collection of high-penetrance monogenic disorders. To date, the only documented monogenic subset is the haploinsufficiency of A20 (HA20), which appears only to comprise a small percentage of sporadic A-BD. The third intriguing finding is that, in comparing A-BD GWAS results with a GWAS of common canker sores (oral aphthae) conducted by the direct-to-consumer genetic testing company 23andMe, there are several susceptibility loci in common, suggesting that A-BD falls on a spectrum that includes a phenotype often considered within the range of normal. The implications are significant, suggesting the eventual reach of autoinflammatory precision medicine into everyday life.

Finally, the fruits of the studies of monogenic autoinflammatory diseases have also begun to extend to genetically complex disorders with an inflammatory component, such as atherosclerosis, type II diabetes, and gout, in which there are other well-documented non-inflammatory pathogenic factors. For several of these diseases, IL-1 has been documented to have an important role in disease progression and severity, leading to clinical trials of IL-1 inhibitors in these illnesses. With proper stratification, such targeted therapies will further extend the scope of autoinflammatory precision medicine.

The publication of this important text is a milestone in the field, permitting even wider dissemination of the key concepts of autoinflammatory diseases into the medical community. The history of the autoinflammatory diseases has featured a highly productive dialogue between clinicians, geneticists, and basic scientists. I am confident that this text will be the catalyst for an even more fruitful discourse in the coming years.

Bethesda, Maryland Dan Kastner, MD, PhD

Preface

Autoinflammatory disease is a newly established and ever-expanding field within the domains of rheumatology and clinical immunology. These inborn disorders of the innate immune system are characterized by episodes of systemic inflammation that are mediated largely by myeloid cells. The field of autoinflammatory diseases was established in 1999, when the tectonic plates of rheumatology moved and a new subfield emerged following the identification of the first genes underlying periodic fever syndromes.

This volume is divided in two parts. The first part deals with the monogenic autoinflammatory diseases, while the polygenic syndromes are addressed in the second part, although the list of the diseases outlined is by no means exhaustive. In order to make this information more accessible and easy-to-use, we selected syndromes that a clinician may encounter in day-to-day practice. This task proved to be challenging in a dynamic and rapidly expanding field where new syndromes and genetic associations are being added with an explosive pace.

The contributing authors were selected because of their expertise and specific interests. Many are widely considered to be international thought leaders in the field of adult and pediatric rheumatology. Beyond being inspirational pioneers in their fields, they are all involved in direct clinical care. Since this publication is aimed toward busy clinicians, the contributors were asked to provide, in concise form, the same practical and clinically relevant information they would convey to physicians who refer patients to them for consultation.

The intended audience for the book is practicing adult and pediatric rheumatologists, clinical immunologists, rheumatology fellows, internists, and pediatricians. However, it is our belief that interested individuals at all levels of medical training may find the content of this book useful and hopefully it will assist them in improving patient care.

New York, NY, USA — Petros Efthimiou

Contents

Contributors

Evangelia Argiriou, MD Department of Physiology, School of Medicine, National and Kapodistrian University of Athens, Athens, Greece

Ezgi Deniz Batu, MD, MSc Department of Pediatrics, Division of Rheumatology, Ankara Training and Research Hospital, University of Health Sciences, Ankara, Turkey

Susanne M. Benseler, MD, PhD Department of Paediatrics, Alberta Children's Hospital, Calgary, AB, Canada

Cumming School of Medicine, University of Calgary, Calgary, AB, Canada

Michael W. Beresford, MD, PhD Department of Women's & Children's Health, Institute of Translational Medicine, University of Liverpool, Liverpool, UK

Department of Paediatric Rheumatology, Alder Hey Children's NHS Foundation Trust Hospital, Liverpool, UK

Fatma Dedeoglu, MD Rheumatology Program/Division of Immunology, Department of Medicine, Boston Children's Hospital, Harvard Medical School, Boston, MA, USA

Selcan Demir, MD Department of Pediatrics, Division of Rheumatology, Hacettepe University Faculty of Medicine, Ankara, Turkey

Arturo Diaz, MD Division of Rheumatology, Beth Israel Deaconess Medical Center, Harvard Medical School, Boston, MA, USA

Petros Efthimiou, MD, FACR New York University School of Medicine, New York, NY, USA

NYU/Langone Health, New York, NY, USA

Christina Maria Flessa, BSc Department of Physiology, School of Medicine, National and Kapodistrian University of Athens, Athens, Greece

Paola Galozzi, PhD Unit of Rheumatology, Department of Medicine – DIMED, University of Padova, Padova, Italy

Marco Gattorno, MD UO Pediatria II, Genoa, Italy

İlkin Elif Günel, MD Department of Pediatrics, Hacettepe University Faculty of Medicine, Ankara, Turkey

Gabriele Hahn, MD Institute of Radiology, Faculty of Medicine Carl Gustav Carus, University of Technology Dresden, Dresden, Germany

Jonathan S. Hausmann, MD Autoinflammatory Diseases Clinic, Boston Children's Hospital, Boston, MA, USA

Autoinflammatory Disease Center, Beth Israel Deaconess Medical Center, Boston, MA, USA

Harvard Medical School, Boston, MA, USA

Christian M. Hedrich, MD, PhD Department of Women's & Children's Health, Institute of Translational Medicine, University of Liverpool, Liverpool, UK

Department of Paediatric Rheumatology, Alder Hey Children's NHS Foundation Trust Hospital, Liverpool, UK

Dirk Holzinger, MD Department of Pediatric Hematology-Oncology, University of Duisburg-Essen, Essen, Germany

María Martha Katsicas, MD Service of Immunology & Rheumatology, Hospital de Pediatría Prof. Dr. Juan P. Garrahan, Buenos Aires, Argentina

Apostolos Kontzias, MD Division of Rheumatology, Allergy and Immunology, Stony Brook University, Stony Brook, NY, USA

Clio P. Mavragani, MD Department of Physiology, School of Medicine, National and Kapodistrian University of Athens, Athens, Greece

Liza McCann, MD Department of Women's & Children's Health, Institute of Translational Medicine, University of Liverpool, Liverpool, UK

Department of Paediatric Rheumatology, Alder Hey Children's NHS Foundation Trust Hospital, Liverpool, UK

Bella Mehta, MBBS Weill Cornell Medicine, New York, NY, USA

Hospital for Special Surgery, New York, NY, USA

Ioannis Mitroulis, MD Institute of Clinical Chemistry and Laboratory Medicine, Technische Universität Dresden, Dresden, Germany

Kitty O'Hare, MD Harvard Medical School, Boston, MA, USA

Transition Medicine for Primary Care, Weitzman Family BRIDGES Adult Transition Program, Boston Children's Hospital, Boston, MA, USA

Pediatric Population Health, Brigham and Women's Hospital, Boston, MA, USA

Karen B. Onel, MD Pediatric Rheumatology, Hospital for Special Surgery/Weill Cornell Medicine, New York, NY, USA

Seza Özen, MD Department of Pediatrics, Division of Rheumatology, Hacettepe University Faculty of Medicine, Ankara, Turkey

Olga Petryna, MD, FACR NYU School of Medicine, Rheumatology Division/ Department of Internal Medicine, New York, NY, USA

Neha Purat, MD, MPH New York Presbyterian Hospital, Department of Internal Medicine, Brooklyn, NY, USA

Andreas Reiff, MD Division Head Rheumatology, Children's Hospital Los Angeles, USC Keck School of Medicine, Los Angeles, CA, USA

Johannes Roth, MD Institute of Immunology, University Hospital Muenster, Muenster, Germany

Ricardo A. G. Russo, MD Service of Immunology & Rheumatology, Hospital de Pediatría Prof. Dr. Juan P. Garrahan, Buenos Aires, Argentina

Grant S. Schulert, MD, PhD Division of Rheumatology, Cincinnati Children's Hospital Medical Center, Cincinnati, OH, USA

Department of Pediatrics, University of Cincinnati, Cincinnati, OH, USA

Petros P. Sfikakis, MD, FACR First Department of Propedeutic & Internal Medicine, National & Kapodistrian University of Athens, Medical School, Athens, Greece

Paolo Sfriso, MD, PhD Unit of Rheumatology, Department of Medicine – DIMED, University of Padova, Padova, Italy

Rebecca Trachtman, MD Icahn School of Medicine at Mount Sinai, New York, NY, USA

Marinka Twilt, MD, MSCE, PhD Alberta Children's Hospital, Calgary, AB, Canada

Athanasios G. Tzioufas, MD Department of Pathophysiology, Medical School, National University of Athens, Athens, Greece

Michael Voulgarelis, MD Department of Pathophysiology, Medical School, National University of Athens, Athens, Greece

Sujani Yadlapati, MD Department of Internal Medicine, Albert Einstein Medical Center, Philadelphia, PA, USA

Qingping Yao, MD, PhD Department of Medicine, Stony Brook University School of Medicine, Stony Brook, NY, USA

Author Biography

Petros Efthimiou is a Board Certified Attending Rheumatologist at NYU Langone Health and Clinical Professor of Medicine and Rheumatology at New York University School of Medicine in New York City, NY, USA.

A *summa cum laude* graduate of the University of Ioannina Medical School in Greece, Dr. Efthimiou became a Research Scholar at Northwestern University College of Medicine in Chicago, Illinois. He then completed his Internal Medicine Residency at Brown University in Providence, Rhode Island, while his Rheumatology Fellowship took place at the Hospital for Special Surgery and New York Presbyterian/Weill Cornell Medicine of Cornell University. The focus of Dr Efthimiou's research has been Adult Autoinflammatory Diseases and, in particular, Adult onset Still's Disease and Macrophage Activation Syndrome.

Chapter 1
Immunology of Auto-inflammatory Syndromes

Grant S. Schulert

Introduction to Innate Immunity and Autoinflammation

Our first line of defense against the microbial world is referred to as the *innate immune system.* Innate immunity represents an ancestrally ancient system that coevolved with microbes and has elements that are remarkably similar to that found in insects, fish, and even plants. Importantly, the innate immune system is distinct from the adaptive immune system, which encompasses effector T cells and antibody producing B cells with a near limitless functional diversity that when dysregulated leads to pathogenic autoimmunity. The primary functions of the innate immune system are to rapidly contain and/or eliminate potential pathogens, remove damaged cells and initiate tissue repair, and activate and regulate specific adaptive immune responses. At the heart of innate immunity are host germline-encoded sensors or *pattern recognition receptors* (Fig. 1.1). During infection, conserved structural moieties or *pathogen-associated molecular patterns* (PAMPs) are recognized by these pattern recognition receptors, which triggers the production of inflammatory chemokines and cytokines including IL-1β, IL-6, TNFα, and type I interferons [1]. Alternatively, signs of tissue injury known as *damage-/danger-associated molecular patterns* (DAMPs) are similarly recognized to further amplify this signaling loop [2]. Innate immune responses lead to the cardinal signs of inflammation: rubor (redness), tumor (swelling), calor (warmth), and dolor (pain), including recruitment of immune effector cells, particularly neutrophils. The paradigm for pattern recognition receptors are the large family of Toll-like receptors (TLR), which are extracellular and intravesicular sensors that evolved from invertebrate

G. S. Schulert
Division of Rheumatology, Cincinnati Children's Hospital Medical Center, Cincinnati, OH, USA

Department of Pediatrics, University of Cincinnati, Cincinnati, OH, USA
e-mail: Grant.Schulert@cchmc.org

P. Efthimiou (ed.), *Auto-Inflammatory Syndromes*,
https://doi.org/10.1007/978-3-319-96929-9_1

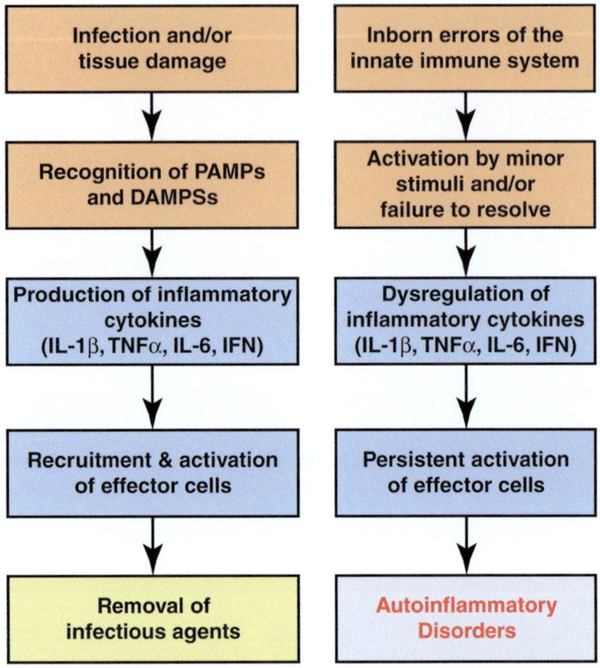

Fig. 1.1 Parallel functions of innate immunity and development of autoinflammation

proteins and recognize an array of bacterial and viral products [3]. In most cases, innate immune responses lead to prompt removal of the infectious agent and resolution of inflammation. In other cases, this innate immune activation serves to initiate an adaptive immune response, ultimately leading to elaboration of T effector cells and specific antibodies directed against the infectious insult.

In contrast, *autoinflammation* represents a disordered and inappropriate innate immune response (Fig. 1.1). Inborn errors in one or more elements of innate immunity lead to chaotic or spontaneous immune activation, with excessive production of inflammatory cytokines. These defects in turn lead to prolonged and persistent activation of immune effector cells, causing the systemic and/or organ-specific features characteristic of autoinflammatory disorders. The concept of autoinflammation was first proposed by Kastner and colleagues in 1999, to describe the hereditary periodic fever syndromes causing systemic inflammation in the absence of classic autoimmune features [4]. It was more formally stated by Masters and colleagues as "seemingly unprovoked, recurrent episodes of fever, serositis, arthritis, and cutaneous inflammation, in the absence of high-titer autoantibodies and antigen-specific T cells" [5] and has since expanded beyond the periodic fever syndromes to include a wide range of monogenic, polygenic, and sporadic diseases.

In this chapter, the innate immune system will be examined, with a particular focus on how defects in these immune sensors and their associated signaling pathways are linked to autoinflammation. This review will focus primarily on the monogenic autoinflammatory syndromes, as their discovery has largely paralleled a revolution in understanding of innate immunity. Genetic diseases can serve as so-called experiments of nature, expanding the understanding of normal host responses while defining disease-specific pathogenic mechanisms. However, similar immune dysfunction likely underlies more complex autoinflammatory disorders discussed throughout this book. It is the hope that this overview of innate immune responses will provide a framework for understanding autoinflammation and inform both clinical diagnosis and rationally directed therapies.

Microbial Sensors: NODs, NOD-Like Receptors, and the Inflammasomopathies

The central molecules of innate immunity are cellular pattern recognition receptors able to sense conserved patterns associated with microbial invaders and/or signs of tissue damage and trigger a rapid inflammatory response. Among these pattern recognition receptors are large families of related intracellular sensors, which are highly conserved evolutionarily, and serve as key mediators in both innate immunity and autoinflammation. These sensors, which include the nucleotide-binding oligomerization domain (NOD) proteins and the NOD-like receptor (NLR) proteins, have been an intense focus of research over the past 15 years [6, 7]. These distinct proteins were recognized to have a shared domain structure, with a variable assembly of so-called pyrin domains, caspase activation and recruitment domains (CARD), and NACHT or NOD domains, suggesting linked roles in inflammation and cell death [8, 9]. These key roles in innate immunity were formally shown in 2002 by Martinon and colleagues, demonstrating that pyrin-domain containing proteins form large, macromolecular complexes able to activate inflammatory caspases and release IL-1β, which they called the *inflammasome*. The subsequent finding that both NOD and NLR proteins can recognize and respond to microbial products [10–12] further defined the emerging paradigm that these molecules represented intracellular pattern recognition receptors with key roles in innate immunity. However, it was also found that dysfunction of these receptors could lead to autoinflammatory diseases. The discovery of the key roles of cytosolic pattern recognition receptors in autoinflammation stems from the initial discovery of *MEFV*, encoding pyrin, as the cause of familial Mediterranean fever (FMF) [13, 14]. This was shortly followed by the linkage of NOD2 mutations to both the monogenic disease Blau syndrome [15] and as risk alleles for inflammatory bowel disease [16, 17] and the discovery of cryopyrin (now referred to as NLRP3) as the causative gene for a family of autoinflammatory conditions now called cryopyrin-associated periodic syndromes (CAPS) [18].

Indeed, many described monogenic autoinflammatory disorders converge at the level of inflammasome assembly and activation (Fig. 1.2). The best characterized of these is NLRP3/cryopyrin, which has key roles in host defense due to its ability to form an inflammasome in response to diverse signals [7]. NLRP3 consists of an N-terminal pyrin domain, a central NOD/NACHT domain, and a C-terminal leucine-rich repeat (LRR) domain. NLRP3 protein expression is rapidly induced in response to proinflammatory stimuli, most notably TLR engagement, often referred

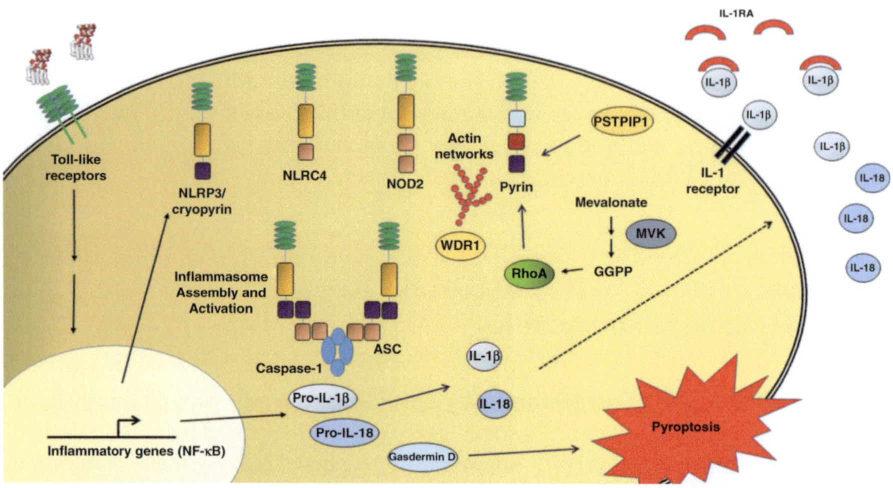

Fig. 1.2 NOD proteins, NLRs, and the inflammasome. Cells express a wide array of innate immune pattern recognition receptors of the NOD and NLR family to recognize pathogens or signs of tissue damage. Upon activation, sensors such as NLRP3/cryopyrin assemble with ASC and caspase-1 into the large inflammasome complex. Inflammasome activation allows for cleavage and release of proinflammatory cytokines including IL-1β and IL-18 and triggers a pro-inflammatory cell death known as pyroptosis. Pyrin also forms an inflammasome, assembly of which involves RhoA inactivation, PSTPIP1, and actin networks including WDR1. Genetic variants in many of these pathways lead to autoinflammation

to as signal 1. Assembly of NLRP3 into an inflammasome is then triggered by a second signal, provided by a diverse array of PAMPs from bacteria, viruses, and parasites, as well as DAMPS such as free ATP and urate crystals [19]. These PAMPs and DAMPs are not believed to directly bind to NLRP3, but rather induce several cellular triggers that collectively release the autoinhibitory LRR domain [20, 21]. Release of autoinhibition allows for NLRP3 oligomerization, mediated by the NOD domain, and binding of the pyrin domain to the inflammasome adapter protein ASC, forming a large filamentous complex. The inflammasome then recruits inactive pro-caspase-1 through homotypic interactions between its CARD domain and that of ASC, forming the inflammasome complex that can be visualized as a so-called speck of nearly 1 μm in size [22]. Activated caspase-1 then mediates the key inflammasome effector functions, namely, proteolytic processing of inactive pro-IL-1β and pro-IL-18 into their bioactive forms, which are released from cells and help initiate host inflammatory responses (Table 1.1). In addition, caspase-1 also activates gasdermin D, a pore-forming protein which leads to a proinflammatory form of cell death known as pyroptosis [23–25]. Collectively, these inflammasome functions and in particular IL-1 lead to endothelial activation, synthesis of acute-phase response proteins by the liver, and initiation of T lymphocyte and natural killer (NK) cells responses, all contributing to successful inflammatory responses to infection or injury [22]. In contrast, autoinflammatory-associated mutations in NLRP3 function in a dominant, gain-of-function manner, leading to spontaneous or

Table 1.1 Cytokines with key roles in innate immunity and autoinflammation

Cytokine	Key functions	Produced by	Targeted therapy
Interleukin-1 (IL-1)	Endothelial activation, fever, acute phase response	Macrophages, endothelial cells	Monoclonal antibodies, recombinant antagonist, inflammasome inhibitors (preclinical)
Interleukin-18 (IL-18)	IFNγ production from NK and T cells	Macrophages	Recombinant antagonist (preclinical)
Tumor necrosis factor (TNFα)	Neutrophil activation, endothelial activation, fever	Macrophages, T cells	Monoclonal antibodies
Interleukin-6 (IL-6)	Acute phase response	Macrophages, T cells, endothelial cells	Monoclonal antibodies
Type I interferon (IFNα/β)	Antiviral state, MHC expression	Macrophages, dendritic cells, fibroblasts	JAK kinase inhibitors
Interleukin-10 (IL-10)	Inhibits cytokine production and costimulatory molecules	Macrophages, regulatory T cells	Recombinant cytokine (preclinical)
Interferon-gamma (IFNγ)	Macrophage activation	NK and T cells	JAK kinase inhibitors, monoclonal antibodies (preclinical)

excessive inflammasome activation. Patients with these variants present as the clinical spectrum of CAPS, with systemic inflammatory episodes of fever, rash, and arthritis/arthralgia, and in some patients more severe symptoms of destructive arthritis, deafness, and CNS inflammation [26].

Several additional NOD and NLR proteins have been linked to autoinflammation (Fig. 1.2). The sensor NLRC4 belongs to a subfamily of receptors which contain N-terminal CARD domains rather than the pyrin domains found in NLRP proteins. NLRC4 detects a variety of bacterial components including flagellin and parts of type 3 secretion systems, through their binding to related Naip proteins. These activated Naips interact with NLRC4, relieving autoinhibition and allowing oligomerization and ultimate inflammasome assembly [19]. Several gain-of-function variants in NLRC4 have recently been described, which likely interrupt the LRR domain and cause constitutive inflammasome activation and release of cytokines, most notably IL-18. Clinically these variants are associated with enterocolitis [27] and recurrent macrophage activation syndrome [28], a life-threatening episode of systemic hyperinflammation causing a cytokine storm [29]. There are also inflammasome-independent roles for NOD proteins in autoinflammation. NOD2 is one of the best characterized PRRs in these families and has a similar structure to NLRC4 but with two N-terminal CARD domains. It senses bacterial muramyl dipeptide through its C-terminal LRR domain; however, it has not been shown to directly form an inflammasome [6]. Rather, NOD2 triggers activation of the kinase RIPK2, which activates NF-κB proinflammatory signaling pathways and release of cytokines, including IL-1β [30, 31]. Mutations in NOD2 near the nucleotide-binding domain are gain-of-function, leading to spontaneous activation and clinically to Blau syndrome and early-onset sarcoidosis [15]. In contrast, variants in the LRR domain of NOD2 are strong genetic risk factors for inflammatory bowel disease [16, 17] and have recently been reported in association with adult-onset autoinflammatory disorders [32]. In addition to these receptors, several additional members of the NLR family including NLRP1, NLRP7, and NLRP12 are linked to inflammatory disorders, further illustrating the central role of these PRRs in linking innate immunity to autoinflammation [7].

Pyrin Inflammasome Dysfunction as a Common Feature of Autoinflammation

An additional inflammasome with key roles in both innate immunity and autoinflammation is the pyrin inflammasome. The pyrin inflammasome is somewhat different, as pyrin is not a member of the NOD/NLR family. Similar to NLRP family members however, pyrin contains its eponymous N-terminal pyrin domain but has an otherwise distinct structure, including a C-terminal B30.2 domain which likely has roles in autorepression [19]. Pyrin also has a novel mechanism of activation, sensing certain bacterial toxins through their ability to inactivate RhoA GTPase [33]. Active RhoA leads to phosphorylation of pyrin, which maintains inhibition of the pyrin inflammasome [34]. Inactivation of RhoA by toxins produced by pathogens such as *Burkholderia*, *Clostridium difficile*, and *C. botulinum* causes dephosphorylation of pyrin and allows for inflammasome assembly [33]. Variants in pyrin cause FMF, the most common monogenic periodic fever syndrome, which occurs primarily in patients with Middle Eastern/Mediterranean background and characterized by episodes of fever, pericarditis, and peritonitis. While originally hypothesized to be recessive and loss-of-function mutations, FMF-associated variants are now felt to be gain-of-function with a gene dosage effect. Pathogenic pyrin variants are primarily in the B30.2 domain and allow for spontaneous inflammasome activation [26], and recent work has confirmed that FMF-associated mutations decrease the activation threshold of pyrin in a dose-dependent manner [35].

Recent work has defined pyrin inflammasome activation as a shared feature in several other autoinflammatory disorders and in the process highlighted key cellular pathways with central roles in regulating innate immune responses. Deficiency of mevalonate kinase was one of the earliest recognized autoinflammatory periodic fever syndromes, and represents a disease spectrum ranging from hyper-IgD syndrome (HIDS) to the severe metabolic disorder mevalonic aciduria [36]. It has been well established that this syndrome is due to a lack of flux through the mevalonate biosynthetic pathway, leading to deficiency in key isoprenoids necessary for proper function of Rho-family GTPases, such as geranylgeranyl pyrophosphate (GGPP), but how this triggered autoinflammation had remained elusive [37]. Recent work highlighting the key role of RhoA in pyrin inflammasome assembly may provide a mechanistic answer (Fig. 1.2). Mutations in mevalonate kinase cause loss of GGPP, which inactivates RhoA and potentiates pyrin inflammasome assembly while also increasing pyrin gene expression [33, 34, 38]. Regulation of pyrin inflammasome assembly underlies other recently described autoinflammatory disorders as well. Mutations in the adapter protein PSTPIP1 have been linked to pyrogenic arthritis with pyoderma gangrenosum and acne (PAPA) syndrome [39], as well as a recently described autoinflammatory syndrome with hyperzincemia and hypercalprotectinemia [40]. PSTPIP1 binds pyrin, releases its autoinhibition, and allows for inflammasome assembly [41]. Pyrin inflammasomes have also been shown to assemble in association with actin [42], and loss of the actin-depolarizing factor WD repeat-containing protein-1 (WDR1) causes excessive pyrin activation in mice [43]. Recently loss-of-function mutations in WDR1 have also been shown to cause an autoinflammatory periodic fever syndrome in humans [44]. These autoinflammatory disorders illustrate the complex cellular pathways that contribute to pyrin inflammasome function.

Cytokines as Key Mediators of Innate Immunity and Autoinflammation

Recognition of PAMPs and DAMPs by sensors including inflammasomes triggers rapid immune responses, mediated in large measure by cytokines (Table 1.1). Cytokines influence cellular function by signaling through their receptors, which include at least five families with broadly similar functional properties. Among these receptors are type I and type II receptors that signal through the Jak/STAT pathways, TNF and IL-1 superfamily that signal through the NF-κB pathway, and IL-17 family leading to activation of multiple pathways including both NF-κB and C/EBP transcription factors [45]. Together, the function of proinflammatory cytokines induced by pattern recognition receptors leads to activation of both leukocytes and endothelial cells, coagulation, fever, and induction of the acute-phase response by the liver. The innate immune system utilizes similarly diverse mechanisms to attenuate and resolve the effects of proinflammatory cytokines. Among these mechanisms are inhibitory and decoy receptors, soluble receptor antagonists, shedding or downregulation of receptors, and functions of anti-inflammatory cytokines such as IL-10 [45]. Regarding IL-1, the central cytokine linked to autoinflammation, there exists a natural cytokine antagonist, IL-1 receptor antagonist (IL-1RA), which neutralizes the cytokine in vivo (Fig. 1.2). Indeed, recombinant IL-1RA (anakinra) is a highly effective treatment for a broad spectrum of autoinflammatory disorders [46]. Genetic loss of IL-1RA leads to a systemic autoinflammatory disorder known as deficiency of IL-1RA (DIRA) [47]. IL-10 is a type II cytokine with key anti-inflammatory functions, signaling through its receptor to decrease expression of proinflammatory cytokines including IL-1β [48]. Patients deficient in IL-10 itself or the two components of its receptor, *IL10RA* and *IL10RB*, present with early-onset inflammatory bowel disease [49, 50], highlighting the key role of this system in regulating innate immunity.

One of the earliest recognized autoinflammatory disorders was termed familial Hibernian fever due to its association with Scottish/Irish families and distinguished from FMF by longer duration episodes of fever, conjunctival and periorbital inflammation, rash, and arthritis [51]. Ultimately familial Hibernian fever was linked to dominantly inherited mutations in the 55 kDa receptor for TNFα, TNFR1 (encoded by *TNFRSF1A*), and renamed TNFα receptor associated periodic syndrome (TRAPS) [4]. The pathophysiology of how mutations in TNRF1 lead to systemic autoinflammation remains unclear. TRAPS patients have a dramatic clinical response to IL-1 blockade therapy [52], but inflammasome dysfunction in this syndrome remains largely unexplored. Patients with TRAPS carry heterozygous missense mutations, typically in the extracellular domain of the receptor, while deletions or frameshift mutations have not been reported, strongly suggesting that TRAPS variants confer a gain-of-function phenotype [53]. These variants do not appear to lead to constitutive receptor activation or increased ligand binding affinity [4]. TRAPS variants may impair the shedding of TNFR1 after ligand binding and causing sustained proinflammatory signaling, but this is not the case for all disease-associated mutations [54, 55]. More recent work has suggested that TRAPS variants can cause impaired intracellular oligomerization of TNFR1, leading to misfolding and retention in the endoplasmic reticulum [56]. Indeed, TRAPS variants have been shown to sensitize cells to PAMPs such as the TLR4 ligand lipopolysaccharide, leading to excessive inflammatory cytokine production [57, 58].

Local effects of cytokines on immune cells and the endothelium have key roles in limiting tissue damage and controlling infections. However, overwhelming and dysregulated cytokine responses on a systemic level can lead to life threatening complications, as seen in sepsis. These states of immunopathology have been termed "cytokine storm syndromes," with massive and deleterious production of proinflammatory cytokines [59]. When such cytokine storms occur in the context of rheumatic diseases or autoinflammation, it is classified as macrophage activation syndrome (MAS). MAS occurs most commonly in patients with systemic juvenile idiopathic arthritis, a chronic childhood arthropathy with features of autoinflammation including uncontrolled IL-1β production [29]. However, MAS has been reported in patients with numerous other rheumatic diseases, including the monogenic periodic fever syndromes [60]. While the underlying mechanisms that trigger MAS are complex and multifactorial [61], patients with MAS display remarkably high levels of numerous cytokines including IL-1, IL-6, IL-10, IL-18, TNFα, and IFNγ, which drive immune dysfunction and lead to end-organ damage [29]. In particular, it is felt that excessive activation of IFNγ, likely due to IL-18, has a central role in MAS pathogenesis [28, 62–64]. While the mainstay of treatment for MAS is high-dose corticosteroids, there is increasing interest in using cytokine-directed therapy against IL-1, IL-18, and IFNγ [65–69].

Type I Interferon Response and Interferonopathies

A distinct innate immune pathway from the inflammasome-induced IL-1 cascade is the type I interferon response (Fig. 1.3). Type I interferons (particularly IFNα and IFNβ) are rapidly induced in response to a wide array of PAMPs but in particular nucleic acids from viral pathogens including both single-stranded and double-stranded RNA and DNA. Type I interferons then elicit a potent antiviral response, signaling through interferon receptors in an autocrine manner to inhibit viral replication in infected cells. In addition, interferons also have paracrine effects to produce an antiviral state in neighboring cells [70]. Interferon receptor activation induces the JAK/STAT signaling pathway, leading to activation of interferon regulatory factor 9 (IRF9) and amplification of this interferon loop [71]. Type I interferon also serves as a key link between innate immunity and effector cells of the adaptive immune system. Type I interferons enhance cytotoxicity of NK cells [72, 73], induce maturation of dendritic cells [74, 75], and impact generation of effector and memory B and T cells [76, 77]. Endogenous RNA and DNA can also serve as DAMPs to activate the interferon response in response to cellular injury. In these settings, interferons are felt to play a key pathogenic role in some autoimmune disease, most notably lupus, where overproduction of type I interferons are central to disease onset and flare [78].

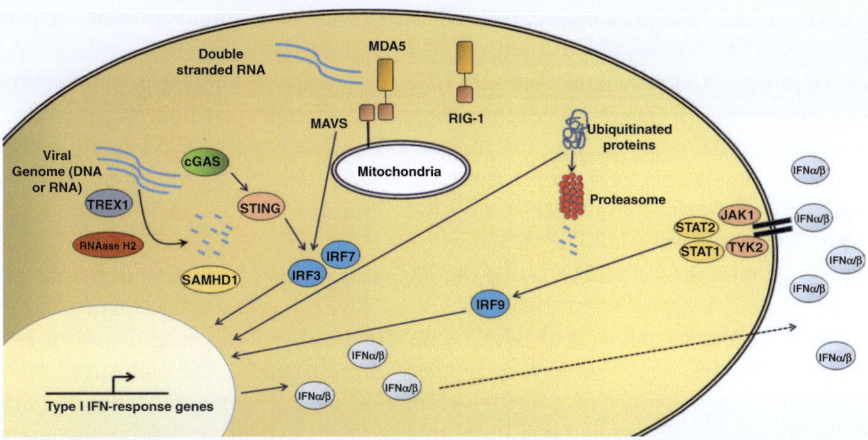

Fig. 1.3 Type I interferon response and the interferonopathies. The innate immune system is triggered by both viral and host-derived cytosolic nucleotides, including RNA and DNA, to initiate the type I interferon response. These nucleotides are detected through several systems, including cGAS activation of STING, as well as RIG-1 and MDA5, which together with MAVS activate IRF3/7. IRF activation produces IFNα and IFNβ, which amplify this loop by signaling through their receptor and JAK/STAT pathways to further enhance interferon production. The type I interferon response is limited by several proteins which degrades cytosolic nucleotides, including TREX1, SAMHD1, and RNAsae H2. Genetic variants in these sensors and regulatory mechanisms cause excessive interferon production, autoinflammation, and in some cases autoimmunity

While the interferon response has been recognized as a potent inflammatory cascade for more than half a century, the specific pattern recognition receptors and molecular pathways that induce interferon have only recently been understood [79]. Central to this response is the stimulator of IFN genes (STING), which was identified as an ER-associated adapter essential for induction of type I interferon by intracellular DNA [80, 81] (Fig. 1.3). STING directly senses cyclic GMP-AMP (cGAMP) [82], which are produced by an intracellular DNA sensor known as cGAMP synthase (cGAS) [83, 84]. STING then triggers activation of IRF3 and production of type I interferons. Recently, de novo variants in STING have been described in patients with systemic inflammation and severe vasculopathy affecting the skin, lungs, and other organs and termed STING-associated vasculopathy of infancy (SAVI) [85]. SAVI variants cause a gain-of-function phenotype, leading to constitutive STING activation and high type I interferon signature. Interferon signaling can be blocked through selective JAK kinase inhibitors [85] and subsequently has been shown that SAVI patients have good clinical response to such treatment [86, 87]. As SAVI involves dysfunctional innate immune mechanisms leading to autoinflammation, but distinct from classic inflammasome-mediated disorders, it was proposed to represent an *autoinflammatory interferonopathy* [88, 89].

Indeed, an expanding class of autoinflammatory conditions involve similar defects in innate immune sensing, leading to excessive type I interferon activation. Viral RNA are recognized by the retinoic acid-inducible (RIG) like receptors including RIG-1 and MDA5, which contain CARD domains as found in NLR proteins (Fig. 1.3). RIG-1 primarily recognizes short, double-stranded RNA, while MDA5 (encoded by *IFIH1*) recognizes longer RNA molecules [90, 91]. Upon activation, RIG-like receptors undergo a conformational change allowing homotypic binding of CARD domains to those in the mitochondrial-localized MAVS1 or interferon promoter stimulator 1 [92]. Interactions with MAVS1 lead to formation of a large functional aggregate that induces type I interferon production [93, 94]. Numerous proteins play key roles in limiting and resolving the cytosolic nucleic acids that are key stimulators for both STING and the RIG-like receptors. Among these mechanisms are DNA repair exonucleases such as TREX1 and ribonucleases such as RNase H2 complex, as well as SAMHD1, which restricts the availability of free deoxynucleotides. Recessive defects in many of these suppressive pathways lead to Aicardi-Goutieres syndrome (AGS), a childhood onset encephalopathy with notably high IFN production and risk for autoimmunity [95–98]. Activating mutations in several of these, including TREX1 and MDA5, can also cause monogenic lupus [99]. Finally, the immunoproteasome has central roles in innate immunity by degrading intracellular proteins tagged for disposal by ubiquitination (Fig. 1.3). PSMB8 is an inducible proteasome catalytic component, mutations in which cause defective assembly and accumulation of ubiquitinated proteins [100, 101]. PSMB8 dysfunction leads to a syndrome known as chronic atypical neutrophilic dermatosis with lipodystrophy and elevated temperature (CANDLE), and additive defects in these subunits lead to activation of the type I interferon pathway through unknown mechanisms [102].

Conclusions and the Road Ahead

Innate immunity represents the host's essential first line of defense against the microbial world, linking recognition of microbial patterns with immediate inflammatory responses. Multicellular organisms have evolved numerous overlapping and redundant families of pattern recognition receptors to detect signs of damage and invasion, potent cytokine messengers to mediate inflammatory responses, and mechanisms to resolve and limit pathogenic inflammation. While an inadequate innate immune response can leave a host vulnerable to possibly fatal infections, excessive or uncontrolled responses also lead to significant pathology that we now recognize as autoinflammation. As the various pattern recognition systems largely converge at the level of cytokine production, cytokine-directed therapies have been greatly beneficial in treating autoinflammation (Table 1.1). Next-generation sequencing and other high-throughput technologies have increased the pace of discovery, with numerous new autoinflammatory conditions identified annually [103]. While newly discovered syndromes allow for better diagnosis and treatment of individual patients, in parallel, they further expand our understanding of the underlying biology of innate immunity.

References

1. Netea MG, Balkwill F, Chonchol M, et al. A guiding map for inflammation. Nat Immunol. 2017;18:826–31. https://doi.org/10.1038/ni.3790.
2. Matzinger P. The danger model: a renewed sense of self. Science. 2002;296:301–5. https://doi.org/10.1126/science.1071059.
3. Pandey S, Kawai T, Akira S. Microbial sensing by Toll-like receptors and intracellular nucleic acid sensors. Cold Spring Harb Perspect Biol. 2014;7:a016246. https://doi.org/10.1101/cshperspect.a016246.
4. McDermott MF, Aksentijevich I, Galon J, et al. Germline mutations in the extracellular domains of the 55 kDa TNF receptor, TNFR1, define a family of dominantly inherited autoinflammatory syndromes. Cell. 1999;97:133–44.
5. Masters SL, Simon A, Aksentijevich I, et al. Horror autoinflammaticus: the molecular pathophysiology of autoinflammatory disease (*). Annu Rev Immunol. 2009;27:621–68. https://doi.org/10.1146/annurev.immunol.25.022106.141627.
6. Philpott DJ, Sorbara MT, Robertson SJ, et al. NOD proteins: regulators of inflammation in health and disease. Nat Rev Immunol. 2014;14:9–23. https://doi.org/10.1038/nri3565.
7. Zhong Y, Kinio A, Saleh M. Functions of NOD-like receptors in human diseases. Front Immunol. 2013;4:333. https://doi.org/10.3389/fimmu.2013.00333.
8. Kastner DL, O'Shea JJ. A fever gene comes in from the cold. Nat Genet. 2001;29:241–2. https://doi.org/10.1038/ng1101-241.
9. Martinon F, Hofmann K, Tschopp J. The pyrin domain: a possible member of the death domain-fold family implicated in apoptosis and inflammation. Curr Biol. 2001;11:R118–20.
10. Mariathasan S, Newton K, Monack DM, et al. Differential activation of the inflammasome by caspase-1 adaptors ASC and Ipaf. Nature. 2004;430:213–8. https://doi.org/10.1038/nature02664.
11. Inohara N, Ogura Y, Fontalba A, et al. Host recognition of bacterial muramyl dipeptide mediated through NOD2. Implications for Crohn's disease. J Biol Chem. 2003;278:5509–12. https://doi.org/10.1074/jbc.C200673200.

12. Girardin SE, Boneca IG, Carneiro LAM, et al. Nod1 detects a unique muropeptide from gram-negative bacterial peptidoglycan. Science. 2003;300:1584–7. https://doi.org/10.1126/science.1084677.
13. Ancient missense mutations in a new member of the RoRet gene family are likely to cause familial Mediterranean fever. The International FMF Consortium. Cell. 1997;90:797–807.
14. French FMF Consortium, Bernot A, Clepet C, et al. A candidate gene for familial Mediterranean fever. Nat Genet. 1997;17:25–31. https://doi.org/10.1038/ng0997-25.
15. Miceli-Richard C, Lesage S, Rybojad M, et al. CARD15 mutations in Blau syndrome. Nat Genet. 2001;29:19–20. https://doi.org/10.1038/ng720.
16. Hugot JP, Chamaillard M, Zouali H, et al. Association of NOD2 leucine-rich repeat variants with susceptibility to Crohn's disease. Nature. 2001;411:599–603. https://doi.org/10.1038/35079107.
17. Ogura Y, Bonen DK, Inohara N, et al. A frameshift mutation in NOD2 associated with susceptibility to Crohn's disease. Nature. 2001;411:603–6. https://doi.org/10.1038/35079114.
18. Hoffman HM, Mueller JL, Broide DH, et al. Mutation of a new gene encoding a putative pyrin-like protein causes familial cold autoinflammatory syndrome and Muckle-Wells syndrome. Nat Genet. 2001;29:301–5. https://doi.org/10.1038/ng756.
19. Mathur A, Hayward JA, Man SM. Molecular mechanisms of inflammasome signaling. J Leukoc Biol. 2017;:jlb.3MR0617-250R. https://doi.org/10.1189/jlb.3MR0617-250R.
20. He Y, Zeng MY, Yang D, et al. NEK7 is an essential mediator of NLRP3 activation downstream of potassium efflux. Nature. 2016;530:354–7. https://doi.org/10.1038/nature16959.
21. Shi H, Wang Y, Li X, et al. NLRP3 activation and mitosis are mutually exclusive events coordinated by NEK7, a new inflammasome component. Nat Immunol. 2016;17:250–8. https://doi.org/10.1038/ni.3333.
22. Franchi L, Muñoz-Planillo R, Núñez G. Sensing and reacting to microbes through the inflammasomes. Nat Immunol. 2012;13:325–32. https://doi.org/10.1038/ni.2231.
23. Kayagaki N, Stowe IB, Lee BL, et al. Caspase-11 cleaves gasdermin D for non-canonical inflammasome signalling. Nature. 2015;526:666–71. https://doi.org/10.1038/nature15541.
24. He W, Wan H, Hu L, et al. Gasdermin D is an executor of pyroptosis and required for interleukin-1β secretion. Cell Res. 2015;25:1285–98. https://doi.org/10.1038/cr.2015.139.
25. Shi J, Zhao Y, Wang K, et al. Cleavage of GSDMD by inflammatory caspases determines pyroptotic cell death. Nature. 2015;526:660–5. https://doi.org/10.1038/nature15514.
26. Manthiram K, Zhou Q, Aksentijevich I, et al. The monogenic autoinflammatory diseases define new pathways in human innate immunity and inflammation. Nat Immunol. 2017;18:832–42. https://doi.org/10.1038/ni.3777.
27. Romberg N, Al Moussawi K, Nelson-Williams C, et al. Mutation of NLRC4 causes a syndrome of enterocolitis and autoinflammation. Nat Genet. 2014;46:1135–9. https://doi.org/10.1038/ng.3066.
28. Canna SW, de Jesus AA, Gouni S, et al. An activating NLRC4 inflammasome mutation causes autoinflammation with recurrent macrophage activation syndrome. Nat Genet. 2014;46:1140–6. https://doi.org/10.1038/ng.3089.
29. Schulert GS, Grom AA. Pathogenesis of macrophage activation syndrome and potential for cytokine- directed therapies. Annu Rev Med. 2015;66:145–59. https://doi.org/10.1146/annurev-med-061813-012806.
30. Maeda S, Hsu L-C, Liu H, et al. Nod2 mutation in Crohn's disease potentiates NF-kappaB activity and IL-1beta processing. Science. 2005;307:734–8. https://doi.org/10.1126/science.1103685.
31. Kobayashi KS, Chamaillard M, Ogura Y, et al. Nod2-dependent regulation of innate and adaptive immunity in the intestinal tract. Science. 2005;307:731–4. https://doi.org/10.1126/science.1104911.
32. Yao Q. Nucleotide-binding oligomerization domain containing 2: structure, function, and diseases. Semin Arthritis Rheum. 2013;43:125–30. https://doi.org/10.1016/j.semarthrit.2012.12.005.

33. Xu H, Yang J, Gao W, et al. Innate immune sensing of bacterial modifications of rho GTPases by the Pyrin inflammasome. Nature. 2014;513:237–41. https://doi.org/10.1038/nature13449.
34. Park YH, Wood G, Kastner DL, et al. Pyrin inflammasome activation and RhoA signaling in the autoinflammatory diseases FMF and HIDS. Nat Immunol. 2016;17:914–21. https://doi.org/10.1038/ni.3457.
35. Jamilloux Y, Lefeuvre L, Magnotti F, et al. Familial Mediterranean fever mutations are hypermorphic mutations that specifically decrease the activation threshold of the Pyrin inflammasome. Rheumatology (Oxford). Published Online First: 12 October 2017. https://doi.org/10.1093/rheumatology/kex373.
36. Favier LA, Schulert GS. Mevalonate kinase deficiency: current perspectives. Appl Clin Genet. 2016;9:101–10. https://doi.org/10.2147/TACG.S93933.
37. van der Burgh R, Ter Haar NM, Boes ML, et al. Mevalonate kinase deficiency, a metabolic autoinflammatory disease. Clin Immunol. 2013;147:197–206. https://doi.org/10.1016/j.clim.2012.09.011.
38. Akula MK, Shi M, Jiang Z, et al. Control of the innate immune response by the mevalonate pathway. Nat Immunol. 2016;17:922–9. https://doi.org/10.1038/ni.3487.
39. Wise CA, Gillum JD, Seidman CE, et al. Mutations in CD2BP1 disrupt binding to PTP PEST and are responsible for PAPA syndrome, an autoinflammatory disorder. Hum Mol Genet. 2002;11:961–9.
40. Holzinger D, Fassl SK, de Jager W, et al. Single amino acid charge switch defines clinically distinct proline-serine-threonine phosphatase-interacting protein 1 (PSTPIP1)-associated inflammatory diseases. J Allergy Clin Immunol. 2015;136:1337–45. https://doi.org/10.1016/j.jaci.2015.04.016.
41. Yu J-W, Fernandes-Alnemri T, Datta P, et al. Pyrin activates the ASC pyroptosome in response to engagement by autoinflammatory PSTPIP1 mutants. Mol Cell. 2007;28:214–27. https://doi.org/10.1016/j.molcel.2007.08.029.
42. Waite AL, Schaner P, Hu C, et al. Pyrin and ASC co-localize to cellular sites that are rich in polymerizing actin. Exp Biol Med (Maywood). 2009;234:40–52. https://doi.org/10.3181/0806-RM-184.
43. Kim ML, Chae JJ, Park YH, et al. Aberrant actin depolymerization triggers the pyrin inflammasome and autoinflammatory disease that is dependent on IL-18, not IL-1β. J Exp Med. 2015;212:927–38. https://doi.org/10.1084/jem.20142384.
44. Standing ASI, Malinova D, Hong Y, et al. Autoinflammatory periodic fever, immunodeficiency, and thrombocytopenia (PFIT) caused by mutation in actin-regulatory gene WDR1. J Exp Med. 2017;214:59–71. https://doi.org/10.1084/jem.20161228.
45. Gadina M, Gazaniga N, Vian L, et al. Small molecules to the rescue: inhibition of cytokine signaling in immune-mediated diseases. J Autoimmun. Published Online First: 1 July 2017. https://doi.org/10.1016/j.jaut.2017.06.006.
46. Goldbach-Mansky R, Kastner DL. Autoinflammation: the prominent role of IL-1 in monogenic autoinflammatory diseases and implications for common illnesses. J Allergy Clin Immunol. 2009;124:1141–9. https://doi.org/10.1016/j.jaci.2009.11.016.
47. Aksentijevich I, Masters SL, Ferguson PJ, et al. An autoinflammatory disease with deficiency of the interleukin-1-receptor antagonist. N Engl J Med. 2009;360:2426–37. https://doi.org/10.1056/NEJMoa0807865.
48. Shouval DS, Biswas A, Kang YH, et al. Interleukin 1β mediates intestinal inflammation in mice and patients with interleukin 10 receptor deficiency. Gastroenterology. 2016;151:1100–4. https://doi.org/10.1053/j.gastro.2016.08.055.
49. Kotlarz D, Beier R, Murugan D, et al. Loss of interleukin-10 signaling and infantile inflammatory bowel disease: implications for diagnosis and therapy. Gastroenterology. 2012;143:347–55. https://doi.org/10.1053/j.gastro.2012.04.045.
50. Glocker E-O, Kotlarz D, Boztug K, et al. Inflammatory bowel disease and mutations affecting the interleukin-10 receptor. N Engl J Med. 2009;361:2033–45. https://doi.org/10.1056/NEJMoa0907206.

51. Williamson LM, Hull D, Mehta R, et al. Familial Hibernian fever. Q J Med. 1982;51:469–80.
52. Gattorno M, Obici L, Cattalini M, et al. Canakinumab treatment for patients with active recurrent or chronic TNF receptor-associated periodic syndrome (TRAPS): an open-label, phase II study. Ann Rheum Dis. 2017;76:173–8. https://doi.org/10.1136/annrheumdis-2015-209031.
53. Cantarini L, Lucherini OM, Muscari I, et al. Tumour necrosis factor receptor-associated periodic syndrome (TRAPS): state of the art and future perspectives. Autoimmun Rev. 2012;12:38–43. https://doi.org/10.1016/j.autrev.2012.07.020.
54. Aganna E, Hammond L, Hawkins PN, et al. Heterogeneity among patients with tumor necrosis factor receptor-associated periodic syndrome phenotypes. Arthritis Rheum. 2003;48:2632–44. https://doi.org/10.1002/art.11215.
55. Aksentijevich I, Galon J, Soares M, et al. The tumor-necrosis-factor receptor-associated periodic syndrome: new mutations in TNFRSF1A, ancestral origins, genotype-phenotype studies, and evidence for further genetic heterogeneity of periodic fevers. Am J Hum Genet. 2001;69:301–14. https://doi.org/10.1086/321976.
56. Lobito AA, Kimberley FC, Muppidi JR, et al. Abnormal disulfide-linked oligomerization results in ER retention and altered signaling by TNFR1 mutants in TNFR1-associated periodic fever syndrome (TRAPS). Blood. 2006;108:1320–7. https://doi.org/10.1182/blood-2005-11-006783.
57. Simon A, Park H, Maddipati R, et al. Concerted action of wild-type and mutant TNF receptors enhances inflammation in TNF receptor 1-associated periodic fever syndrome. Proc Natl Acad Sci U S A. 2010;107:9801–6. https://doi.org/10.1073/pnas.0914118107.
58. Bulua AC, Simon A, Maddipati R, et al. Mitochondrial reactive oxygen species promote production of proinflammatory cytokines and are elevated in TNFR1-associated periodic syndrome (TRAPS). J Exp Med. 2011;208:519–33. https://doi.org/10.1084/jem.20102049.
59. Behrens EM, Koretzky GA. Review: cytokine storm syndrome: looking toward the precision medicine era. Arthritis Rheumatol. 2017;69:1135–43. https://doi.org/10.1002/art.40071.
60. Rigante D, Emmi G, Fastiggi M, et al. Macrophage activation syndrome in the course of monogenic autoinflammatory disorders. Clin Rheumatol. 2015;34:1333. https://doi.org/10.1007/s10067-015-2923-0.
61. Schulert GS, Canna SW. Convergent pathways of the hyperferritinemic syndromes. Int Immunol. 2018;30:195–203. https://doi.org/10.1093/intimm/dxy012.
62. Bracaglia C, de Graaf K, Pires Marafon D, et al. Elevated circulating levels of interferon-γ and interferon-γ-induced chemokines characterise patients with macrophage activation syndrome complicating systemic juvenile idiopathic arthritis. Ann Rheum Dis. 2017;76:166–72. https://doi.org/10.1136/annrheumdis-2015-209020.
63. Shimizu M, Nakagishi Y, Yachie A. Distinct subsets of patients with systemic juvenile idiopathic arthritis based on their cytokine profiles. Cytokine. 2013;61:345–8. https://doi.org/10.1016/j.cyto.2012.11.025.
64. Put K, Avau A, Brisse E, et al. Cytokines in systemic juvenile idiopathic arthritis and haemophagocytic lymphohistiocytosis: tipping the balance between interleukin-18 and interferon-γ. Rheumatology (Oxford). 2015;54:1507–17. https://doi.org/10.1093/rheumatology/keu524.
65. Canna SW, Girard C, Malle L, et al. Life-threatening NLRC4-associated hyperinflammation successfully treated with IL-18 inhibition. J Allergy Clin Immunol. 2017;139:1698–701. https://doi.org/10.1016/j.jaci.2016.10.022.
66. Durand M, Troyanov Y, Laflamme P, et al. Macrophage activation syndrome treated with anakinra. J Rheumatol. 2010;37:879–80. https://doi.org/10.3899/jrheum.091046.
67. Kelly A, Ramanan AV. A case of macrophage activation syndrome successfully treated with anakinra. Nat Clin Pract Rheumatol. 2008;4:615–20. https://doi.org/10.1038/ncprheum0919.
68. Kahn PJ, Cron RQ. Higher-dose Anakinra is effective in a case of medically refractory macrophage activation syndrome. J Rheumatol. 2013;40:743–4. https://doi.org/10.3899/jrheum.121098.
69. Prencipe G, Caiello I, Pascarella A, et al. Neutralization of IFN-γ reverts clinical and laboratory features in a mouse model of macrophage activation syndrome. J Allergy Clin Immunol. 2017. Published Online First: 12 August 2017. https://doi.org/10.1016/j.jaci.2017.07.021.

70. Fuertes MB, Woo S-R, Burnett B, et al. Type I interferon response and innate immune sensing of cancer. Trends Immunol. 2013;34:67–73. https://doi.org/10.1016/j.it.2012.10.004.
71. Darnell JE, Kerr IM, Stark GR. Jak-STAT pathways and transcriptional activation in response to IFNs and other extracellular signaling proteins. Science. 1994;264:1415–21.
72. Lee CK, Rao DT, Gertner R, et al. Distinct requirements for IFNs and STAT1 in NK cell function. J Immunol. 2000;165:3571–7.
73. Nguyen KB, Salazar-Mather TP, Dalod MY, et al. Coordinated and distinct roles for IFN-alpha beta, IL-12, and IL-15 regulation of NK cell responses to viral infection. J Immunol. 2002;169:4279–87.
74. Montoya M, Schiavoni G, Mattei F, et al. Type I interferons produced by dendritic cells promote their phenotypic and functional activation. Blood. 2002;99:3263–71.
75. Spadaro F, Lapenta C, Donati S, et al. IFN-α enhances cross-presentation in human dendritic cells by modulating antigen survival, endocytic routing, and processing. Blood. 2012;119:1407–17. https://doi.org/10.1182/blood-2011-06-363564.
76. Fink K, Lang KS, Manjarrez-Orduno N, et al. Early type I interferon-mediated signals on B cells specifically enhance antiviral humoral responses. Eur J Immunol. 2006;36:2094–105. https://doi.org/10.1002/eji.200635993.
77. Kolumam GA, Thomas S, Thompson LJ, et al. Type I interferons act directly on CD8 T cells to allow clonal expansion and memory formation in response to viral infection. J Exp Med. 2005;202:637–50. https://doi.org/10.1084/jem.20050821.
78. Shrivastav M, Niewold TB. Nucleic acid sensors and type I interferon production in systemic lupus erythematosus. Front Immunol. 2013;4:319. https://doi.org/10.3389/fimmu.2013.00319.
79. Jensen KE, Neal AL, Owens RE, et al. Interferon responses of Chick embryo fibroblasts to nucleic acids and related compounds. Nature. 1963;200:433–4.
80. Ishikawa H, Ma Z, Barber GN. STING regulates intracellular DNA-mediated, type I interferon-dependent innate immunity. Nature. 2009;461:788–92. https://doi.org/10.1038/nature08476.
81. Ishikawa H, Barber GN. STING is an endoplasmic reticulum adaptor that facilitates innate immune signalling. Nature. 2008;455:674–8. https://doi.org/10.1038/nature07317.
82. Burdette DL, Monroe KM, Sotelo-Troha K, et al. STING is a direct innate immune sensor of cyclic di-GMP. Nature. 2011;478:515–8. https://doi.org/10.1038/nature10429.
83. Wu J, Sun L, Chen X, et al. Cyclic GMP-AMP is an endogenous second messenger in innate immune signaling by cytosolic DNA. Science. 2013;339:826–30. https://doi.org/10.1126/science.1229963.
84. Sun L, Wu J, Du F, et al. Cyclic GMP-AMP synthase is a cytosolic DNA sensor that activates the type I interferon pathway. Science. 2013;339:786–91. https://doi.org/10.1126/science.1232458.
85. Liu Y, Jesus AA, Marrero B, et al. Activated STING in a vascular and pulmonary syndrome. N Engl J Med. 2014;371:507–18. https://doi.org/10.1056/NEJMoa1312625.
86. König N, Fiehn C, Wolf C, et al. Familial chilblain lupus due to a gain-of-function mutation in STING. Ann Rheum Dis. 2017;76:468–72. https://doi.org/10.1136/annrheumdis-2016-209841.
87. Melki I, Rose Y, Uggenti C, et al. Disease-associated mutations identify a novel region in human STING necessary for the control of type I interferon signaling. J Allergy Clin Immunol. 2017;140:543–552.e5 Published Online First: 3 January 2017. https://doi.org/10.1016/j.jaci.2016.10.031.
88. Moghaddas F, Masters SL. Monogenic autoinflammatory diseases: Cytokinopathies. Cytokine. 2015;74:237–46. https://doi.org/10.1016/j.cyto.2015.02.012.
89. Crow YJ. Type I interferonopathies: a novel set of inborn errors of immunity. Ann N Y Acad Sci. 2011;1238:91–8. https://doi.org/10.1111/j.1749-6632.2011.06220.x.
90. Kato H, Takeuchi O, Sato S, et al. Differential roles of MDA5 and RIG-I helicases in the recognition of RNA viruses. Nature. 2006;441:101–5. https://doi.org/10.1038/nature04734.
91. Hornung V, Ellegast J, Kim S, et al. 5′-Triphosphate RNA is the ligand for RIG-I. Science. 2006;314:994–7. https://doi.org/10.1126/science.1132505.

92. Kawai T, Akira S. Innate immune recognition of viral infection. Nat Immunol. 2006;7:131–7. https://doi.org/10.1038/ni1303.
93. Loo Y-M, Gale M. Immune signaling by RIG-I-like receptors. Immunity. 2011;34:680–92. https://doi.org/10.1016/j.immuni.2011.05.003.
94. Hou F, Sun L, Zheng H, et al. MAVS forms functional prion-like aggregates to activate and propagate antiviral innate immune response. Cell. 2011;146:448–61. https://doi.org/10.1016/j.cell.2011.06.041.
95. Rice GI, Bond J, Asipu A, et al. Mutations involved in Aicardi-Goutières syndrome implicate SAMHD1 as regulator of the innate immune response. Nat Genet. 2009;41:829–32. https://doi.org/10.1038/ng.373.
96. Grieves JL, Fye JM, Harvey S, et al. Exonuclease TREX1 degrades double-stranded DNA to prevent spontaneous lupus-like inflammatory disease. Proc Natl Acad Sci U S A. 2015;112:5117–22. https://doi.org/10.1073/pnas.1423804112.
97. Crow YJ, Hayward BE, Parmar R, et al. Mutations in the gene encoding the 3′-5' DNA exonuclease TREX1 cause Aicardi-Goutières syndrome at the AGS1 locus. Nat Genet. 2006;38:917–20. https://doi.org/10.1038/ng1845.
98. Crow YJ, Leitch A, Hayward BE, et al. Mutations in genes encoding ribonuclease H2 subunits cause Aicardi-Goutières syndrome and mimic congenital viral brain infection. Nat Genet. 2006;38:910–6. https://doi.org/10.1038/ng1842.
99. Volpi S, Picco P, Caorsi R, et al. Type I interferonopathies in pediatric rheumatology. Pediatr Rheumatol. 2016;14:35. https://doi.org/10.1186/s12969-016-0094-4.
100. Arima K, Kinoshita A, Mishima H, et al. Proteasome assembly defect due to a proteasome subunit beta type 8 (PSMB8) mutation causes the autoinflammatory disorder, Nakajo-Nishimura syndrome. Proc Natl Acad Sci U S A. 2011;108:14914–9. https://doi.org/10.1073/pnas.1106015108.
101. Kitamura A, Maekawa Y, Uehara H, et al. A mutation in the immunoproteasome subunit PSMB8 causes autoinflammation and lipodystrophy in humans. J Clin Invest. 2011;121:4150–60. https://doi.org/10.1172/JCI58414.
102. Brehm A, Liu Y, Sheikh A, et al. Additive loss-of-function proteasome subunit mutations in CANDLE/PRAAS patients promote type I IFN production. J Clin Invest. 2015;125:4196–211. https://doi.org/10.1172/JCI81260.
103. de Jesus AA, Canna SW, Liu Y, et al. Molecular mechanisms in genetically defined autoinflammatory diseases: disorders of amplified danger signaling. Annu Rev Immunol. 2015;33:823–74. https://doi.org/10.1146/annurev-immunol-032414-112227.

Part I
Monogenic Autoinflammatory Diseases

Chapter 2
Mevalonate Kinase Deficiency (MKD)/ Hyperimmunoglobulin D Syndrome (HIDS)

Olga Petryna and Neha Purat

Introduction

Mevalonate kinase deficiency (MKD)/hyperimmunoglobulin D syndrome (HIDS) is a rare autoinflammatory disease which was first discovered by Rowe and Fahey in 1965 [1]. Being an autosomal recessive disease, it is believed to result from a mutation in mevalonate kinase (MVK) gene – an enzyme involved in the phosphorylation of mevalonic acid, a component in the isoprenoid and cholesterol biosynthesis pathway [2]. Isoprenoids, including farnesyl, geranyl, and ubiquinone, are essential compounds in diverse cellular functions, and isoprenoid compounds affect the stability and maturation of MVK [3].

On the more severe end of the spectrum, mevalonic aciduria (MVA) usually occurs in childhood, during the first decade of life, and is often fatal, whereas HIDS manifestations are much milder and not life-threatening. There have been cases of adult onset HIDS described in literature. Observational study by Durel et al. [4] describes 23 patients with adult HIDS with mean age at diagnosis being 40 years. In this study significant amount of adult patients (65%) presented with abating severity and frequency of attacks with age, but only 35% were able to achieve remission.

Because of extreme rarity of the condition, with only close to 300 cases reported worldwide, very little has been published about incidence and prevalence of MKD and HIDS in particular. With the largest cohorts of patient registered in Northern Europe, some studies report prevalence of 5 cases of HIDS per 1,000,000 in the

O. Petryna (✉)
NYU School of Medicine, Rheumatology Division/Department of Internal Medicine, New York, NY, USA
e-mail: olga.petryna@nyulangone.org

N. Purat
New York Presbyterian Hospital, Department of Internal Medicine, Brooklyn, NY, USA

P. Efthimiou (ed.), *Auto-Inflammatory Syndromes*,
https://doi.org/10.1007/978-3-319-96929-9_2

whole population in the Netherlands [5]. Highest prevalence of HIDS was observed in patients of Dutch and French descent.

The symptoms can be very nonspecific; hence, it becomes challenging to differentiate with other periodic fever syndromes. Wide spectrum of disease severity is defined by the severity of the enzymatic defect stemming from a variety of MVK gene mutations [6].

Increased levels of immunoglobulin D (IgD) as well as high levels of the cytokines, mainly IL 1, IL 6, and tumor necrosis factor-α (TNFα) are usually observed in majority of the patients.

Differential diagnoses include tumor necrosis factor (TNF) receptor-associated periodic syndrome (TRAPS), juvenile systemic granulomatosis, juvenile idiopathic arthritis, familial Mediterranean fever (FMF), and Behçet disease.

Pathophysiology and Genetics

HIDS is considered a classic monogenic recessively inherited disease resulting from a defect in the gene encoding mevalonate kinase (MVK), an enzyme in which the end products include cholesterol, protein isoprenylates (including the prenylated Ras/Rho proteins), dolichol, and ubiquinone [7].

The most common mutation in MKD is p.V377I (G1129A); this mutation is observed primarily among heterozygous individuals with HIDS [8]. Less frequently observed mutations are I268T, H20PIN, and P167L, but their associations with the frequency or severity of febrile attacks have not been demonstrated (Table 2.1). One study found that the vast majority of V377I alleles from MKD patients who were geographically clustered in Western Europe shared a common ancestral origin [9]. The carrier frequency of any MVK mutation in the Dutch population is 1:65 [10]. Although MKD is a recessive disorder, it may also exhibit a pseudodominant pattern of inheritance; in one study, a mother and her two monozygotic twins had MKD [11].

The exact pathogenesis of HIDS still remains unclear. However, several of the isoprenoid end products have been involved in posttranslational events affecting lipid synthesis, protein degradation, and apoptosis [14]. A link between the isoprenoid pathway and apoptosis was also suggested by Nagashima et al. [15] who also showed that inhibition of this pathway by statins induced apoptosis in rheumatoid arthritis

Table 2.1 Most common MVK mutations

Most common MVK gene mutations from van der Hilst registry [12]	Most common MVK gene mutations from Eurofever registry [13]
V377I	p.V377I + p.V377I
I268T	p.V377I + p.I268T
H20P/N	p.V377I + p.G335A
P167L	p.V377I + p.G336S
H380R	p.V377I + p.L264F
R215Q	p.V377I + p.L265R
W188X	p.V377I + p.P165L

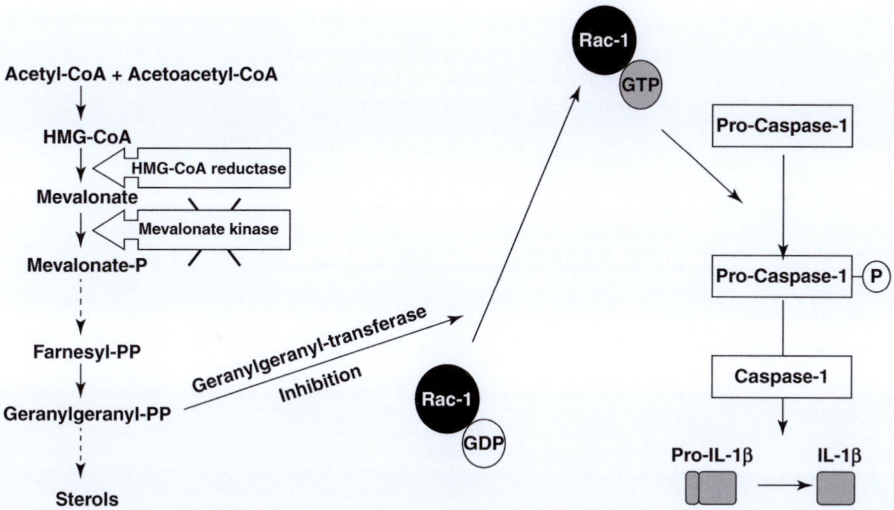

Fig. 2.1 Hypothetical pathogenesis of HIDS. Adapted from Normand et al. [35]. HMG-CoA 3′-hydroxy-3′-methylglutaryl coenzyme A; PP pyrophosphate, GDP guanosine diphosphate, GTP guanosine triphosphate, IL interleukin. (Adapted from Kostjukovits et al. [18])

synoviocytes. This finding also mirrored in MVD and could offer an explanation for the beneficial effect of statins seen in patients with HIDS as well [16].

A deficiency of MVK resulting in shortage of the isoprenoid downstream compounds leads to systemic inflammation through mediation by interleukin (IL)-1β [17]. Lack of geranylgeranyl phosphate leads to caspase-1 activation through Rac1 signaling and subsequent conversion of pre-IL-1β to an active IL-1β (Fig. 2.1) [18].

In another observational study, it was determined that the increased cytokine response in HIDS patients is specific for TLR4, TLR2, and NOD2 ligation and involves other pro-inflammatory cytokines along with IL-1b. Exposing PBMCs from patients with HIDS to LPS (TLR4 ligand) for 24 h in this study resulted in increased IL-1α and IL-1β secretion, while stimulation with TLR2 (Pam3Cys) and NOD2 (MDP) ligands lead to increased IL-1α, IL-1β, IL-6, and TNF secretion. Authors assumed that more easier secretion of IL-1b resulted in the increased ratio between active and inactive caspase-1 protein in HIDS patients. The study favored multi-cytokine mechanism in HIDS pathophysiology [19].

Organ Manifestations

The most common clinical characteristics of the disease are fever above 103F which can last up to 3–7 days with periods of well-being between the cycles, lymphadenopathy mainly in cervical region, aphthous ulcers, gastrointestinal symptoms (nausea,

Table 2.2 Frequency of most common clinical manifestations of HIDS from three largest cohorts

Symptoms	% of patients 103 patient cohort by van der Hilst et al. [12]	% of patients 114 patients by Ter Haar et al. [13]	% of patients 23 patients by Durel et al. [4]
Skin lesions	68.9	Maculopapular rash 39 Urticarial rash 15	82.6
Lymphadenopathy	87.4	85	82.6
Hepato/ splenomegaly	Hepatomegaly 21.6 Splenomegaly 32.4	38	47.8
Arthralgia	83.5	71	87.0
Arthritis	55.3	28	47.8
Abdominal pain	85.4	88	82.6
Diarrhea	71.6	84	47.8
Vomiting	70.9	69	30.4
Headache	63.3	38	34.8
Aphthous ulcers	48.5	60	30.4

vomiting), maculopapular rash, and arthralgias. Other symptoms such as headache, shortness of breath, chest pain, and splenomegaly have been reported [12].

The most common manifestations outlined in Table 2.2 can be grouped by organ systems as follows:

Systemic Complains Periodic febrile attacks lasting up to a week at a time are more common in childhood. Even though severity and frequency of attacks may subside with age with very few or no attacks off treatment in some cases, in majority of the patients, fevers rarely resolve completely [12]. Most of the time, patients remain symptomatic, experiencing more than six febrile attacks per year. A French and Belgian study reported nearly 55% of their patients surviving into adulthood with severe disease (disease activity scores of 2), characterized by frequent severe febrile episodes with major organ involvement [20].

Skin and Mucous Membranes Skin manifestations of HIDS vary from most commonly reported maculopapular eruption, urticaria, and periorbital erythema to rare cases of erythema nodosum and purpura. Aphthous ulcers and pharyngitis are typical during the attacks.

Lymphadenopathy Lymphadenopathy is seen in almost 90% of the patients during attacks. The enlarged lymph nodes were generally located primarily in the cervical region. Axillary and inguinal lymphadenopathy is less frequent [13].

Splenomegaly and Hepatomegaly Hepatosplenomegaly is highly prevalent in majority of HIDS patients. From the published reports, it was found in >30% of cases, with majority of the patient experiencing accompanying lymphadenopathy. International HIDS database reports 22% of patient experiencing isolated hepatomegaly. A few pediatric cases report cholestatic hepatitis.

Gastrointestinal Symptoms Most common GI symptoms of HIDS are flares of abdominal pain, vomiting, and/or diarrhea happening in parallel with febrile attacks and occasionally resembling acute abdomen in most severe cases. Occasional cases of aseptic peritonitis and abdominal adhesions have been reported.

Musculoskeletal Involvement Inflammatory polyarthritis and arthralgia affecting predominantly large peripheral joints and hand joints in RA distribution (MCPs and PIPs) are highly prevalent in HIDS. In some larger published reviews, inflammatory polyarthritis was observed in over 50% of the patients and arthralgia was present in 83.5% of HIDS cases [12].

A handful of cases of osteitis, contractures, and bone deformities have been reported [13].

Myalgias are not uncommon and were described in close to 50% of HIDS patients. No cases of inflammatory myopathy were reported to date.

Neurologic Manifestations CNS involvement is not uncommon in MVD. Cases of mental retardation, retinitis pigmentosa, and cerebellar disease that are more prevalent in severe phenotypes (MVA) where disease manifested in childhood [13, 21].

In HIDS cases headaches, dizziness, and mood disorders are common during the attacks, and in some 25% tend to happen in periods between the attacks. Etiology of mood disorders remains obscure, although psychological impact of the disease tends to play a role.

Rare Manifestations

Macrophage activation syndrome and AA amyloidosis tend to be uncommon in HIDS and were described in only a handful of case reports. The first patient with amyloidosis in HIDS was described by Obici et al. [22] in a case report of a 27-year-old male of Italian descent. In this case the patient presented with proteinuria accompanied by febrile attacks which lasted 3–7 days, lymphadenopathy and abdominal symptoms. Kidney biopsy with Congo red stain confirmed AA amyloidosis. In this patient, two mutations in the mevalonate kinase gene were identified, one of which, the leucine-to-arginine substitution at codon 265, was novel.

Pseudotumors are very uncommon to HIDS but nonetheless described in a few cases. One of the case studies reported an 11-year-old patient with several hypoechoic pseudotumoral hepatosplenic masses. Similar nodular lesions, suggestive of metastases, disseminated in the liver and spleen as well as lung consolidations were detected with the thoracoabdominal CT (T1-weighted). Extensive screening for infection was nevertheless negative and empiric antibiotic therapy unsuccessful. The lesions were completely reversible with corticosteroids [23].

A few reports of *pneumonia and interstitial lung disease* were described but not widely prevalent in HIDS.

Another rare complication reported in HIDS was pauci-immune crescentic glomerulonephritis [24]. Glomerular inflammation was believed to be induced by HIDS-related cytokine release. Larger cohort studies did not observe glomerular disease in HIDS.

Pregnancy

HIDS in pregnancy has not been described vastly, mostly because based on available data, HIDS does not cause any complication during pregnancy, labor, and postpartum, nor it is known to cause disturbance in fetal outcome. Interestingly enough frequency of febrile attacks tends to subside during pregnancy. Nausea and vomiting were described in certain cases, which can make differential with hyperemesis gravidarum difficult. Immunoglobulin D levels tend to remain high in pregnant women with HIDS. Due to relatively mild manifestations during this time, HIDS rarely requires treatment during pregnancy [25].

Laboratory parameters although nonspecific include increased level of acute-phase reactants (ESR, CRP, ferritin, SAA) during febrile attacks. High-serum interleukin-1 and interleukin-6 and TNFa and increased level of IgD (>140 mg/dl) along with high level of mevalonic acid in the urine during the attacks comprise more specific laboratory findings. Increase in Ig A levels was noted in some cases as well [26].

Genetic confirmation of the defect in the protein coding for mevalonate kinase enzyme is a gold standard in diagnosis of HIDS [26]. Less commonly used immunoblot analysis was performed in some cases and demonstrated a deficiency of MK protein in patient fibroblasts, indicating a protein-destabilizing effect of the mutations [27].

Treatment

There is no standard therapy for MKD/HIDS and treatment protocols have changed since the last decade. Conventional DMARDS, such as methotrexate, azathioprine, tacrolimus, dapsone, and intravenous immunoglobulins, demonstrated very limited success in HIDS.

Corticosteroids are useful in management of acute febrile attacks but demonstrate suboptimal efficacy in prevention subsequent flares. One larger cohort reports only 24.4% patients with good response and 37.8% with some response in reduction in severity and duration of attacks with continuous use of steroids [12].

Observational study by Durel et al. showed limited efficacy of colchicine, NSAIDs, and HMG-CoA reductase inhibitors in treatment of HIDS [4]. In some milder cases, zaragozic acid A demonstrated efficacy, suggesting a role for modulation of isoprenoid biosynthesis in treatment of HIDS [28].

Published reports have suggested notable decrease in disease activity and decrease in inflammatory markers with a TNF receptor blocker etanercept. Data varies from report to report and no large trials are available. It is known that onset of action of etanercept may be delayed up to 36 h, and even though severity of the attacks decreases, etanercept does help achieve full remission in many instances. The retrospective analysis of data on both adult and pediatric cases form the Eurofever registry revealed more patients responded to IL-1 inhibitor anakinra (89%) than to etanercept (65%) [29].

IL-1 blocking agent should be preferred in patients with frequent attacks and in patients with chronic active disease and long-term complications. Some studies suggest dose escalation of IL-1 agents should be tried first before switching to other biologic therapies [30].

Anakinra (a recombinant, human IL-1 receptor antagonist) was first described to reduce the overall number and severity of febrile attacks in a 7-year-old girl with MKD in 2006 [31]. Two prospective trials and others series confirm the effectiveness of anakinra in MKD [20]. In retrospective analysis of 67 MKD patients from Eurofever cohort anakinra therapy resulted in impressive responses in 89% of the patients. However, complete remission was observed in much smaller percentage of the patients (22%).

Canakinumab, a human immunoglobulin G1 monoclonal antibody directed against IL-1b, has been extensively studied in the treatment of HIDS in the last decade. There have been studies showing improvement of the febrile attacks and also some cases of complete remission.

Most recently phase 2 open-label single-arm study with two treatment phases and one withdrawal phase has demonstrated complete response (physician's global assessment of disease activity score of 0 or 1 and C-reactive protein levels less than 10 mg/liter) to canakinumab in all nine patients enrolled in the study [32].

Recent literature suggests targeting the IL-6 pathway being effective in HIDS. Larger studies are lacking, but there have been a few reports supporting use of humanized monoclonal antibody against IL-6R tocilizumab in HIDS patients with inadequate response to IL-1 [beta] or TNF-[alpha] [33, 34].

Conclusion

MKD, a rare monogenic autosomal recessive auto-inflammatory disease resulting from loss of function mutation in MVK gene, presents with the spectrum of disorders from milder HIDS to severe and often life-threatening mevalonic aciduria (MVA). While MVA can lead to death in early childhood, HIDS in general does not reduce life expectancy. Regardless of spectrum of the disease, MKD has negative impact on patient's daily activities, education, and employment. Early diagnosis and treatment may improve quality of life and prevent long-term complications and irreversible organ damage. Development of effective targeted therapies remains one of the main unmet needs in management of MKD.

References

1. Rowe DS, Fahey JL. A New Class of Human Immunoglobulins. I. A Unique Myeloma Protein. J Exp Med. 1965;121:171–84.
2. Drenth JP, et al. Location of the gene causing hyperimmunoglobulinemia D and periodic fever syndrome differs from that for familial Mediterranean fever. International Hyper-IgD Study Group. Hum Genet. 1994;94(6):616–20.
3. Church LD, et al. Hereditary auto-inflammatory disorders and biologics. Springer Semin Immunopathol. 2006;27(4):494–508.
4. Durel CA, et al. Observational study of a French and Belgian multicenter cohort of 23 patients diagnosed in adulthood with mevalonate kinase deficiency. Medicine (Baltimore). 2016;95(11):e3027.
5. Toplak N, et al. Periodic fever syndromes in Eastern and Central European countries: results of a pediatric multinational survey. Pediatr Rheumatol Online J. 2010;8:29.
6. Stoffels M, Simon A. Hyper-IgD syndrome or mevalonate kinase deficiency. Curr Opin Rheumatol. 2011;23(5):419–23.
7. Drenth JP, van der Meer JW. Hereditary periodic fever. N Engl J Med. 2001;345(24):1748–57.
8. Caso F, et al. Working the endless puzzle of hereditary autoinflammatory disorders. Mod Rheumatol. 2014;24(3):381–9.
9. Simon A, et al. A founder effect in the hyperimmunoglobulinemia D and periodic fever syndrome. Am J Med. 2003;114(2):148–52.
10. Houten SM, et al. Carrier frequency of the V377I (1129G>A) MVK mutation, associated with Hyper-IgD and periodic fever syndrome, in the Netherlands. Eur J Hum Genet. 2003;11(2):196–200.
11. Hospach T, et al. Pseudodominant inheritance of the hyperimmunoglobulinemia D with periodic fever syndrome in a mother and her two monozygotic twins. Arthritis Rheum. 2005;52(11):3606–10.
12. van der Hilst JC, et al. Long-term follow-up, clinical features, and quality of life in a series of 103 patients with hyperimmunoglobulinemia D syndrome. Medicine (Baltimore). 2008;87(6):301–10.
13. Ter Haar NM, et al. The phenotype and genotype of mevalonate kinase deficiency: a series of 114 cases from the Eurofever registry. Arthritis Rheumatol. 2016;68(11):2795–805.
14. Edwards PA, Ericsson J. Sterols and isoprenoids: signaling molecules derived from the cholesterol biosynthetic pathway. Annu Rev Biochem. 1999;68:157–85.
15. Nagashima T, et al. Apoptosis of rheumatoid synovial cells by statins through the blocking of protein geranylgeranylation: a potential therapeutic approach to rheumatoid arthritis. Arthritis Rheum. 2006;54(2):579–86.
16. Simon A, et al. Simvastatin treatment for inflammatory attacks of the hyperimmunoglobulinemia D and periodic fever syndrome. Clin Pharmacol Ther. 2004;75(5):476–83.
17. Henneman L, et al. Compromised geranylgeranylation of RhoA and Rac1 in mevalonate kinase deficiency. J Inherit Metab Dis. 2010;33(5):625–32.
18. Kostjukovits S, et al. Treatment of hyperimmunoglobulinemia D syndrome with biologics in children: review of the literature and Finnish experience. Eur J Pediatr. 2015;174(6):707–14.
19. Stoffels M, et al. TLR2/TLR4-dependent exaggerated cytokine production in hyperimmunoglobulinaemia D and periodic fever syndrome. Rheumatology (Oxford). 2015;54(2):363–8.
20. Bader-Meunier B, et al. Mevalonate kinase deficiency: a survey of 50 patients. Pediatrics. 2011;128(1):e152–9.
21. Balgobind B, Wittebol-Post D, Frenkel J. Retinitis pigmentosa in mevalonate kinase deficiency. J Inherit Metab Dis. 2005;28(6):1143–5.
22. Obici L, et al. First report of systemic reactive (AA) amyloidosis in a patient with the hyperimmunoglobulinemia D with periodic fever syndrome. Arthritis Rheum. 2004;50(9):2966–9.
23. Damian LO, et al. Ultrasonographic findings in hyperimmunoglobulin D syndrome: a case report. Med Ultrason. 2017;19(2):224–7.

24. Tsimaratos M, et al. Crescentic glomerulonephritis in hyper IgD syndrome. Pediatr Nephrol. 1999;13(2):132–4.
25. de Hullu JA, et al. Hyper-IgD syndrome and pregnancy. Eur J Obstet Gynecol Reprod Biol. 1996;68(1–2):223–5.
26. Drenth JP, Haagsma CJ, van der Meer JW. Hyperimmunoglobulinemia D and periodic fever syndrome. The clinical spectrum in a series of 50 patients. International Hyper-IgD Study Group. Medicine (Baltimore). 1994;73(3):133–44.
27. Houten SM, et al. Mutations in MVK, encoding mevalonate kinase, cause hyperimmunoglobulinaemia D and periodic fever syndrome. Nat Genet. 1999;22(2):175–7.
28. Schneiders MS, et al. Manipulation of isoprenoid biosynthesis as a possible therapeutic option in mevalonate kinase deficiency. Arthritis Rheum. 2006;54(7):2306–13.
29. Ter Haar N, et al. Treatment of autoinflammatory diseases: results from the Eurofever registry and a literature review. Ann Rheum Dis. 2013;72(5):678–85.
30. Ozen S, Demir S. Monogenic periodic fever syndromes: treatment options for the pediatric patient. Paediatr Drugs. 2017;19(4):303–11.
31. Bodar EJ, et al. Effect of etanercept and anakinra on inflammatory attacks in the hyper-IgD syndrome: introducing a vaccination provocation model. Neth J Med. 2005;63(7):260–4.
32. Arostegui JI, et al. Open-label, phase II study to assess the efficacy and safety of Canakinumab treatment in active Hyperimmunoglobulinemia D with periodic fever syndrome. Arthritis Rheumatol. 2017;69(8):1679–88.
33. Shendi HM, Devlin LA, Edgar JD. Interleukin 6 blockade for hyperimmunoglobulin D and periodic fever syndrome. J Clin Rheumatol. 2014;20(2):103–5.
34. Musters A, et al. Anti-interleukin 6 receptor therapy for hyper-IgD syndrome. BMJ Case Rep. 2015;2015. ISSN 1757-790X.

Chapter 3
The TNF Receptor-Associated Autoinflammatory Syndrome (TRAPS)

Marco Gattorno

Introduction

The *TNF receptor-associated autoinflammatory syndrome* (TRAPS, MIM 142680), formerly known as familial Hibernian fever [1], is a rare dominantly inherited disorder, caused by mutations in the p55 TNF receptor (or TNFR1), encoded by the TNF superfamily receptor 1A (*TNFRSF1A*) gene [2]. The disease was originally identified in families of Northern European ancestry but has been described in almost all ethnic groups, including those living in Mediterranean countries and Asia. Fever is often prolonged and can be accompanied by serositis, arthritis, a skin rash with underlying fasciitis and periorbital oedema.

Pathogenesis

A total of 158 sequence variants of the *TNFRSF1A* have been recorded so far; of these 75 are associated with a TRAPS phenotype [3] (http://fmf.igh.cnrs.fr/infevers/).

The first TRAPS-related mutations analysed were missense mutations resulting in single amino acid substitutions in the cysteine-rich domains (CRD), CRD1, CRD2 or CRD3 of the ectodomain of the mature TNFR1 (also called p55 TNFR) protein [3–5]. These CRDs are involved in disulphide bond formation and in the folding of the extracellular portion of the protein. Here hence mutations resulting in cysteine substitutions demonstrate a higher penetrance being usually associated with a more aggressive phenotype (see below). In contrast, other variants, such as R92Q and P46L, that are associated with a milder phenotype have a less severe impact on the structure of the protein [4].

M. Gattorno
UO Pediatria II, Genoa, Italy
e-mail: marcogattorno@ospedale-gaslini.ge.it

P. Efthimiou (ed.), *Auto-Inflammatory Syndromes*,
https://doi.org/10.1007/978-3-319-96929-9_3

In some patients, plasma concentrations of the soluble form of the receptor are low or paradoxically normal during attacks and may also be low in between [2]. This suggested a quantitative or qualitative abnormality of the soluble form of the receptor. The shedding of free TNFRs from the membrane produces a pool of soluble receptors that may scavenge circulating TNF by competing with membrane-bound receptors. This latter phenomenon was considered as a possible strategy for the regulation of the effect of circulating free TNF during acute inflammation. In fact some *TNFRSF1A* mutations display a defect of shedding [2] leading to a lack of appropriate TNF inhibition and therefore to uncontrolled inflammation (Fig. 3.1a).

At variance with the p75 receptor, p55 TNFR is also able to induce cell apoptosis, via activation of the caspase cascade. In fact, TNFR1 can trigger cellular activation via NF-kB or apoptosis via activation of pro-apoptotic caspases. A defect of TNF-induced apoptosis has been identified in TRAPS patients [6, 7].

The transfection of the mutant form of TNFRI protein in different cell types allowed to identify an additional relevant pathogenic mechanism related to the disease. In fact the mutated TNFRI display a defect of trafficking to the cell membrane with a clear accumulation in the endoplasmic reticulum [8] (Fig. 3.1b). As a consequence, elevated levels of mitochondrial reactive oxygen species (ROS) lead to an overactivation of some intracellular pro-inflammatory pathways such as mitogen-activated protein kinase (MAPK) [9, 10] (Fig. 3.1c). These data coming from

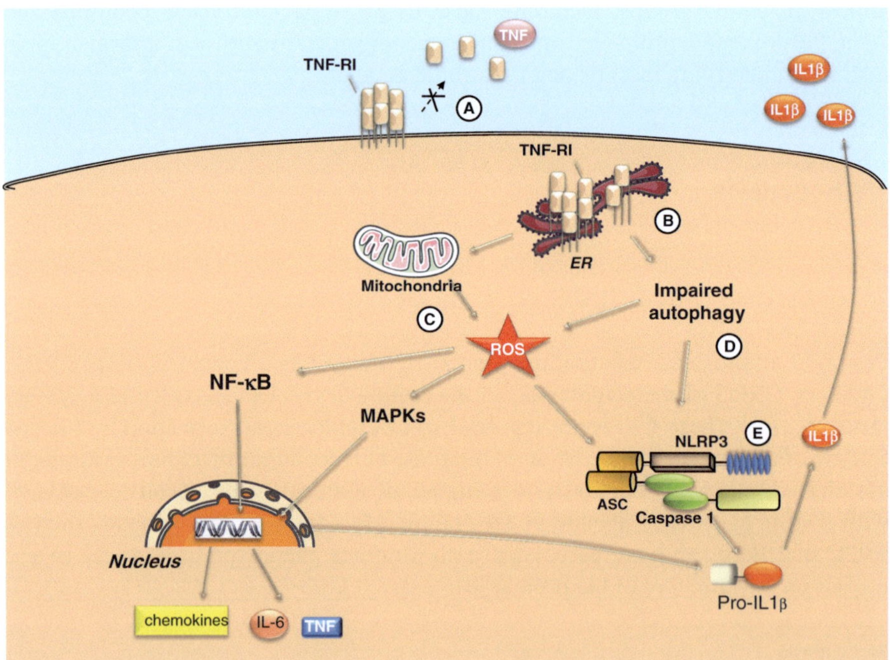

Fig. 3.1 Possible pathogenic mechanisms related to TRAPS (see also text). (Adapted from Gattorno and Martini, A&R, 2013)

TRAPS confirm therefore that the accumulation of unfolded proteins in ER may represent a relevant trigger for the activation of inflammation [11].

In a recent study, the gene expression signature in blood of active TRAPS patients was compared to healthy controls [12]. The disease-causing gene TNFRSF1A was upregulated in TRAPS patients by 1.4-fold compared to the healthy volunteers. Other genes relevant to inflammation were also upregulated among TRAPS patients including MAPK14 (2-fold), NFKB1 (1.3-fold), TLR5 (2.4-fold) and MMP9 (2.4-fold), among others. The upregulation of genes in the apoptosis and survival, endoplasmic reticulum stress response pathway and autophagy pathway maps was also observed [12].

TRAPS monocytes try to override the accumulation of unfolded with a process called autophagy [13]. Autophagy is the main mechanism responsible for elimination of both damaged cellular compartments in physiological conditions and insoluble aggregates of mutant proteins which accumulate under pathological circumstances. Interestingly, downregulation of autophagy has been observed to enhance the inflammatory response, such as in mice lacking autophagy-related proteins [14], thus suggesting that an autophagy defect may be a common pathogenic event underlying a number of autoinflammatory syndromes.

TRAPS patients display an exhaustion of the autophagy system due to the overload of the unfolded mutated protein that represents a further "stress signal" for the cells [13]. This may lead to the activation of the NLRP3 inflammasome [15] (Fig. 3.1d), consistent with the oversecretion of active IL-1β observed in TRAPS patents [13]. In the meanwhile, it is possible that ROS and the consequent antioxidant response could represent a further stimuli for the activation of NLRP3 inflammasome [16, 17] (Fig. 3.1e). Of note, IL-1β and other four genes in the IL-1 immune response signalling were upregulated at the gene expression level in TRAPS patients when compared to healthy controls [12].

These observations may explain the apparent paradox of a better response to anti-IL-1 rather than to anti-TNF treatment observed in TRAPS patients (see below).

Clinical Presentation

Disease onset is usually reported during the paediatric age but is often misdiagnosed. Data from an international registry (Eurofever, www.printo.it/eurofever) shows a mean delay of diagnosis in TRAPS patients of 18 years [18]. On the other hand, in a relevant percentage of patients (almost 20%), disease onset is reported in adult age [19].

The main differential diagnosis of TRAPS is against the other periodic fevers (Table 3.1). The classical disease presentation of TRAPS in childhood is characterized by fever attacks lasting from 1 to 3 weeks. However, shorter episodes can be observed in up to 20% of patients [5, 19]. Fever onset is often abrupt and associated with shiver. Fever episodes are spaced by variable intervals of complete well-being. No clear periodicity is usually observed [5, 7, 19].

Table 3.1 Autoinflammatory diseases presenting as periodic or recurrent fever: differential diagnosis

Disease (year of identification)	Gene (year of identification)	Protein	Inheritance	Main clinical features
FMF **(1945)**	*MEFV* **(1997)**	Pyrin	AR	Short duration of fever episodes: 24–48 h. Severe serositis with abdominal and chest pain. Erysipelas-like erythema. Good response to colchicine
Hyper-IgD **(1984)**	*MVK* **(1998)**	MVK	AR	Very early onset (usually <12 months). Mean duration of episodes: 4–5 days. Poor conditions during fever episodes. Abdominal pain, vomiting and diarrhoea. Splenomegaly. Variable response to steroids on demand
TRAPS **(1982)**	*TNFRSF1A* **(1999)**	TNFR1	AD	Prolonged fever episodes: 1–3 weeks. Periorbital oedema, monocytic fasciitis. Incidence of renal amyloidosis: 15–25%. Better response to IL-1 rather than to TNF blockade
FCAS, MWS, CINCA **(1940, 1962, 1982)**	*NLRP3* **(2000)**	Cryopyrin	AD	FCAS: rash, fever and arthralgia after cold exposure. MWS: recurrent or subchronic urticaria-like lesions, sensorineural hearing loss, amyloidosis. CINCA: as above + mental retardation, chronic aseptic meningitis and bone deformities, with a chronic course. All: dramatic response to IL-1 blockade
FCAS 2 **(2008)**	*NLRP12* **(2008)**	NLPR12	AD	Mild inflammatory phenotype. Periodic fever and rash after cold exposure. Possible hearing loss
PFAPA **(1987)**	*n/a*	n/a	n/a	Early onset (<5 years). Clear periodicity. Predominance of pharyngotonsillitis and latero-cervical lymph node involvement. Good response to steroids on demand and tonsillectomy

FMF familial Mediterranean fever, *FCAS* familial cold autoinflammatory syndrome, *MWS* Muckle-Wells syndrome, *CINCA* chronic infantile neurological cutaneous and articular syndrome, *TRAPS* TNF receptor-associated autoinflammatory syndrome, *PFAPA* periodic fever, aphthous stomatitis, pharyngitis and adenitis, *AR* autosomal recessive, *AD* autosomal dominant, *n/a* not applicable (multifactorial)

Limb pain is frequently observed and is more prominent than arthritis, which may involve large joints (hips, knees, ankles). Abdominal and chest pain are frequently observed and are due to acute peritoneal or pleural inflammation. Ocular involvement, characterized by periorbital oedema and conjunctivitis, is frequent, especially in children [5, 19].

The cutaneous manifestations associated with TRAPS are extremely variable. A wide spectrum of skin rashes can be observed in most patients: urticaria-like, plaques and patches [20, 21].

The most distinctive lesion is an erythematous, swollen, warm and tender plaque of various sizes with hazy edges. It rather involves the upper and lower limbs but can be observed at the chest. Usually, the rash has a migratory course from the root to the extremity of the limbs [21].

This pseudo-cellulitis is often accompanied by painful myalgias due to a monocytic fasciitis, which constitute one of the most distinctive manifestations of TRAPS attacks. These cutaneous lesions are histologically characterized by deep perivascular infiltrates of mononuclear cells [22].

Attacks are associated with important rise in acute-phase reactants (ESR, CRP), increased neutrophils' count and variable degree of hypochromic anaemia.

In adulthood, fever episodes may become less frequent, and patients may experience a subchronic disease course characterized by flares of abdominal pain, arthro-myalgia, ocular manifestations and a slight but persistent elevation of acute-phase reactants, including serum amyloid A (SAA). Renal AA amyloidosis represents the most serious long-term complication, with a prevalence ranging from 14 to 25% [5, 20].

Evidence-based classification criteria for TRAPS and other monogenic recurrent fevers have been recently developed on the basis of data coming from the Eurofever Registry [23]. According to these criteria, either "positive" or "negative" (presence or absence of a given variable) are associated with each inherited recurrent fever, with a high accuracy. The presence of a positive family history, long-lasting fever episodes, periorbital oedema, migratory rash and myalgia together with the absence of vomiting and aphthosis is strongly associated with TRAPS (Table 3.2) [23].

Mutations of the *TNFRSF1A* gene that result in cysteine substitutions demonstrate a higher penetrance of the clinical phenotype and are characterized by a severe disease course and by an increased probability of developing renal amyloidosis. In contrast, other low-penetrance mutations (such as the R92Q and P46L mutations)

Table 3.2 The Eurofever classification criteria for TRAPS (Ref. [23])

Presence	**Score**
Periorbital oedema	21
Duration of episodes >6 days	19
Migratory rash^	18
Myalgia	6
Relatives affected	7
Absence	
Vomiting	14
Aphthous stomatitis	15
Cut-off	**≥43**

^Centrifugal migratory, erythematous patches most typically overlying a local area of myalgia, usually on the limbs or trunk

are usually associated with a more heterogeneous clinical presentation, with a milder disease course and lower prevalence of amyloidosis [5].

This observation was confirmed also in study conducted on a paediatric population of 21 TRAPS patients [7]. Children carrying a R92Q substitution displayed a milder disease course in term of duration of flares (mean duration 4.1 days) and intensity of disease-associated symptoms. The majority of these patients respond well to steroid on demand and do not need continuous biologic treatment to control disease activity. As observed in other studies, the allele frequency in normal population ranges from 2% to 4%. Interestingly, in most of paediatric R92Q patients, the mutation is inherited from one asymptomatic parent, thus confirming the low penetrance of this substitution [7].

Treatment

Corticosteroids, when given at the onset of an attack, can attenuate its length and severity. This strategy is used in a relevant percentage of patients, especially if few episodes per year are experienced by the patients [24].

In the most severe forms of the disease, clinical signs of inflammation are extremely frequent or permanent and require daily use of corticosteroids, leading to dependency and requiring the use of other anti-inflammatory drugs. Colchicine does not seem to prevent recurrences of TRAPS attacks, even if some effect has been reported in patients with low-penetrance mutations [24].

The use of immunosuppressive drugs has been reported to be ineffective [20, 24]. Since the molecular defect of p55 TNFR is associated with an impaired shedding of the receptor from the membrane surface, the use of etanercept (Enbrel), fusion protein of the soluble TNF receptor 2 and the Fc component of human immunoglobulin, has been proposed [2]. However, although there is anecdotal evidence of the efficacy of etanercept in the prevention of disease flares and in the treatment of long-term renal complications [20, 25–28], others have shown that this biological agent is ineffective in some patients and unable to completely control inflammation in others [29–33].

Bulua et al. reported the experience of 15 TRAPS patients enrolled in a prospective, open-label, dose escalation study using etanercept. The treatment significantly attenuated the total symptom score, as well as reduced the frequency of symptoms and reduced acute-phase reactants during asymptomatic periods. However, during a 10-year follow-up period, most of the patients discontinued treatment (with a median of treatment of 3.3 years). The main reasons for discontinuation were injection reactions and lack of efficacy [34].

Of note, the use of anti-TNF monoclonal antibodies (infliximab and adalimumab) has been shown to worsen the inflammatory manifestations in TRAPS patients [33, 35, 36].

On the other hand, after these disappointing experiences with anti-TNF blockers, some preliminary anecdotic observations showed the excellent response to anti-IL-1 treatments, such as IL-1anakinra in some patients [30, 36].

In a preliminary study, four children and one adult with TRAPS were treated with anakinra due to the high frequency of fever episodes or the development of a chronic disease course [37]. All patients had a dramatic response, with disappearance of symptoms and normalization of acute-phase reactants. In all paediatric patients, anakinra was withdrawn after 15 days of treatment. After a few days, a disease relapse occurred, with a prompt new response to the reintroduction of anakinra. During the following year, the patients were treated continuously with anakinra and did not experience any disease-related clinical manifestations or any increase in acute-phase reactants [37].

Data from Eurofever Registry has supported the better performance of IL-1 blockade on anti-TNF treatment in TRAPS patients. In fact, even if etanercept was beneficial in 32 of the 37 patients, only 11 (30%) experienced a complete response. Conversely anakinra was able to induce a complete response (absence of clinical manifestations and normalization of acute-phase reactants) in 26 of 33 patients (79%) and a partial response in 5 others [24]. The same good results have been preliminary reported in one patients treated with the anti-IL-1 monoclonal antibody (canakinumab) [38].

Canakinumab is a fully human monoclonal selective anti-IL-1β antibody with a half-time of 4 weeks. Interim data of open-label 4-month canakinumab therapy and 5-month follow-up involving 20 active TRAPS patients has been recently presented [39]. A 4-month open-label 150 mg (2 mg/kg) of canakinumab every 4 weeks followed by up to 5-month treatment withdrawal was performed. On day 8, 16 (80%) achieved complete/almost complete response, and 18 (90%) achieved clinical remission. Clinical remission was maintained by all patients from day 15 onwards. After withdrawal of treatment at month 4, the patients presented a relapse of the disease after a median period of 3 months. All patients regained complete/almost complete response 8–27 days after canakinumab redose. All patients completed the following 24-month open-label period. Only two serious adverse events, an upper respiratory infection and a TRAPS relapse, were reported [39].

These latter data supported the pivotal role of IL-1β in the pathogenesis of TRAPS and prompted the elaboration of a large registrative trial. Indeed, a randomized, double-blind, placebo-controlled trial recently confirmed the efficacy of canakinumab in TRAPS and in other two monogenic periodic fevers (colchicine-resistant FMF and mevalonate kinase deficiency) [40].

In all the diseases, canakinumab has demonstrated highly significant differences vs placebo in the primary outcome (resolution of the index flare by day 15 and no subsequent flares up to week 16) in the first phase of the trial, after randomization. Most of the TRAPS patients displayed a complete response at the dose of 150 or 300 mg every 4 week. Moreover, in the subsequent 40-week phase of the study, patients were further randomized in order to evaluate canakinumab at a prolonged dosing interval (every 8 weeks) [40].

Notably 53% of the TRAPS patients randomized with a prolonged dosing interval (150 mg q8w) maintained a complete control of the disease [40]. This drug is now registered for these three new indications in the USA and Europe.

Among other possible alternative treatments, some anecdotal reports have recently showed the good response to anti-IL-6 treatment in some TRAPS patients (refs).

References

1. Williamson LM, Hull D, Mehta R, Reeves WG, Robinson BH, Toghill PJ. Familial Hibernian fever. Q J Med. 1982;51(204):469–80.
2. McDermott MF, Aksentijevich I, Galon J, McDermott EM, Ogunkolade BW, Centola M, et al. Germline mutations in the extracellular domains of the 55 kDa TNF receptor, TNFR1, define a family of dominantly inherited autoinflammatory syndromes. Cell. 1999;97(1):133–44.
3. Touitou I, Lesage S, McDermott M, Cuisset L, Hoffman H, Dode C, et al. Infevers: an evolving mutation database for auto-inflammatory syndromes. Hum Mutat. 2004;24(3):194–8.
4. Aksentijevich I, Galon J, Soares M, Mansfield E, Hull K, Oh HH, et al. The tumor-necrosis-factor receptor-associated periodic syndrome: new mutations in TNFRSF1A, ancestral origins, genotype-phenotype studies, and evidence for further genetic heterogeneity of periodic fevers. Am J Hum Genet. 2001;69(2):301–14.
5. Aganna E, Hammond L, Hawkins PN, Aldea A, McKee SA, van Amstel HK, et al. Heterogeneity among patients with tumor necrosis factor receptor-associated periodic syndrome phenotypes. Arthritis Rheum. 2003;48(9):2632–44.
6. Siebert S, Amos N, Fielding CA, Wang EC, Aksentijevich I, Williams BD, et al. Reduced tumor necrosis factor signaling in primary human fibroblasts containing a tumor necrosis factor receptor superfamily 1A mutant. Arthritis Rheum. 2005;52(4):1287–92.
7. D'Osualdo A, Ferlito F, Prigione I, Obici L, Meini A, Zulian F, et al. Neutrophils from patients with TNFRSF1A mutations display resistance to tumor necrosis factor-induced apoptosis – Pathogenetic and clinical implications. Arthritis Rheum. 2006;54(3):998–1008.
8. Lobito AA, Kimberley FC, Muppidi JR, Komarow H, Jackson AJ, Hull KM, et al. Abnormal disulfide-linked oligomerization results in ER retention and altered signaling by TNFR1 mutants in TNFR1-associated periodic fever syndrome (TRAPS). Blood. 2006;108(4):1320–7.
9. Simon A, Park H, Maddipati R, Lobito AA, Bulua AC, Jackson AJ, et al. Concerted action of wild-type and mutant TNF receptors enhances inflammation in TNF receptor 1-associated periodic fever syndrome. Proc Natl Acad Sci U S A. 2010;107(21):9801–6.
10. Bulua AC, Simon A, Maddipati R, Pelletier M, Park H, Kim KY, et al. Mitochondrial reactive oxygen species promote production of proinflammatory cytokines and are elevated in TNFR1-associated periodic syndrome (TRAPS). J Exp Med. 2011;208(3):519–33.
11. Hasnain SZ, Lourie R, Das I, Chen AC, McGuckin MA. The interplay between endoplasmic reticulum stress and inflammation. Immunol Cell Biol. 2012;90(3):260–70.
12. Torene R, Nirmala N, Obici L, Cattalini M, Tormey V, Caorsi R, et al. Canakinumab reverses overexpression of inflammatory response genes in tumour necrosis factor receptor-associated periodic syndrome. Ann Rheum Dis. 2017;76(1):303–9.
13. Bachetti T, Chiesa S, Castagnola P, Bani D, Di ZE, Omenetti A, et al. Autophagy contributes to inflammation in patients with TNFR-associated periodic syndrome (TRAPS). Ann Rheum Dis. 2013;72(6):1044–52. https://doi.org/10.1136/annrheumdis-2012-201952. Epub 2012 Oct 31.
14. Saitoh T, Fujita N, Jang MH, Uematsu S, Yang BG, Satoh T, et al. Loss of the autophagy protein Atg16L1 enhances endotoxin-induced IL-1beta production. Nature. 2008;456(7219):264–8.
15. Nakahira K, Haspel JA, Rathinam VA, Lee SJ, Dolinay T, Lam HC, et al. Autophagy proteins regulate innate immune responses by inhibiting the release of mitochondrial DNA mediated by the NALP3 inflammasome. Nat Immunol. 2011;12(3):222–30.
16. Tassi S, Carta S, Delfino L, Caorsi R, Martini A, Gattorno M, et al. Altered redox state of monocytes from cryopyrin-associated periodic syndromes causes accelerated IL-1beta secretion. Proc Natl Acad Sci U S A. 2010;107(21):9789–94.
17. Rubartelli A, Gattorno M, Netea MG, Dinarello CA. Interplay between redox status and inflammasome activation. Trends Immunol. 2011;32(12):559–66.
18. Toplak N, Dolezalova P, Constantin T, Sediva A, Pasic S, Ciznar P, et al. Periodic fever syndromes in Eastern and Central European countries: results of a pediatric multinational survey. Pediatr Rheumatol Online J. 2010;8:29.

19. Lachmann HJ, Meini A, Touitou I, Obici L, Finetti M, Minden K, et al. Demographic and Genetic Results From the EUROFEVERS/EUROTRAPS Consortia in the Largest Series of Patients with TRAPS Yet Reported. Arthritis Rheum. 2011;63(10):S386–7.
20. Hull KM, Drewe E, Aksentijevich I, Singh HK, Wong K, McDermott EM, et al. The TNF receptor-associated periodic syndrome (TRAPS): emerging concepts of an autoinflammatory disorder. Medicine (Baltimore). 2002;81(5):349–68.
21. Yao Q, Englund KA, Hayden SP, Tomecki KJ. Tumor necrosis factor receptor associated periodic fever syndrome with photographic evidence of various skin disease and unusual phenotypes: case report and literature review. Semin Arthritis Rheum. 2012;41(4):611–7.
22. Hull KM, Wong K, Wood GM, Chu WS, Kastner DL. Monocytic fasciitis: a newly recognized clinical feature of tumor necrosis factor receptor dysfunction. Arthritis Rheum. 2002;46(8):2189–94.
23. Federici S, Sormani MP, Ozen S, Lachmann HJ, Amaryan G, Woo P, et al. Evidence-based provisional clinical classification criteria for autoinflammatory periodic fevers. Ann Rheum Dis. 2015;74(5):799–805.
24. Ter Haar N, Lachmann H, Ozen S, Woo P, Uziel Y, Modesto C, et al. Treatment of autoinflammatory diseases: results from the Eurofever Registry and a literature review. Ann Rheum Dis. 2013;72(5):678–85. https://doi.org/10.1136/annrheumdis-2011-201268. Epub 2012 Jun 29. Review.
25. Drewe E, McDermott EM, Powell PT, Isaacs JD, Powell RJ. Prospective study of anti-tumour necrosis factor receptor superfamily 1B fusion protein, and case study of anti-tumour necrosis factor receptor superfamily 1A fusion protein, in tumour necrosis factor receptor associated periodic syndrome (TRAPS): clinical and laboratory findings in a series of seven patients. Rheumatology. 2003;42(2):235–9.
26. Drewe E, Huggins ML, Morgan AG, Cassidy MJ, Powell RJ. Treatment of renal amyloidosis with etanercept in tumour necrosis factor receptor-associated periodic syndrome. Rheumatology (Oxford). 2004;43(11):1405–8.
27. Kallinich T, Briese S, Roesler J, Rudolph B, Sarioglu N, Blankenstein O, et al. Two familial cases with tumor necrosis factor receptor-associated periodic syndrome caused by a non-cysteine mutation (T50M) in the TNFRSF1A gene associated with severe multiorganic amyloidosis. J Rheumatol. 2004;31(12):2519–22.
28. Jesus AA, Oliveira JB, Aksentijevich I, Fujihira E, Carneiro-Sampaio MM, Duarte AJ, et al. TNF receptor-associated periodic syndrome (TRAPS): description of a novel TNFRSF1A mutation and response to etanercept. Eur J Pediatr. 2008;167(12):1421–5.
29. Weyhreter H, Schwartz M, Kristensen TD, Valerius NH, Paerregaard A. A new mutation causing autosomal dominant periodic fever syndrome in a Danish family. J Pediatr. 2003;142(2):191–3.
30. Simon A, Bodar EJ, van der Hilst JC, van der Meer JW, Fiselier TJ, Cuppen MP, et al. Beneficial response to interleukin 1 receptor antagonist in traps. Am J Med. 2004;117(3):208–10.
31. Arostegui JI, Solis P, Aldea A, Cantero T, Rius J, Bahillo P, et al. Etanercept plus colchicine treatment in a child with tumour necrosis factor receptor-associated periodic syndrome abolishes auto-inflammatory episodes without normalising the subclinical acute phase response. Eur J Pediatr. 2005;164(1):13–6.
32. Jacobelli S, Andre M, Alexandra JF, Dode C, Papo T. Failure of anti-TNF therapy in TNF Receptor 1-Associated Periodic Syndrome (TRAPS). Rheumatology (Oxford). 2007;46:1211.
33. Drewe E, Powell RJ, McDermott EM. Comment on: Failure of anti-TNF therapy in TNF receptor 1-associated periodic syndrome (TRAPS). Rheumatology (Oxford). 2007;46(12):1865–6.
34. Bulua AC, Mogul DB, Aksentijevich I, Singh H, He D, Muenz L, et al. Efficacy of etanercept in the tumor necrosis factor receptor-associated periodic syndrome (TRAPS). Arthritis Rheum. 2012;64(3):908–13. https://doi.org/10.1002/art.33416.
35. Siebert S, Amos N, Lawson TM. Comment on: Failure of anti-TNF therapy in TNF receptor 1-associated periodic syndrome (TRAPS). Rheumatology (Oxford). 2008;47(2):228–9.

36. Sacre K, Brihaye B, Lidove O, Papo T, Pocidalo MA, Cuisset L, et al. Dramatic improvement following interleukin 1beta blockade in tumor necrosis factor receptor-1-associated syndrome (TRAPS) resistant to anti-TNF-alpha therapy. J Rheumatol. 2008;35(2):357–8.
37. Gattorno M, Pelagatti MA, Meini A, Obici L, Barcellona R, Federici S, et al. Persistent efficacy of anakinra in patients with tumor necrosis factor receptor-associated periodic syndrome. Arthritis Rheum. 2008;58(5):1516–20.
38. Brizi MG, Galeazzi M, Lucherini OM, Cantarini L, Cimaz R. Successful treatment of tumor necrosis factor receptor-associated periodic syndrome with canakinumab. Ann Intern Med. 2012;156(12):907–8.
39. Gattorno M, Obici L, Cattalini M, Tormey V, Abrams K, Davis N, et al. Canakinumab treatment for patients with active recurrent or chronic TNF receptor-associated periodic syndrome (TRAPS): an open-label, phase II study. Ann Rheum Dis. 2017;76(1):173–8.
40. De Benedetti F, Anton J, Gattorno M, Lachmann H, Kone-Paut I, Ozen S, et al. A phase III pivotal umbrella trial of canakinumab in patients with autoinflammatory periodic fever syndromes (Colchicine Resistant FMF, HIDS/MKD and TRAPS). Ann Rheum Dis. 75(Suppl 2):615–6.

Chapter 4
PAPA Syndrome and the Spectrum of PSTPIP1-Associated Inflammatory Diseases

Dirk Holzinger and Johannes Roth

Introduction

PAPA syndrome (OMIM #604416) was initially described by two different groups a couple of years apart. In 1997, a new autosomal dominant disorder of pyogenic arthritis, pyoderma gangrenosum, and acne was described in a multigenerational family [1], whereas a second group described the disease as "familial recurrent arthritis" in 2000 [2]. In both families the symptom complex of recurrent arthritis, sterile but purulent synovial fluid, and cutaneous manifestations such as pyoderma gangrenosum (large, open purulent lesions) and severe cystic acne was described.

Also in 2000, the disease locus was mapped to chromosome 15 [3], and finally mutations (p.A230T and p.E250Q) in proline-serine-threonine phosphatase-interacting protein 1 (PSTPIP1, also known as CD2BP1) were identified as the cause of PAPA syndrome [4]. PSTPIP1 interacts with a PEST [rich in proline (P), glutamic acid (E), serine (S), and threonine (T)]-type protein tyrosine phosphatase (PTP-PEST). Initially, it was shown that the mutations that cause PAPA syndrome diminish the interaction of PSTPIP1 with PTP-PEST, but the relevance of this finding for the promotion of autoinflammation was unclear [4].

PSTPIP1 is a cytoskeleton-associated adaptor protein that modulates T-cell activation [5], phagocyte activation, cytoskeletal organization, and interleukin (IL)-1ß release [6]. Initial experimental approaches helped to localize PAPA within the spectrum of autoinflammatory diseases. It could be shown that mutated PSTPIP1 markedly increased pyrin-binding and IL-1ß production by peripheral

---

D. Holzinger (✉)
Department of Pediatric Hematology-Oncology, University of Duisburg-Essen, Essen, Germany

J. Roth
Institute of Immunology, University Hospital Muenster, Muenster, Germany

P. Efthimiou (ed.), *Auto-Inflammatory Syndromes*,
https://doi.org/10.1007/978-3-319-96929-9_4

blood leukocytes (PBMCs) from a PAPA patient and in cell lines transfected with PAPA-associated mutants [6]. Moreover, PAPA-associated PSTPIP1 mutants promote the interaction of pyrin with apoptosis-associated speck-like protein containing a carboxy-terminal CARD (ASC) promoting ASC oligomerization into an active ASC pyroptosome [7]. Despite identifying the genetic background of PAPA and first insights into its pathogenesis, the treatment of the disease is still difficult, as therapeutic approaches with tumor necrosis factor (TNF) [8–10] or IL-1 [11] inhibition have been reported with varying success.

In the last years, the spectrum of autoinflammatory diseases due to mutations in *PSTPIP1* with distinct clinical phenotypes has been expanded [12–14] indicating that the PAPA syndrome is only one clinical entity within the spectrum of *PSTPIP1*-associated inflammatory diseases (PAID). The identification of endogenous Toll-like receptor (TLR) 4 ligands as hallmark of PAPA and PSTPIP1-associated myeloid-related proteinemia inflammatory (PAMI) syndrome [13], the association of PSTPIP1 with the cytoskeleton, the modulation of cell motility, and finally the results from mice ectopically expressing human PSTPIP1 mutant proteins [15] offer new insights in the pathogenesis of PAID.

Spectrum of PSTPIP1-Associated Inflammatory Diseases

PSTPIP1 mutations are associated with periodic inflammatory flares reflected by systemic symptoms like fever or an acute phase response and local inflammation of the skin, joints, and in many cases other internal organs (Table 4.1). Until now 25 sequence variants have been reported for the *PSTPIP1* gene in the Infevers database (see the Infevers website: http://fmf.igh.enrs.fr/ISSAID/infevers/). PAID are rare diseases, and the systematic registration of cases in Eurofever shows a prevalence of 16 cases in Europe (see the Eurofever website: https://www.printo.it/eurofever/correlation.asp).

Pyogenic Arthritis, Pyoderma Gangrenosum, and Acne (PAPA) Syndrome

PAPA syndrome has been described as first PAID characterized by pyogenic arthritis, pyoderma gangrenosum, and acne [1]. However, in this initial report, the syndrome was already characterized as pleiotropic disorder and manifested in ten affected family members with variable expression of an arthritis that began in childhood, whereas pyoderma gangrenosum and severe cystic acne began in adolescence and beyond [1]. Thirty-six more cases are reported in the literature demonstrating a high variability in clinical presentation and penetrance of PAPA syndrome with heterozygous mutations p.A230T and p.E250Q (Table 4.1). Meanwhile, p.D246N [17], pE256G [18], and p.D266N have been identified as additional PAPA-causing mutations [19].

Table 4.1 Spectrum of PSTPIP1-associated inflammatory diseases (PAID)

Syndrome	Pyogenic arthritis, pyoderma gangrenosum, and acne syndrome	PSTPIP1-associated myeloid-related proteinemia inflammatory syndrome	Pyogenic arthritis, pyoderma gangrenosum, acne, and hidradenitis suppurativa syndrome	Pyogenic arthritis, pyoderma gangrenosum, and acne syndrome	Pyoderma gangrenosum, acne, and ulcerative colitis syndrome
Acronym	PAPA	PAMI	PAPASH	PAPA-like	PAC
Mutation	p.A230T (*n* = 23) p.E250Q (*n* = 24) p.E256G (*n* = 2) p.D246N (*n* = 1) p.D266N (*n* = 1) not specified (*n* = 2)	p.E250K (*n* = 17) p.E257K (*n* = 1)	p.E277D	p.G258A homozygous	p.G403R
Reported cases (*n*)	53	18	1	1	1
Rheumatic symptoms	Arthritis (total 78%; 53% reported as pyogenic) Arthralgia (13%) Tendinitis (2%) Periostitis with osteolytic lesion (2%)	Arthritis (total *n* = 61%; 17% reported as pyogenic) Arthralgia (11%) Morning stiffness (6%) Osteomyelitis (17%)	Pyogenic arthritis	Arthralgia	

(continued)

Table 4.1 (continued)

Syndrome	Pyogenic arthritis, pyoderma gangrenosum, and acne syndrome	PSTPIP1-associated myeloid-related proteinemia inflammatory syndrome	Pyogenic arthritis, pyoderma gangrenosum, acne, and hidradenitis suppurativa syndrome	Pyogenic arthritis, pyoderma gangrenosum, and acne syndrome	Pyoderma gangrenosum, acne, and ulcerative colitis syndrome
Acronym	PAPA	PAMI	PAPASH	PAPA-like	PAC
Dermatological symptoms	Acne (56%) PG (27%) Ulcers (13%) Pustulosis (11%) Abscesses (16%) EP (8%) Psoriasis (6%) Cutaneous edema (4%) Hidradenitis (3%) Rosacea (2%) TP (2%) Urticaria (2%)	PG (39%) Ulcerative /necrotic lesion (33%) Acne (28%) Pustular rash (17%) Abscesses (13%) Rash (11%) EM (6%)	Mild acne Abscesses PG HS	Acne PG	Acne PG Recalcitrant Pustular rash
HSM	–	89%	–	–	–
Cytopenia	Anemia (8%)	Neutropenia (94%) Anemia (89%) Thrombocytopenia (44%)	–	Anemia	–
Additional Findings	Elevated MRP8/ MRP814 (116 ± 74 μg/mL) (21%)	Hypercalprotectinemia (MRP8/ MRP814 2070 ± 1190 μg/mL) (89%) Hyperzincemia (>50 μmol/l) (89%)			

Adapted and updated from Holzinger and Roth [16]

Clinical symptoms and laboratory findings in PAID. Patients reported in multiple studies have only been included once

EM erythema multiforme, *EP* erythematous plaques, *HSM* hepatosplenomegaly, *HS* hidradenitis suppurativa, *PG* pyoderma gangrenosum, *TP* thrombophlebitis

PAPA syndrome is characterized by autosomal dominant inheritance of early-onset, destructive, recurrent inflammation of the joints, skin, and muscle. It typically presents with recurrent sterile, erosive arthritis in childhood, occurring spontaneously or after minor trauma. The arthritis is oligoarticular, affecting one to three joints at a time, and is characterized by recurring inflammatory episodes that resemble septic arthritis and lead to accumulation of pyogenic, neutrophil-rich material within the affected joints, which ultimately results in significant synovial and cartilage destruction. Episodic inflammatory arthritis typically does not resolve spontaneously and must be treated with intraarticular steroids or surgical drainage of the infiltrate. An associated infectious or environmental agent responsible for triggering these flares could not be identified [1, 4, 16].

By puberty, joint symptoms tend to subside, and cutaneous symptoms increase. Dermatologic manifestations are also episodic and recurrent with onset usually during the second decade of life and are characterized by debilitating, aggressive, and ulcerative skin lesions, usually of the lower extremities. Cutaneous manifestations include pathergy, frequently with abscesses at the sites of injections, severe cystic acne, and recurrent non-healing sterile ulcers, often diagnosed as pyoderma gangrenosum. Cultures of the skin and joints of these patients are sterile. Synovial tissue biopsy reveals massive polymorphonuclear infiltrate without the presence of immunoglobulin or complement deposits [1, 2, 20].

Standard laboratory findings typically reflect systemic inflammation but are otherwise non-diagnostic; however, elevated levels of proinflammatory cytokines and especially high levels of proinflammatory alarmins myeloid-related protein (MRP) 8/14 within the range of familial Mediterranean fever (FMF) and systemic juvenile idiopathic arthritis (SJIA) have been reported [13]. Some individuals report significant psychosocial impairment due to physical disability, steroid-induced cushingoid appearance, and permanent, widespread cutaneous scarring [20].

PSTPIP1-Associated Myeloid-Related Proteinemia Inflammatory (PAMI) Syndrome

In 2015 it could be shown that a single amino acid charge switch defines clinically distinct (PSTPIP1)-associated inflammatory diseases. Patients with a p.E250K and p.E257K mutations showed a distinct clinical phenotype when compared to patients with classical PAPA syndrome. Conclusively, PAMI syndrome was defined as distinct autoinflammatory disorder presenting clinical and biochemical features not found in patients with classical PAPA syndrome. In addition to prominent skin inflammation and arthralgia/arthritis, PAMI is characterized by severe chronic systemic inflammation, hepatosplenomegaly, pancytopenia, and failure to thrive. In addition to the presence of a severe course and early-onset disease, hepatosplenomegaly, failure to thrive, cytopenia, hyperzincemia, and extremely high levels of MRP8/MRP14 separate PAMI syndrome from PAPA. Interestingly, in the control cohort of patients with PAPA syndrome ($n = 11$), the most relevant clinical findings of anemia, neutropenia, thrombocytopenia (hepato)splenomegaly, and failure to thrive were absent [13].

The mutations p.E250K and p.E257K result in charge reversal in the y-domain of *PSTPIP1* (E → K) and increased interaction with pyrin compared to p.E250Q mutants. 12 of 14 patients had a de novo mutation, and only in the two rare familial cases variable expressivity of disease was noted as described in PAPA syndrome [13]. Both mutants, p.E250K and p.E257K, substantially affect a negative patch on wild-type PSTPIP1 protein, whereas the influence of PAPA mutant p.E250Q upon the electrostatic potential is much less pronounced. Functionally, relative to the E250Q mutation, the E250K mutant exhibits markedly increased binding to pyrin [13]. In addition to the clinical symptoms, PAMI can be distinguished from PAPA and healthy controls by serum protein expression levels [13]. Interestingly, many of these proteins play a role in positive inflammatory feedback mechanisms between innate immune cells and the epithelium [21–23].

Besides this cohort three other cases with de novo p.E250K mutation were described which presented with a different and more complex phenotype compared to cases of classical PAPA syndrome [24–26]. Additionally, another familial case was reported with a phenotype distinct from classical PAPA. The patient had a milder phenotype, with no skin features, minor episodes of arthritis with no sequelae, and normal growth [27]. Compared to the patients with de novo mutations, the two familial cases seem to have a milder phenotype. Furthermore a cerebral arterial vasculopathy or vasculitis and a posterior cerebral artery dissecting aneurysm have been reported in a patient with p.E257K mutation, which have never been found before in a patient with PAID [28].

Pyoderma Gangrenosum, Acne, and Ulcerative Colitis (PAC); Pyogenic Arthritis, Pyoderma Gangrenosum, Acne, and Hidradenitis Suppurativa (PAPASH); and PAPA-Like Syndrome

In the last years, the spectrum of PAID has been expanded, and three other phenotypes with PSTPIP1 mutations have been described.

In a 33-year-old man with a long-standing history of ulcerative colitis, severe acne and recurrent skin ulcerations, and recalcitrant pustular rash, the mutation p.G403R in *PSTIPIP1* was detected, and the term pyoderma gangrenosum, acne, and ulcerative colitis (PAC) syndrome was suggested. Treatment with a human IL-1 receptor antagonist IL-1Ra (anakinra) led to a dramatic improvement in the patient's condition [29].

In a 16-year-old patient with the PSTPIP1 mutation p.E277D, a pyogenic arthritis, pyoderma gangrenosum, acne, and hidradenitis suppurativa (PAPASH) syndrome was defined as a new entity [14]. This term has been chosen because of its resemblance to pyoderma gangrenosum, acne, and hidradenitis suppurativa

(PASH) syndrome that has been described in two unrelated patients as autoinflammatory diseases of the skin [30]. Despite mutations in *PSTPIP1* could be excluded initially, an increased repetition of the CCTG microsatellite motif was present in the *PSTPIP1* promotor on one allele in both patients with PASH syndrome [30]. Additionally, a p.A405C mutation could be identified in a PASH patient. However, the same study reported 12 PASH syndrome cases without mutations in *PSTPIP1* [31].

Finally, "PAPA-like syndrome" was defined in a 22-year-old male who presented with skin ulcers and acne lesions since the age of 14 as well as recurrent episodes of arthralgia and fever that did not respond to the administration of high-dose antibiotics from early childhood. The patient was diagnosed as having features of a "PAPA-like syndrome" in which cutaneous manifestations, such as pyoderma gangrenosum and acne fulminans, predominated. Here, a homozygous p.G258A mutation could be identified, and the skin lesions responded well to canakinumab treatment. Two of nine family members carrying the mutant allele heterozygously exhibit active acne-like lesions [12]. The patient was treated with canakinumab, a human anti-interleukin 1β monoclonal antibody, which led to rapid remission of the symptoms. "PAPA-like syndrome" is the only entity within PAID with an autosomal recessive heredity.

Interestingly, a heterozygous p.G258A mutation, which may affect the structure and function of the PSTPIP1 protein, was described before in 1 of 14 patients with pyoderma gangrenosum [32] indicating that this mutation might have a pathophysiological relevance.

At the moment it is still uncertain whether PAC, PAPASH, and PAPA-like syndrome are only single observations or part of an expanding spectrum of PAID in contrast to classical PAPA and PAMI syndrome that have been characterized by different groups and in larger patient cohort.

Pathogenetic Mechanisms

PSTPIP1 is a protein with complex functions and interactions. Therefore, the underlying molecular mechanism of the inflammatory processes in PAID is currently not clear, but there is experimental evidence for a complex pathogenesis of this autoinflammatory entity.

Structure and Functions of PSTPIP1

PSTPIP1 is a cytoskeletal adaptor protein that was originally identified in the mouse through its interaction with PEST (rich in proline (P), glutamic acid (E), serine (S), and threonine (T) residues)-type protein tyrosine phosphatase (PTP-PEST, also known as PTPN12) [33]. Its human homolog, called CD2BP1, was identified by interaction with the T-cell surface protein CD2 [34]. Meanwhile the gene and protein are now generally cited as PSTPIP1.

The structure of PSTPIP1 consists of a N-terminal Fer-CIP4 homology (FCH) domain, a central coiled-coil region, through which it binds to PEST-type phosphatases [35, 36] and a C-terminal SH3 domain that is important for the binding of several PEST phosphatase substrates, including c-abl and WASP [36, 37]. PSTPIP1 and several related proteins share an extended region containing a coiled-coil downstream of the FCH domain. Proteins with these shared domains comprise the F-BAR (FCHBAR) class of the BAR domain superfamily (BAR is named for Bin-Amphiphysin-Rvs). The BAR domain proteins function to link cellular membranes to the actin cytoskeleton and are involved in endocytosis [38].

Interestingly, all mutations of PAID cluster in the coiled-coil region of PSTPIP1 suggest that the PTP-PEST interaction mediated through this domain is central to pathology.

Indeed, the p.E250Q and p.A230T variants of PSTPIP1 found in PAPA severely abrogated binding to PTP-PEST leading to hyperphosphorylation of PSTPIP1 itself [4]. This hyperphosphorylated state was also demonstrated for the p.E250K mutation of PAMI [13]. Accordingly it could be shown that binding of PTP-PEST to PSTPIP1 is essential for its dephosphorylation and tyrosine 344 is the primary phosphorylation site of PSTPIP1 [6, 39, 40].

PSTPIP1 interacts through its SH3 domain with other immune-related proteins such as WASP, c-Abl kinase, and Fas ligand (FasL) [35, 40, 41]. These proteins bind primarily via the PSTPIP1 SH3 domain to be delivered to PTP-PEST for dephosphorylation [5, 42, 43]. Until now there are no conclusive studies demonstrating whether PAID mutations in PSTPIP1 may directly alter these interactions or may mediate effects due to hyperphosphorylation of these proteins or of PSTPIP1 itself. In case of the PSTPIP1/WASP interaction, it could be shown that this is phosphorylation-dependent and PAPA mutations consequently predict reduced interaction in vivo. Thus WASP-mediated cytoskeletal reorganization events might be implicated in PAPA pathogenesis via posttranslational mechanisms [4, 40].

In summary, multiple functions for a PSTPIP1/PTP-PEST complex in hematopoietic cells are discussed that may have direct consequences for immune cell adhesion, invasion, and migration [5, 35, 40, 41, 43–45]. Besides that PSTPIP1 also interacts with other PTP-PEST homologs such as PTP hematopoietic stem cell factor (HSCF) [33], which might be a link to pancytopenia, as observed in PAMI patients [13].

Finally, PSTIPIP1 forms homodimers and generates membrane-associated cytosolic filamentous structures. The F-BAR region is necessary and sufficient for its self-aggregation. This PSTPIP1 filament network is dependent upon an intact tubulin cytoskeleton, and the distribution of this network can be modulated by pyrin, indicating that this is a dynamic structure. However, p.A230T and p.E250Q did not alter the self-binding capacity of PSTPIP1 [46].

Interaction with Pyrin and the Inflammasome

Interestingly PSTPIP1 directly interacts with pyrin, which is mutated in another autoinflammatory disease, FMF, thus suggesting potential molecular mechanisms for the inflammatory mechanisms of PAID. Interestingly, FMF shows some clinical similarities to PAID, including a neutrophil-rich sterile infiltrate of the joints and neutrophilic dermatoses. The relationship of FMF and PAPA was clarified by the discovery of molecular interaction, when a pyrin bait identified PSTPIP1 in yeast two hybrid screens of a monocyte library [20]. PAPA-associated p.A230T and p.E250Q mutations in PSTPIP1 significantly increase binding of PSTPIP1 to pyrin [6]. The increased interaction with pyrin is most likely because the PSTPIP1 variants bind PTP-PEST less avidly and are therefore hyperphosphorylated and because the avidity of PSTPIP1 for pyrin varies with PSTPIP1 phosphorylation status. This binding is even increased with p.E250K mutant proteins and might be due to the charge switch of the PSTPIP1 surface caused by the mutation [13]. There is now increasing experimental evidence that this PSTPIP1-pyrin interaction has significant consequences for the innate immune response. Pyrin has been described to form an alternative inflammasome and that mutations in pyrin may lead to an uncontrolled activation of this pathway resulting in an overwhelming production of active IL-1ß [47]. In a cellular model, it has been shown that this process can be triggered by the interaction of PSTPIP1 with pyrin. PSTPIP1 mutants found in PAPA show a stronger effect on pyrin-inflammasome activation than wild-type PSTPIP1 [7]. This mechanism is regulated by p38 mitogen-activated protein kinases (MAPK) signaling and depends on an intact microtubule network [48]. While PAPA mutations affect pyrin-mediated pathways, the reverse is apparently not the case since FMF causal mutations do not affect binding to PSTPIP1. This is explained by the fact that causal mutations for FMF almost always occur outside the PSTPIP1-binding site of pyrin, a B-box domain that mediates pyrin autoinhibition in the absence of PSTPIP1 [49].

In a mouse model ectopic expression of human PSTPIP1 p.A230T mutant protein induced an inflammatory phenotype with a strong induction of IL-1 and TNF expression [15].

Increased Interleukin (IL)-1β Secretion

Due to variable methodologies and limited case numbers in different studies, the relevance of IL-1β secretion in PAPA has not been clarified yet [6, 24]. In different studies both in vitro and ex vivo, PAPA-associated mutations were associated with increased IL-1β production. This could be due to increased sequestration and impairment of pyrin function, thereby diminishing its inhibition of inflammation [6]. On the other hand, the domain of pyrin to which PSTPIP1 binds (the B box) is an autoinhibitory domain that constrains ASC binding [7]. Another study analyzed

IL-1β secretion from monocytes isolated from 13 patients at baseline and following activation. The IL-1β secretion in PAPA was increased, required NLRP3, and correlated with disease activity. Consistent with the literature, IL-1β assessments were heterogeneous, and the analysis failed to disclose any significant difference between active PAPA and HC for released IL-1a, IL-18, IL-6, and TNF-a [50]. Interestingly Il-1ß secretion was only apparent after stimulation with the exogenous TLR-4 ligand lipopolysaccharide (LPS), which points to a putative role of endogenous TLR-4 ligands like MRP8 and MRP14 (see below) for the release of IL-1ß from PAPA monocytes.

Role of Myeloid-Related Proteins (MRP) 8 and 14

Another hallmark of PAID is a very high (PAPA: 116 ± 74 μg/mL vs. 0.5 ± 0.1 μg/mL in healthy controls (HC)) or exorbitant (PAMI: 2070 ± 1190 μg/mL) expression of two proinflammatory proteins of the S100 family, MRP8 (S100A8) and MRP14 (S100A9) [13]. These proteins belong to the family of so-called alarmins or danger-associated molecular patterns (DAMPs), which are released during cell stress or damage at local sites of inflammation [51, 52]. Hypersecretion of S100 proteins can result in a sterile inflammatory environment, which triggers proinflammatory cytokine as well as further S100 expression [53, 54]. During inflammatory attacks, serum levels of S100 proteins are massively elevated in FMF, and the excessive amount of these proteins suggests its involvement in the pathogenesis [13, 53]. MRP8 and MRP14 promote inflammation via activation of TLR4, and knockout of this molecular system has an inhibitory effect in many inflammatory conditions [52, 55, 56]. MRP8 and MRP14 are lacking structural elements required for secretion via the classical endoplasmic reticulum and Golgi-dependent secretory pathway. Thus, one of the primary, though passive, release "mechanisms" involves necrotic cell death. Further, there is evidence for active cytoskeleton-dependent nonclassical secretion [57–59] (Fig. 4.1), which are similarly used by cytokines such as interleukin (IL)-1 [60].

Recently, a genome-wide expression analysis revealed that the MRP-induced response in human monocytes is mainly related to immune cell activation, NF-kB signaling, cell migration, as well as leukocyte activation and signal transduction which fits very well to the clinical picture of PAID patients [61]. Beside phagocytes keratinocytes seem to be a major source of MRPs in PAMI patients [13]. Although the exact role of these molecules in the pathogenesis of PAID is yet not clear, there are several interesting links to the molecular processes described above for PSTPIP1 and pyrin, and MRP8 and MRP14 show a high overexpression and release in FMF (110 ± 82 μg/mL) as well [13].

Like PSTPIP1, MRP8 and MRP14 are highly expressed in phagocytes. Both proteins bind to both the subcellular actin network and microtubules in a calcium-

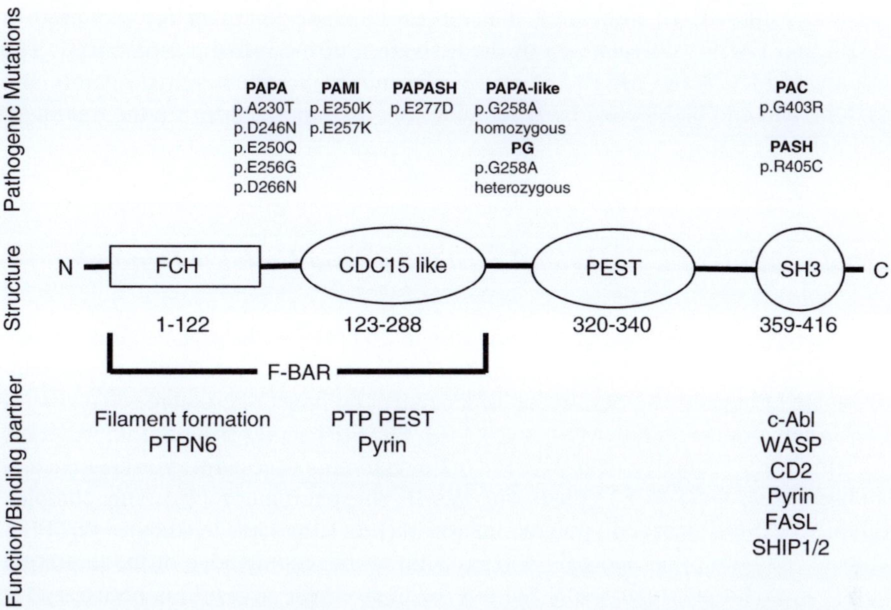

Fig. 4.1 Location of mutations in PSTPIP1 and its clinical manifestations. Mutations causing pyogenic arthritis, pyoderma gangrenosum (PG), and acne syndrome (PAPA); PSTPIP1-associated myeloid-related proteinemia inflammatory (PAMI) syndrome; pyogenic arthritis, pyoderma gangrenosum, acne, and hidradenitis suppurativa (PAPASH) syndrome; and PAPA-like syndrome mutations reported in pyoderma gangrenosum (PG) are located within the CDC15 domain, whereas the pyoderma gangrenosum, acne, and ulcerative colitis (PAC) syndrome-causing mutation and the mutation reported in pyoderma gangrenosum, acne, and hidradenitis suppurativa (PASH) syndrome are located within the SH3 domain. Interaction partners of each domain are indicated. c-Abelson tyrosine kinase (c-Abl); cluster of differentiation 2 (CD2); Fas ligand (FASL); Fes/CIP4 homology (FCH); protein tyrosine phosphatase non-receptor type 6 (PTPN6); protein tyrosine phosphatase with C-terminal rich in proline (P), glutamic acid (E), serine (S), and threonine (T) residue-type motif (PTP PEST); Src-homology 3 (SH3); Wiskott-Aldrich syndrome protein (WASP)

dependent manner. Knock-out of these molecules induces a migratory phenotype in phagocytes with reduced recruitment of phagocytes in a wound model [58]. Extracellular MRP8 and MRP14 form a positive inflammatory feedback loop with IL-1ß, and all three proteins seem to play a significant role in the autoinflammatory process of PAPA, PAMI, and FMF as well [13, 62]. Interestingly, the mechanism of release of IL-1ß and MRP8 and MRP14 show some striking similarities. All three molecules lack a leader sequence necessary for the classical secretory pathway via endoplasmic reticulum and Golgi complex. The release of these proteins follows a so-called alternative pathway, which is purely characterized so far. However, MRP8 and MRP14 are not processed by the inflammasome/

caspase 1 like IL-1ß indicating that the mechanism dominant for secretion in PAPA and FMF is downstream of the activation of the inflammasome [63]. The release of MRP8 and MRP14 is energy dependent, needs an active microtubule system, and can be blocked by colchicine, the first-choice drug for the treatment of FMF [57, 63].

Organization of Cytoskeletal Structures and Cellular Dynamics

Several reports point to a more general role of PSTPIP1 in the organization of cytoskeletal structures and cellular dynamics in leukocytes. PSTPIP1 forms a membrane-associated filament network, which is dependent on intact microtubules. Dynamics of this network are modulated by pyrin [46]. PSTPIP1 serves as a scaffold molecule for a molecular complex with WASP, a main regulator of the actin cytoskeleton, and a phosphatase (PST-PEST) regulating WASP phosphorylation [40]. This complex inhibits WASP-driven actin polymerization [44]. In stimulated leukocytes PSTPIP1 colocalized with pyrin and polymerized actin at the leading edge of the migrating cell [64]. Actin polymerization, but not the microtubule network, is necessary for the polarized distribution of PSTPIP1 [45]. Consequently mutations of PSTPIP1 lead to a complex migratory phenotype in phagocytes regulating the balance of the formation of podosomes and filopodia [65, 66].

Regulation of Osteoclast Activity

As mentioned above PSTPIP1 plays an important role in podosome formation. Just recently the impact of PSTPIP1 and PSTPIP2 on podosome dynamics specifically in osteoclasts has been addressed. Bone resorption relies on the ability of osteoclasts to assemble F-actin-rich podosomes that condense into podosomal belts, forming sealing zones. Sealing zones segregate bone-facing ruffled membranes from other membrane domains and disassemble when osteoclasts migrate to new areas. Whereas PSTPIP2 regulates podosome and sealing zone assembly, PSTPIP1 regulates their disassembly. PSTPIP1 recruits, through its F-BAR domain, the protein tyrosine phosphatase non-receptor type 6 (PTPN6) that dephosphorylates the phosphatidylinositol 5-phosphatases SHIP1/SHIP2 bound to the SH3 domain of PSTPIP1. Depletion of any component of this complex prevents sealing zone disassembly and increases osteoclast activity. In conclusion, a PSTPIP1-/PTPN6-/SHIP1-/SHIP2-dependent negative feedback mechanism controls osteoclast cell polarity and activity during bone resorption [67]. The impact of PAID mutations has not been tested in this setting. However, it is imaginable that an increase of osteoclast activity by mutated pyrin might cause bone damage as seen in sterile osteomyelitis in some of these patients.

Interactions with the Adaptive Immune System

Although clinical and laboratory signs of autoimmunity are not dominant in the pathogenesis of PAID, there are some reports indicating that PSTPIP1 has an additional function in the formation of the immunological synapse in T cells in a WASP-dependent manner [42]. In addition, PSTPIP1 interacts with CD2 and Fas ligand (FasL) [5, 41, 42]. PSTPIP1 binding inhibits WASP phosphorylation, which is required for activated T-cell transcriptional activity and immunologic synapse formation. However, PSTPIP1 p.A230T and p.E250Q mutations did not affect WASP binding in yeast. Whether such mutations may decrease binding and increase T-cell activation in mammalian cells is still unclear [4]. Although the effect of PAID-associated PSTPIP1 mutants on T-cell function in vivo is unknown, the adaptive immune response could provide at least a trigger for PAPA flares. Interestingly in some individuals with PAMI, an autoimmune neutropenia has been noted [13]. The interaction with T-cell proteins is obviously dependent on the SH3 domain of PSTPIP1 indicating that this effect does not involve interaction with the PST-PEST phosphatase described above [68].

Treatment

PAID are due to their rarity, clinical heterogeneity, and the complex pathogenesis difficult to treat. Physicians are dealing not only with different phenotypes of PAID but also interindividually differences within one syndrome. Furthermore, as in PAPA, clinical symptoms might change with age, and therefore another therapeutic target, e.g., arthritis or pyoderma gangrenosum, has to be addressed. In contrast to other autoinflammatory diseases with a straightforward treatment concept as IL-1 blockade in CAPS, patients with PAID still lack an evidence-based therapeutic approach. More clinical experience with PAID should help to clarify and prioritize best treatment options in the face of varying symptoms in specific target organs.

Until now, steroids, anti-TNF-a [8, 10, 69], and anti-IL-1 agents [11, 24] have been proposed for the treatment especially of PAPA. The recombinant IL1 receptor antagonist anakinra has proven to be effective in controlling flares for PAPA syndrome patients [11, 70] and seems to be effective in resolving joint inflammation at least for some patients. On the other side, the anti-TNF monoclonal antibody, infliximab, induces dramatic resolution of severe pyoderma gangrenosum in some PAPA patients [8–10]. In contrast, cystic acne, the second cutaneous symptom of PAPA syndrome, does not seem as responsive to IL1 and TNF blockade [20].

In Table 4.2 used agents and reported effects in almost all published cases with PAID are summarized and might give an orientation about the efficacy and target of different therapeutic options. Significant variability in response has been observed, and biologics have not been consistently effective in all cases and do not necessarily

Table 4.2 Therapeutic approaches to PSTPIP1-associated inflammatory diseases (PAID)

Acronym	Response	PAPA	PAMI	PAPASH	PAPA-like	PAC
Cases (n)		25	18	1	1	1
Steroids	–	Steroids i.a. ($n = 1$)	pred p.o. ($n = 2$)			
	+	pred p.o. ($n = 8$): arthritis, PG, abscesses Steroids topical ($n = 1$): pustulosis Steroids i.v. ($n = 1$): PG Steroids i.a. ($n = 4$): arthritis	pred p.o. ($n = 9$): PG anemia, systemic inflammation, arthritis, HSM, LP	pred p.o. ($n = 1$): PG	pred p.o. ($n = 1$): PG, acne	pred p.o. ($n = 1$): PG, acne
Anti-IL1	–	Anakinra ($n = 3$)	Anakinra ($n = 4$) Canakinumab ($n = 2$) Secukinumab ($n = 1$)			
	+	Anakinra ($n = 10$): arthritis, PG, acne, osteolytic lesions, systemic inflammation Canakinumab ($n = 1$): arthritis	Anakinra ($n = 5$): systemic inflammation, arthritis, anemia, thrombocytopenia, skin lesions; weight and grow gain Canakinumab ($n = 2$): arthritis, anemia, HSM, systemic inflammation, PG	Anakinra ($n = 1$): arthritis, acne, PG, HS	Canakinumab ($n = 1$): acne, PG	Anakinra ($n = 1$): rash, PG
Anti-TNF	–	Etanercept ($n = 2$) Infliximab ($n = 1$)	Etanercept ($n = 1$) Adalimumab ($n = 1$) Infliximab ($n = 1$)			Infliximab, adalimumab ($n = 1$)
	+	Infliximab ($n = 3$): PG Adalimumab ($n = 2$) (+pred+MTX $n = 1$) ($n = 2$): PG Etanercept ($n = 1$): PG	Adalimumab ($n = 2$): systemic inflammation, PG, acne Infliximab ($n = 1$): skin lesions arthritis			

Other anti-inflammatory drugs	–	Thalidomide ($n = 1$) IVIG ($n = 1$) Colchicine ($n = 1$) MTX ($n = 2$) HCQ ($n = 2$) Tacrolimus topical ($n = 1$) CsA ($n = 1$) MMF ($n = 1$) Dapsone ($n = 2$)	IVIG ($n = 2$) MTX ($n = 1$) Colchicine ($n = 1$) Tacrolimus ($n = 1$)			
	+	Tacrolimus ($n = 1$) MMF (+pred) ($n = 1$): PG Leflunomide ($n = 1$) AZA ($n = 1$ + pred): PG	CsA ($n = 5$ (4 + pred)): arthritis, anemia, systemic inflammation, skin lesions, HM, PG Tacrolimus ($n = 2$): arthritis, anemia, systemic inflammation, skin lesions Tocilizumab ($n = 1$): arthritis, proteinuria, and hematuria Colchicine ($n = 1$ + pred): arthritis, systemic inflammation GM-CSF ($n = 1$): skin lesions AZA ($n = 1$ + pred): vasculitis	Dapsone ($n = 1$): HS Tacrolimus locally ($n = 1$): PG		
Co-medication	–	Plasmapheresis ($n = 1$)				
	+	Isoretinoin ($n = 2$): acne	Isoretinoin ($n = 2$): acne	Azithromycin ($n = 1$): acne		Isoretinoin ($n = 1$): acne

Adapted and updated from Holzinger and Roth [16]

Medications applied in patients with PAID with no (–) or good (+) response and symptoms that have been affected by the therapy. Patients reported in multiple studies have only been included once

AZA azathioprine, *CsA* cyclosporine A, *GM-CSF* granulocyte macrophage colony-stimulating factor, *HSM* hepatosplenomegaly, *HS* hidradenitis suppurativa, *HCQ* hydroxychloroquine, *IVIG* intravenous immunoglobulins, *LP* lymphadenopathy, *MTX* methotrexate, *MMF* mycophenolate mofetil, *pred* prednisolone, *PG* pyoderma gangrenosum

induce remission of all the disease manifestations. Reflecting the evidence that PSTPIP1 functions in multiple pathways and in several immune-related cells, this is not surprising.

Three reports reviewed treatment of PAPA and PAMI in the largest cohorts described so far [13, 24, 50]. In the first report, five patients (four PAPA and one PAMI) were presented. Infliximab showed efficacy in two of three treated patients. Treatment with adalimumab was successful in two patients, whereas response to anakinra varied. Of the four patients who received anakinra, two patients (one with PAMI) had inadequate responses to the treatment, and one discontinued the therapy due to adverse effects. The fourth patient exhibited a good response to anakinra [24].

In the second report, the pattern of IL-1β secretion in PAPA patients was analyzed in an attempt to provide evidence-based insights supporting the application of an anti-IL-1 regimen. The long-term efficacy of anti-IL-1 treatment in PAPA patients was retrospectively investigated in five PAPA patients (four patients received anakinra and one patient anakinra, followed by canakinumab), three of them had already been unresponsive to treatment with anti-TNFα mAb for a mean follow-up of 28 months without benefit. All patients showed a significant decrease in frequency of disease flares and normalization of acute phase reactants. Three patients displayed a complete resolution of the clinical manifestations and could withdraw steroids. Interestingly, one PAMI patient with p.E250K was included, who displayed a response to anakinra with an incomplete control of severe pyoderma gangrenosum, and shift to canakinumab led to a complete resolution [50].

In the third report, response to treatment was evaluated in 10 PAMI patients. Interestingly, no consistently effective therapy was observed. Best responses were noted when using IL-1 inhibitors, either anakinra (n = 4) or canakinumab (n = 1), but there were also five patients who were unresponsive to this therapy. Treatment with cyclosporine A (CsA) (n = 4) or prednisolone (n = 5) resulted in a partial response. Anti-TNF showed a response in one patient (infliximab), whereas it was ineffective in two patients (adalimumab and etanercept). Of note, cutaneous symptoms, arthritis, anemia, and systemic inflammation improved, but neutropenia persisted in all patients following treatment. In three patients (hepato)splenomegaly resolved with treatment [13]. Response to CsA was also reported in the first study in a PAMI patient [24] and was the most effective treatment in a recent report about a PAMI patient with severe pyoderma gangrenosum. Infliximab, canakinumab, and secukinumab were ineffective, but introduction of CsA almost completely healed the PG [25].

Based on all observations anti-IL-1, and in some cases with PG as main symptom, anti-TNF treatment seems to be a therapeutic option (Table 4.2). Nevertheless, IL-1 inhibition is probably not as effective in PAID as for cryopyrin-associated periodic syndrome (CAPS) patients underlying the fact that PSTPIP1 mutations have additional pathophysiologic effects like induction of inflammatory alarmins.

Summary

PSTPIP1-associated diseases are associated with a range of clinical phenotypes and show variable expressivity. Therefore, the term PSTPIP1-associated inflammatory diseases (PAID) encompasses PAPA (p.A230T, p.E250Q, p.E256G, p.D246N, p.D266N) and PAMI (p.E250K, p.E257K) [13] syndrome and possibly PAPASH (p.E277D) [14], PAC (p.G403R) [29], and PAPA-like syndrome (homozygous p.G258A) [12] if these phenotypes can be confirmed in other patients [16].

Interestingly, all mutations despite p.G403R are located within the region, which interacts with pyrin and PTP PEST (Fig. 4.1) indicating the pathophysiological relevance of these interactions. However, PSTPIP1 functions are complex and include interaction with pyrin and the inflammasome, organization of cytoskeletal structures and cellular dynamics, interactions with the adaptive immune system, and regulation of osteoclast activity. In particular, monocytes from PAPA patients show an oversecretion of IL-1ß during the active phase of the disease, which seems to be dependent on the NLRP3 inflammasome [50]. However, this finding was not consistent in all patients, and despite anti-IL-1 treatment-induced control of clinical manifestations in PAPA patients, therapies targeting IL1 lack efficacy in some individuals with PAID. Recent data indicate that a complex dysregulation of the innate immune system leads to an uncontrolled release of cytokines as IL-1 and IL-18 and DAMPs/alarmins as MRP8 and MRP14 driving the autoinflammatory process responsible for the clinical picture of PAID patients.

These findings and the complex interactions of PSTPIP1 with other proteins involved in the immune response (e.g., WASP, FASL, CD3) might explain the clinical peculiarity of PAID in terms of variability in clinical presentation and response to treatment.

References

1. Lindor NM, Arsenault TM, Solomon H, Seidman CE, McEvoy MT. A new autosomal dominant disorder of pyogenic sterile arthritis, pyoderma gangrenosum, and acne: PAPA syndrome. Mayo Clin Proc. 1997;72(7):611–5.
2. Wise CA, Bennett LB, Pascual V, Gillum JD, Bowcock AM. Localization of a gene for familial recurrent arthritis. Arthritis Rheum. 2000;43(9):2041–5.
3. Yeon HB, Lindor NM, Seidman JG, Seidman CE. Pyogenic arthritis, pyoderma gangrenosum, and acne syndrome maps to chromosome 15q. Am J Hum Genet. 2000;66(4):1443–8.
4. Wise CA, Gillum JD, Seidman CE, Lindor NM, Veile R, Bashiardes S, et al. Mutations in CD2BP1 disrupt binding to PTP PEST and are responsible for PAPA syndrome, an autoinflammatory disorder. Hum Mol Genet. 2002;11(8):961–9.
5. Yang H, Reinherz EL. CD2BP1 modulates CD2-dependent T cell activation via linkage to protein tyrosine phosphatase (PTP)-PEST. J Immunol. 2006;176(10):5898–907.
6. Shoham NG, Centola M, Mansfield E, Hull KM, Wood G, Wise CA, et al. Pyrin binds the PSTPIP1/CD2BP1 protein, defining familial Mediterranean fever and PAPA syndrome as disorders in the same pathway. Proc Natl Acad Sci U S A. 2003;100(23):13501–6.

7. Yu JW, Fernandes-Alnemri T, Datta P, Wu J, Juliana C, Solorzano L, et al. Pyrin activates the ASC pyroptosome in response to engagement by autoinflammatory PSTPIP1 mutants. Mol Cell. 2007;28(2):214–27.
8. Cortis E, De Benedetti F, Insalaco A, Cioschi S, Muratori F, D'Urbano LE, et al. Abnormal production of tumor necrosis factor (TNF) – alpha and clinical efficacy of the TNF inhibitor etanercept in a patient with PAPA syndrome [corrected]. J Pediatr. 2004;145(6):851–5.
9. Edrees AF, Kaplan DL, Abdou NI. Pyogenic arthritis, pyoderma gangrenosum, and acne syndrome (PAPA syndrome) associated with hypogammaglobulinemia and elevated serum tumor necrosis factor-alpha levels. J Clin Rheumatol. 2002;8(5):273–5.
10. Stichweh DS, Punaro M, Pascual V. Dramatic improvement of pyoderma gangrenosum with infliximab in a patient with PAPA syndrome. Pediatr Dermatol. 2005;22(3):262–5.
11. Dierselhuis MP, Frenkel J, Wulffraat NM, Boelens JJ. Anakinra for flares of pyogenic arthritis in PAPA syndrome. Rheumatology (Oxford). 2005;44(3):406–8.
12. Geusau A, Mothes-Luksch N, Nahavandi H, Pickl WF, Wise CA, Pourpak Z, et al. Identification of a homozygous PSTPIP1 mutation in a patient with a PAPA-like syndrome responding to canakinumab treatment. JAMA Dermatol. 2013;149(2):209–15.
13. Holzinger D, Fassl SK, de Jager W, Lohse P, Rohrig UF, Gattorno M, et al. Single amino acid charge switch defines clinically distinct proline-serine-threonine phosphatase-interacting protein 1 (PSTPIP1)-associated inflammatory diseases. J Allergy Clin Immunol. 2015;136(5):1337–45.
14. Marzano AV, Trevisan V, Gattorno M, Ceccherini I, De Simone C, Crosti C. Pyogenic arthritis, pyoderma gangrenosum, acne, and hidradenitis suppurativa (PAPASH): a new autoinflammatory syndrome associated with a novel mutation of the PSTPIP1 gene. JAMA Dermatol. 2013;149(6):762–4.
15. Wang D, Hoing S, Patterson HC, Ahmad UM, Rathinam VA, Rajewsky K, et al. Inflammation in mice ectopically expressing human Pyogenic Arthritis, Pyoderma Gangrenosum, and Acne (PAPA) Syndrome-associated PSTPIP1 A230T mutant proteins. J Biol Chem. 2013;288(7):4594–601.
16. Holzinger D, Roth J. Alarming consequences – autoinflammatory disease spectrum due to mutations in proline-serine-threonine phosphatase-interacting protein 1. Curr Opin Rheumatol. 2016;28(5):550–9.
17. Fathalla BM, Al-Wahadneh AM, Al-Mutawa M, Kambouris M, El-Shanti H. A novel de novo PSTPIP1 mutation in a boy with pyogenic arthritis, pyoderma gangrenosum, acne (PAPA) syndrome. Clin Exp Rheumatol. 2014;32(6):956–8.
18. Toplak N, Frenkel J, Ozen S, Lachmann HJ, Woo P, Kone-Paut I, et al. An international registry on autoinflammatory diseases: the Eurofever experience. Ann Rheum Dis. 2012;71(7):1177–82.
19. Touitou I, Lesage S, McDermott M, Cuisset L, Hoffman H, Dode C, et al. Infevers: an evolving mutation database for auto-inflammatory syndromes. Hum Mutat. 2004;24(3):194–8.
20. Smith EJ, Allantaz F, Bennett L, Zhang D, Gao X, Wood G, et al. Clinical, molecular, and genetic characteristics of PAPA syndrome: a review. Curr Genomics. 2010;11(7):519–27.
21. Schroder K, Hertzog PJ, Ravasi T, Hume DA. Interferon-gamma: an overview of signals, mechanisms and functions. J Leukoc Biol. 2004;75(2):163–89.
22. Song X, Zhu S, Shi P, Liu Y, Shi Y, Levin SD, et al. IL-17RE is the functional receptor for IL-17C and mediates mucosal immunity to infection with intestinal pathogens. Nat Immunol. 2011;12(12):1151–8.
23. Zindl CL, Lai JF, Lee YK, Maynard CL, Harbour SN, Ouyang W, et al. IL-22-producing neutrophils contribute to antimicrobial defense and restitution of colonic epithelial integrity during colitis. Proc Natl Acad Sci U S A. 2013;110(31):12768–73.
24. Demidowich AP, Freeman AF, Kuhns DB, Aksentijevich I, Gallin JI, Turner ML, et al. Brief report: genotype, phenotype, and clinical course in five patients with PAPA syndrome (pyogenic sterile arthritis, pyoderma gangrenosum, and acne). Arthritis Rheum. 2012;64(6):2022–7.

25. Klotgen HW, Beltraminelli H, Yawalkar N, van Gijn ME, Holzinger D, Borradori L. The expanding spectrum of clinical phenotypes associated with PSTPIP1 mutations: from PAPA to PAMI syndrome and beyond. Br J Dermatol. 2018;178:982–3.
26. Lindwall E, Singla S, Davis WE, Quinet RJ. Novel PSTPIP1 gene mutation in a patient with pyogenic arthritis, pyoderma gangrenosum and acne (PAPA) syndrome. Semin Arthritis Rheum. 2015;45(1):91–3.
27. Belelli E, Passarelli C, Pardeo M, Holzinger D, De Benedetti F, Insalaco A. Haematological involvement associated with a mild autoinflammatory phenotype, in two patients carrying the E250K mutation of PSTPIP1. Clin Exp Rheumatol. 2017;35(Suppl 108(6)):113–5.
28. Khatibi K, Heit JJ, Telischak NA, Elbers JM, Do HM. Cerebral vascular findings in PAPA syndrome: cerebral arterial vasculopathy or vasculitis and a posterior cerebral artery dissecting aneurysm. J Neurointerv Surg. 2016;8(8):e29.
29. Zeeli T, Padalon-Brauch G, Ellenbogen E, Gat A, Sarig O, Sprecher E. Pyoderma gangrenosum, acne and ulcerative colitis in a patient with a novel mutation in the PSTPIP1 gene. Clin Exp Dermatol. 2015;40(4):367–72.
30. Braun-Falco M, Kovnerystyy O, Lohse P, Ruzicka T. Pyoderma gangrenosum, acne, and suppurative hidradenitis (PASH)--a new autoinflammatory syndrome distinct from PAPA syndrome. J Am Acad Dermatol. 2012;66(3):409–15.
31. Calderon-Castrat X, Bancalari-Diaz D, Roman-Curto C, Romo-Melgar A, Amoros-Cerdan D, Alcaraz-Mas LA, et al. PSTPIP1 gene mutation in a pyoderma gangrenosum, acne and suppurative hidradenitis (PASH) syndrome. Br J Dermatol. 2016;175(1):194–8.
32. Nesterovitch AB, Hoffman MD, Simon M, Petukhov PA, Tharp MD, Glant TT. Mutations in the PSTPIP1 gene and aberrant splicing variants in patients with pyoderma gangrenosum. Clin Exp Dermatol. 2011;36(8):889–95.
33. Spencer S, Dowbenko D, Cheng J, Li W, Brush J, Utzig S, et al. PSTPIP: a tyrosine phosphorylated cleavage furrow-associated protein that is a substrate for a PEST tyrosine phosphatase. J Cell Biol. 1997;138(4):845–60.
34. Li J, Nishizawa K, An W, Hussey RE, Lialios FE, Salgia R, et al. A cdc15-like adaptor protein (CD2BP1) interacts with the CD2 cytoplasmic domain and regulates CD2-triggered adhesion. EMBO J. 1998;17(24):7320–36.
35. Cong F, Spencer S, Cote JF, Wu Y, Tremblay ML, Lasky LA, et al. Cytoskeletal protein PSTPIP1 directs the PEST-type protein tyrosine phosphatase to the c-Abl kinase to mediate Abl dephosphorylation. Mol Cell. 2000;6(6):1413–23.
36. Wu Y, Spencer SD, Lasky LA. Tyrosine phosphorylation regulates the SH3-mediated binding of the Wiskott-Aldrich syndrome protein to PSTPIP, a cytoskeletal-associated protein. J Biol Chem. 1998;273(10):5765–70.
37. Tian L, Nelson DL, Stewart DM. Cdc42-interacting protein 4 mediates binding of the Wiskott-Aldrich syndrome protein to microtubules. J Biol Chem. 2000;275(11):7854–61.
38. Dawson JC, Legg JA, Machesky LM. Bar domain proteins: a role in tubulation, scission and actin assembly in clathrin-mediated endocytosis. Trends Cell Biol. 2006;16(10):493–8.
39. Angers-Loustau A, Cote JF, Charest A, Dowbenko D, Spencer S, Lasky LA, et al. Protein tyrosine phosphatase-PEST regulates focal adhesion disassembly, migration, and cytokinesis in fibroblasts. J Cell Biol. 1999;144(5):1019–31.
40. Cote JF, Chung PL, Theberge JF, Halle M, Spencer S, Lasky LA, et al. PSTPIP is a substrate of PTP-PEST and serves as a scaffold guiding PTP-PEST toward a specific dephosphorylation of WASP. J Biol Chem. 2002;277(4):2973–86.
41. Baum W, Kirkin V, Fernandez SB, Pick R, Lettau M, Janssen O, et al. Binding of the intracellular Fas ligand (FasL) domain to the adaptor protein PSTPIP results in a cytoplasmic localization of FasL. J Biol Chem. 2005;280(48):40012–24.
42. Badour K, Zhang J, Shi F, McGavin MK, Rampersad V, Hardy LA, et al. The Wiskott-Aldrich syndrome protein acts downstream of CD2 and the CD2AP and PSTPIP1 adaptors to promote formation of the immunological synapse. Immunity. 2003;18(1):141–54.

43. Qian J, Chen W, Lettau M, Podda G, Zornig M, Kabelitz D, et al. Regulation of FasL expression: a SH3 domain containing protein family involved in the lysosomal association of FasL. Cell Signal. 2006;18(8):1327–37.
44. Badour K, Zhang J, Shi F, Leng Y, Collins M, Siminovitch KA. Fyn and PTP-PEST-mediated regulation of Wiskott-Aldrich syndrome protein (WASp) tyrosine phosphorylation is required for coupling T cell antigen receptor engagement to WASp effector function and T cell activation. J Exp Med. 2004;199(1):99–112.
45. Cooper KM, Bennin DA, Huttenlocher A. The PCH family member proline-serine-threonine phosphatase-interacting protein 1 targets to the leukocyte uropod and regulates directed cell migration. Mol Biol Cell. 2008;19(8):3180–91.
46. Waite AL, Schaner P, Richards N, Balci-Peynircioglu B, Masters SL, Brydges SD, et al. Pyrin Modulates the Intracellular Distribution of PSTPIP1. PLoS One. 2009;4(7):e6147.
47. Chae JJ, Cho YH, Lee GS, Cheng J, Liu PP, Feigenbaum L, et al. Gain-of-function Pyrin mutations induce NLRP3 protein-independent interleukin-1beta activation and severe autoinflammation in mice. Immunity. 2011;34(5):755–68.
48. Yu JW, Farias A, Hwang I, Fernandes-Alnemri T, Alnemri ES. Ribotoxic stress through p38 mitogen-activated protein kinase activates in vitro the human pyrin inflammasome. J Biol Chem. 2013;288(16):11378–83.
49. Ryan JG, Masters SL, Booty MG, Habal N, Alexander JD, Barham BK, et al. Clinical features and functional significance of the P369S/R408Q variant in pyrin, the familial Mediterranean fever protein. Ann Rheum Dis. 2010;69(7):1383–8.
50. Omenetti A, Carta S, Caorsi R, Finetti M, Marotto D, Lattanzi B, et al. Disease activity accounts for long-term efficacy of IL-1 blockers in pyogenic sterile arthritis pyoderma gangrenosum and severe acne syndrome. Rheumatology (Oxford). 2016;55(7):1325–35.
51. Chan JK, Roth J, Oppenheim JJ, Tracey KJ, Vogl T, Feldmann M, et al. Alarmins: awaiting a clinical response. J Clin Invest. 2012;122(8):2711–9.
52. Ehrchen JM, Sunderkotter C, Foell D, Vogl T, Roth J. The endogenous Toll-like receptor 4 agonist S100A8/S100A9 (calprotectin) as innate amplifier of infection, autoimmunity, and cancer. J Leukoc Biol. 2009;86(3):557–66.
53. Gohar F, Orak B, Kallinich T, Jeske M, Lieber M, von Bernuth H, et al. Correlation of secretory activity of neutrophils with genotype in patients with familial Mediterranean fever. Arthritis Rheumatol (Hoboken, NJ). 2016;68(12):3010–22.
54. Kessel C, Holzinger D, Foell D. Phagocyte-derived S100 proteins in autoinflammation: putative role in pathogenesis and usefulness as biomarkers. Clin Immunol. 2013;147(3):229–41.
55. Vogl T, Stratis A, Wixler V, Völler T, Thurainayagam S, Jorch SK, Zenker S, Dreiling A, Chakraborty D, Fröhling M, Paruzel P, Wehmeyer C, Hermann S, Papantonopoulou O, Geyer C, Loser K, Schäfers M, Ludwig S, Stoll M, Leanderson T, Schultze JL, König S, Pap T, Roth J. Autoinhibitory regulation of S100A8/S100A9 alarmin activity locally restricts sterile inflammation. J Clin Invest. 2018;128(5):1852–66.
56. Vogl T, Tenbrock K, Ludwig S, Leukert N, Ehrhardt C, van Zoelen MA, et al. Mrp8 and Mrp14 are endogenous activators of Toll-like receptor 4, promoting lethal, endotoxin-induced shock. Nat Med. 2007;13(9):1042–9.
57. Rammes A, Roth J, Goebeler M, Klempt M, Hartmann M, Sorg C. Myeloid-related protein (MRP) 8 and MRP14, calcium-binding proteins of the S100 family, are secreted by activated monocytes via a novel, tubulin-dependent pathway. J Biol Chem. 1997;272(14):9496–502.
58. Vogl T, Ludwig S, Goebeler M, Strey A, Thorey IS, Reichelt R, et al. MRP8 and MRP14 control microtubule reorganization during transendothelial migration of phagocytes. Blood. 2004;104(13):4260–8.
59. Foell D, Wittkowski H, Kessel C, Luken A, Weinhage T, Varga G, et al. Proinflammatory S100A12 can activate human monocytes via Toll-like receptor 4. Am J Respir Crit Care Med. 2013;187(12):1324–34.
60. Rubartelli A, Cozzolino F, Talio M, Sitia R. A novel secretory pathway for interleukin-1 beta, a protein lacking a signal sequence. EMBO J. 1990;9(5):1503–10.

61. Fassl SK, Austermann J, Papantonopoulou O, Riemenschneider M, Xue J, Bertheloot D, et al. Transcriptome assessment reveals a dominant role for TLR4 in the activation of human monocytes by the alarmin MRP8. J Immunol. 2015;194(2):575–83.
62. Frosch M, Ahlmann M, Vogl T, Wittkowski H, Wulffraat N, Foell D, et al. The myeloid-related proteins 8 and 14 complex, a novel ligand of toll-like receptor 4, and interleukin-1beta form a positive feedback mechanism in systemic-onset juvenile idiopathic arthritis. Arthritis Rheum. 2009;60(3):883–91.
63. Frosch M, Roth J. New insights in systemic juvenile idiopathic arthritis--from pathophysiology to treatment. Rheumatology (Oxford). 2008;47(2):121–5.
64. Akkaya-Ulum YZ, Balci-Peynircioglu B, Purali N, Yilmaz E. Pyrin-PSTPIP1 colocalises at the leading edge during cell migration. Cell Biol Int. 2015;39(12):1384–94.
65. Cortesio CL, Wernimont SA, Kastner DL, Cooper KM, Huttenlocher A. Impaired podosome formation and invasive migration of macrophages from patients with a PSTPIP1 mutation and PAPA syndrome. Arthritis Rheum. 2010;62(8):2556–8.
66. Starnes TW, Bennin DA, Bing X, Eickhoff JC, Grahf DC, Bellak JM, et al. The F-BAR protein PSTPIP1 controls extracellular matrix degradation and filopodia formation in macrophages. Blood. 2014;123(17):2703–14.
67. Sztacho M, Segeletz S, Sanchez-Fernandez MA, Czupalla C, Niehage C, Hoflack B. BAR Proteins PSTPIP1/2 Regulate Podosome Dynamics and the Resorption Activity of Osteoclasts. PLoS One. 2016;11(10):e0164829.
68. Marcos T, Ruiz-Martin V, de la Puerta ML, Trinidad AG, Rodriguez Mdel C, de la Fuente MA, et al. Proline-serine-threonine phosphatase interacting protein 1 inhibition of T-cell receptor signaling depends on its SH3 domain. FEBS J. 2014;281(17):3844–54.
69. Tofteland ND, Shaver TS. Clinical efficacy of etanercept for treatment of PAPA syndrome. J Clin Rheumatol. 2010;16(5):244–5.
70. Brenner M, Ruzicka T, Plewig G, Thomas P, Herzer P. Targeted treatment of pyoderma gangrenosum in PAPA (pyogenic arthritis, pyoderma gangrenosum and acne) syndrome with the recombinant human interleukin-1 receptor antagonist anakinra. Br J Dermatol. 2009;161(5):1199–201.

Chapter 5
Blau Syndrome

Rebecca Trachtman and Karen B. Onel

Introduction

In 1985, Blau syndrome was initially described simultaneously by both Blau and Jabs. Based on studies of two distinct families, they described a phenotype consisting of arthritis, uveitis, and dermatitis with neuropathy [1, 2]. Similar to sarcoidosis, on pathology patients are found to have non-caseating granulomas, with epithelioid and giant cells. In 2001, NOD2 mutations were discovered to be the genetic defect in Blau syndrome, differentiating Blau syndrome from sporadic early-onset sarcoidosis (EOS) [3]. Although Blau syndrome classically involves a clinical triad of (1) dermatitis, (2) arthritis, and (3) uveitis, other manifestations may be present (Table 5.1). Here, we will describe the clinical characteristics, pathophysiology, diagnosis, management, and prognosis of Blau syndrome.

Clinical Features

Dermatitis

Rash is typically the presenting feature of Blau, occurring within the first year of life. Classically, this rash is a fine, erythematous, maculopapular, scaly exanthem on the trunk and extremities [4]. Given that these findings can be indistinct, this

R. Trachtman
Icahn School of Medicine at Mount Sinai, New York, NY, USA

K. B. Onel (✉)
Pediatric Rheumatology, Hospital for Special Surgery/Weill Cornell Medicine,
New York, NY, USA
e-mail: onelk@hss.edu

P. Efthimiou (ed.), *Auto-Inflammatory Syndromes*,
https://doi.org/10.1007/978-3-319-96929-9_5

Table 5.1 Major clinical manifestations

Clinical manifestations	Approximate prevalence (%)
Arthritis	96
Dermatitis	81
Uveitis	81

rash is often misdiagnosed initially as atopic dermatitis. Later, this rash remains scaly but tends to become more tan-colored in appearance. This often helps in making a diagnosis, as the findings are more specific; however, skin biopsy can be very useful when the diagnosis remains unclear. Skin biopsy findings typically reveal granulomatous inflammation.

Arthritis

The arthritis of Blau syndrome tends to present in the first 2–4 years of life, following the development of rash. Classically, arthritis tends to be polyarticular and boggy (approximately 96% and 75%, respectively), due to deposition of granulomas in the articular spaces [5]. Arthritis tends to affect peripheral joints, especially the wrists, knees, ankles, and proximal interphalangeal joints, and involves both synovitis and tenosynovitis [6]. Although this arthritis can be deforming, it tends to be nonerosive, and joint destruction is rare. However, contractures over affected joints are common long-term sequelae. In addition, dysplastic bony changes have been noted in many patients with Blau syndrome-associated arthropathy, although the etiology for this finding remains unknown [6].

Uveitis

Of the classical triad of symptoms, uveitis is typically the last to present, often occurring around 4–5 years of age. Approximately 80% of patients with Blau syndrome develop uveitis; of these, 75% develop panuveitis, with posterior uveitis and multifocal choroiditis. The uveitis of Blau syndrome tends to be insidious in onset and is usually bilateral in nature. This uveitis is severe and requires intensive treatment, with resulting high rates of blindness without treatment. Of note, nodules representing granulomas are often seen on slit lamp examination, differentiating it from other types of uveitis that present in children.

Other Manifestations

The triad described above encompasses the classical findings in Blau syndrome. However, many other clinical manifestations have been noted, including fever, lymphadenopathy, and splenomegaly in upwards of 30% of all patients. Although the rash described above is classic, other rashes have been associated with Blau syndrome, especially erythema nodosum, which is the second most common cutaneous manifestation. In addition, neuropathy, especially of the facial nerve, has been described in association with Blau syndrome.

Additional manifestations have been described in very small numbers of patients, including leukocytoclastic vasculitis and arteritis, granulomatous nephritis, pericarditis, granulomatous hepatitis, hypertension, and pulmonary hypertension [4]. However, as the syndrome has been described relatively recently, additional manifestations may become apparent over time.

Pathophysiology

Genetic Mutations

It has been established that NOD2 is the causative mutation in Blau syndrome [3]. NOD2, also known as CARD15, is located on chromosome 16q12 and encodes the NOD2 protein [7]. The NOD2 protein belongs to the family of pattern recognition molecules that is expressed on many myeloid cells and is important for pathogen recognition by cells of the innate immune system [8, 9]. The NOD2 protein has

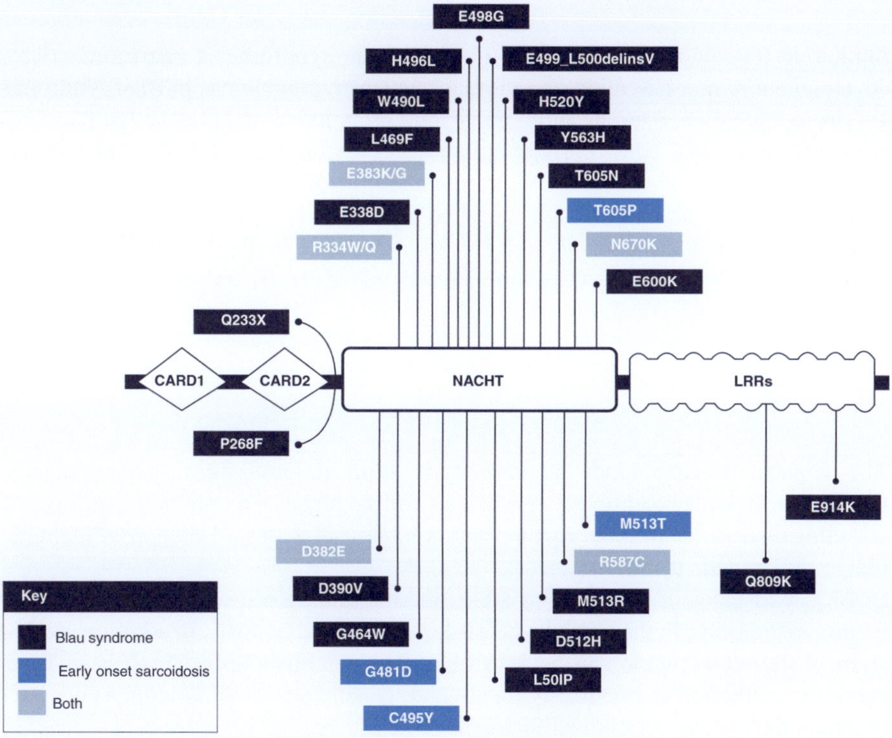

Fig. 5.1 Known NOD2 mutations and their locations [10]

three domains: (1) the CARD domain for caspase activation and recruitment, (2) the NOD/NACHT domain for central binding, and (3) the C-terminal region [10].

Multiple different causative mutations have been discovered in NOD2, and more are continuing to be found (Fig. 5.1) [11–16]. Most studies and registries have found mutations in 90–100% of patients and families; however, some affected families do not have known NOD2 mutations [6, 17, 18]. Although mutations are varied, most are found within or near the NOD/NACHT domain of the NOD2 protein [14]. These NOD2 mutations are thought to involve gain of function, likely through hyperactivation of NFκB, although this mechanism remains incompletely understood [19, 20]. This results in an autoinflammatory disease with a pronounced and exuberant inflammatory response. This is in contrast to the mutations that are seen in inflammatory bowel disease that are associated with loss-of-function mutations, despite the location being very close.

It is also interesting to note that despite high expression of the NOD2 protein, there is incomplete penetrance of disease secondary to NOD2 mutations suggesting the mutation to be necessary but not sufficient. As discovered by Saulsbury et al., some members of a family with a NOD2 mutation were asymptomatic and did not develop the Blau syndrome phenotype, while other members developed overt disease [21].

Histology and Morphology

Similar to sarcoidosis and Crohn's disease, Blau syndrome is characterized by development of non-caseating granulomas. However, granulomas in Blau syndrome are distinct, characterized by large polycyclic granulomas with dense lymphocytic coronas or halos [4]. These coronal lymphocytes are largely of the Th17 phenotype [6]. This is thought to reflect the vigorous inflammatory response that is associated with the gain-of-function NOD2 mutation that exists in Blau syndrome [22]. In addition, Janssen et al. observed high levels of multiple cytokines, including the type 2 interferon IFN-γ and the pro-inflammatory cytokines IL-6, TGF-β, and IL-17 [22].

Diagnosis

The diagnosis of Blau syndrome is primarily clinical, based on history, especially family history and presenting symptoms, as well as physical examination consistent with this disease. Additional testing that is most useful toward diagnosis includes biopsy and genetic testing.

Biopsy of the skin is most accessible, and the finding of granulomatous inflammation in the skin can therefore be helpful in making a diagnosis. In addition, evaluation of the NOD2 gene can be very helpful in establishing a diagnosis of Blau syndrome, although as previously mentioned, genetic abnormality alone is not sufficient in the absence of clinical features.

Management

As described above, mutations in a single gene have been implicated in the etiology of Blau syndrome, and these mutations lead to dysregulated inflammation and granuloma formation. As a result, Blau syndrome has been classified as one of the monogenic autoinflammatory disorders and is generally treated as such.

There is little evidence regarding appropriate and effective treatment strategies for Blau syndrome, largely because this disease remains rare. The primary goal of treatment is prevention of progression of eye disease and resulting vision loss and blindness. One important secondary goal of treatment is avoidance of joint deformation and development of dysplastic bone changes.

Treatment with nonsteroidal anti-inflammatory drugs has been tried, although symptomatic relief is usually temporary, and disease progression is not affected [23]. Corticosteroids are often used for management of disease flares, as well as maintenance of a quiescent state; however, steroid sequelae are unfavorable, and steroid-sparing agents are preferred [24]. To date, mainstays of therapy include methotrexate, azathioprine, and thalidomide [24, 25]. Recently anti-TNF medications have been used with increasing frequency, especially to avoid ocular complications, and these medications have had some success [23, 26, 27, 28]. Most recently, with the recognition that IL-1 plays a role in disease activity in Blau syndrome, IL-1 inhibition has become a treatment goal for management of specific and systemic manifestations of Blau syndrome, also with some success [29, 30]. However, it is important to note that some studies so far do not support this claim for excessive IL-1 activity in Blau syndrome [31].

Prognosis

The natural history and disease course of Blau syndrome are not well known. Recently, registries of patients with Blau syndrome have been started, with the goal of determining natural history of disease. It is understood that mortality from Blau syndrome is low, while morbidity from disease can be high, especially in the form of vision loss and joint contractures. High rates of ophthalmologic complications have been noted in patients followed prospectively, with approximately 67% developing significant vision loss. In addition, over 50% of patients develop joint deformities with time. Health and pain assessments also reveal significant morbidity and disability as a result of Blau syndrome. Using the Health Assessment Questionnaire and the Childhood Health Assessment Questionnaire, approximately 33% of patients reported mild impairment, and 33% reported moderate to severe impairment. There were also high rates of pain in these cohorts and high scores for impact of disease on global health and quality of life.

Summary

Blau syndrome is a monogenic, familial form of early-onset sarcoidosis, caused by multiple different mutations on the NOD2 gene. This disease entity is characterized by the triad of granulomatous uveitis, arthritis, and skin disease. The most problematic long-term manifestations are ocular disease and profound vision loss and joint contractures, which both carry significant morbidity and stress the need for more effective treatments. Therapeutic management remains a primary area for further study, as treatment continues to be varied and based on little evidence.

References

1. Blau EB. Familial granulomatous arthritis, iritis, and rash. J Pediatr. 1985;107(5):689–93.
2. Jabs DA, et al. Familial granulomatous synovitis, uveitis, and cranial neuropathies. Am J Med. May 1985;78(5):801–4.
3. Miceli-Richard C, et al. CARD15 mutations in Blau syndrome. Nat Genet. 2001;29(1):15. https://doi.org/10.1038/ng720.
4. Wouters CH, et al. Blau syndrome, the prototypic auto-inflammatory granulomatous disease. Pediatr Rheumatol Online J. 2014;12:33. https://doi.org/10.1186/1546-0096-12-33.
5. Rosé CD, et al. Pediatric granulomatous arthritis: an international registry. Arthritis Rheum. 2006;54(10):3337–44. https://doi.org/10.1002/art.22122.
6. Rosé CD, et al. Blau syndrome: cross-sectional data from a multicentre study of clinical, radiological and functional outcomes. Rheumatology (Oxford, England). 2015;54(6):1008–16. https://doi.org/10.1093/rheumatology/keu437.
7. Tromp G, et al. Genetic linkage of familial granulomatous inflammatory arthritis, skin rash, and uveitis to chromosome 16. Am J Hum Genet. 1996;59(5):1097–107.
8. Ogura Y, et al. Nod2, a Nod1/Apaf-1 family member that is restricted to monocytes and activates NF-kappaB. J Biol Chem. 2001;276(7):4812–8. https://doi.org/10.1074/jbc.M008072200.
9. Lecat A, Piette J, Legrand-Poels S. The protein Nod2: an innate receptor more complex than previously assumed. Biochem Pharmacol. 2010;80(12):2021–31. https://doi.org/10.1016/j.bcp.2010.07.016.
10. Caso F, et al. Caveats and truths in genetic, clinical, autoimmune and autoinflammatory issues in Blau syndrome and early onset sarcoidosis. Autoimmun Rev. 2014;13(12):1220–9. https://doi.org/10.1016/j.autrev.2014.08.010.
11. Rose CD, Martin TM, Wouters CH. Blau syndrome revisited. Curr Opin Rheumatol. 2011;23(5):411–8. https://doi.org/10.1097/BOR.0b013e328349c430.
12. Milman N, et al. A novel mutation in the NOD2 gene associated with Blau syndrome: a Norwegian family with four affected members. Scand J Rheumatol. 2009;38(3):190–7. https://doi.org/10.1080/03009740802464194.
13. Okada S, et al. Cardiac infiltration in early-onset sarcoidosis associated with a novel heterozygous mutation, G481D, in CARD15. Rheumatology (Oxford, England). 2009;48(6):706–7. https://doi.org/10.1093/rheumatology/kep061.
14. Sakai H, et al. A case of early-onset sarcoidosis with a six-base deletion in the NOD2 gene. Rheumatology (Oxford, England). 2010;49(1):194–6. https://doi.org/10.1093/rheumatology/kep315.
15. van Duist MM, et al. A new CARD15 mutation in Blau syndrome. Eur J Hum Genet: EJHG. 2005;13(6):742–7. https://doi.org/10.1038/sj.ejhg.5201404.

16. Villanueva-Mendoza C, et al. Familial case of Blau syndrome associated with a CARD15/NOD2 mutation. Ophthalmic Genet. 2010;31(3):155–8. https://doi.org/10.3109/13816810.2010.492818.
17. Kanazawa N, et al. Early-onset sarcoidosis and CARD15 mutations with constitutive nuclear factor-kappaB activation: common genetic etiology with Blau syndrome. Blood. 2005;105(3):1195–7. https://doi.org/10.1182/blood-2004-07-2972.
18. Wang X, et al. CARD15 mutations in familial granulomatosis syndromes: a study of the original Blau syndrome kindred and other families with large-vessel arteritis and cranial neuropathy. Arthritis Rheum. 2002;46(11):3041–5. https://doi.org/10.1002/art.10618.
19. Barnich N, et al. Membrane recruitment of NOD2 in intestinal epithelial cells is essential for nuclear factor-{kappa}B activation in Muramyl dipeptide recognition. J Cell Biol. 2005;170(1):21–6. https://doi.org/10.1083/jcb.200502153.
20. Tattoli I, et al. The nodosome: Nod1 and Nod2 control bacterial infections and inflammation. Semin Immunopathol. 2007;29(3):289–301. https://doi.org/10.1007/s00281-007-0083-2.
21. Saulsbury FT, et al. Incomplete penetrance of the NOD2 E383K substitution among members of a pediatric granulomatous arthritis pedigree. Arthritis Rheum. 2009;60(6):1804–6. https://doi.org/10.1002/art.24532.
22. Janssen CEI, et al. Morphologic and immunohistochemical characterization of granulomas in the nucleotide oligomerization domain 2-related disorders Blau syndrome and Crohn disease. J Allergy Clin Immunol. 2012;129(4):1076–84. https://doi.org/10.1016/j.jaci.2012.02.004.
23. Vitale A, et al. Biological treatments: new weapons in the management of monogenic autoinflammatory disorders. Mediat Inflamm. 2013;2013:939847. https://doi.org/10.1155/2013/939847.
24. Sfriso P, et al. Blau syndrome, clinical and genetic aspects. Autoimmun Rev. 2012;12(1):44–51. https://doi.org/10.1016/j.autrev.2012.07.028.
25. Yasui K, et al. Thalidomide dramatically improves the symptoms of early-onset sarcoidosis/Blau syndrome: its possible action and mechanism. Arthritis Rheum. 2010;62(1):250–7. https://doi.org/10.1002/art.25035.
26. Chauhan K, Michet C. A case of Blau syndrome. Case Rep Rheumatol. 2014;2014:216056. https://doi.org/10.1155/2014/216056.
27. Milman N, et al. Favourable effect of TNF-alpha inhibitor (infliximab) on Blau syndrome in monozygotic twins with a de novo CARD15 mutation. APMIS. 2006;114(12):912–9. https://doi.org/10.1111/j.1600-0463.2006.apm_522.x.
28. Otsubo Y, et al. A long-term follow-up of Japanese mother and her daughter with Blau syndrome: effective treatment of anti-TNF inhibitors and useful diagnostic tool of joint ultrasound examination. Mod Rheumatol. 2017;27(1):169–73. https://doi.org/10.3109/14397595.2014.964388.
29. Aróstegui JI, et al. NOD2 gene-associated pediatric granulomatous arthritis: clinical diversity, novel and recurrent mutations, and evidence of clinical improvement with interleukin-1 blockade in a Spanish cohort. Arthritis Rheum. 2007;56(11):3805–13. https://doi.org/10.1002/art.22966.
30. Simonini G, et al. Clinical and transcriptional response to the long-acting Interleukin-1 blocker canakinumab in Blau syndrome-related uveitis. Arthritis Rheum. February 2013;65(2):513–8. https://doi.org/10.1002/art.37776.
31. Martin TM, et al. The NOD2 defect in Blau syndrome does not result in excess interleukin-1 activity. Arthritis Rheum. 2009;60(2):611–8. https://doi.org/10.1002/art.24222.

Chapter 6
Deficiency of the Interleukin-1 Receptor Antagonist (DIRA)

Arturo Diaz

DIRA is a rare autosomal recessive autoinflammatory disease that may have been first clinically described by Leung in 1985 [1] as a syndrome of infantile cortical hyperostosis and intramedullary lesions suggestive of osteomyelitis, and by Ivker in 1993 [2] as a syndrome of unknown etiology characterized by infantile pustular psoriasis associated with bone lytic lesions. The phenotype and genotype of DIRA, also called osteomyelitis, sterile multifocal, with periostitis and pustulosis OMIM:612852, were defined in 2009 by two groups reporting 10 patients that linked the disease to homozygous loss of function germ line mutations in *IL1RN*, the gene encoding the interleukin-1 (IL-1) receptor antagonist (IL-1Ra) [3, 4]. The unopposed effect of IL-I1α and IL-1β leads to increased IL-1 signaling and systemic inflammation.

Clinical Manifestations

Most patients with DIRA have presented with the first manifestations of the disease from birth to 8 weeks of age. The latest onset of disease has been reported in one case at 1 year of age [5]. Thirty percent of pregnancies had resulted in premature births, the infants may be small for gestational age, and some have had evidence of fetal distress suggesting that the disease may start in utero. A single case of an aborted fetus with manifestations of DIRA has given support to an intrauterine onset of disease [6].

Characteristic clinical features are localized to the skin, oral mucosa, joints, and bone (Fig. 6.1). Patients present with growth retardation and failure to thrive, but unlike other autoinflammatory diseases, most patients with DIRA do not have fever.

A. Diaz (✉)
Division of Rheumatology, Beth Israel Deaconess Medical Center, Harvard Medical School, Boston, MA, USA
e-mail: adiaz3@bidmc.harvard.edu

P. Efthimiou (ed.), *Auto-Inflammatory Syndromes*,
https://doi.org/10.1007/978-3-319-96929-9_6

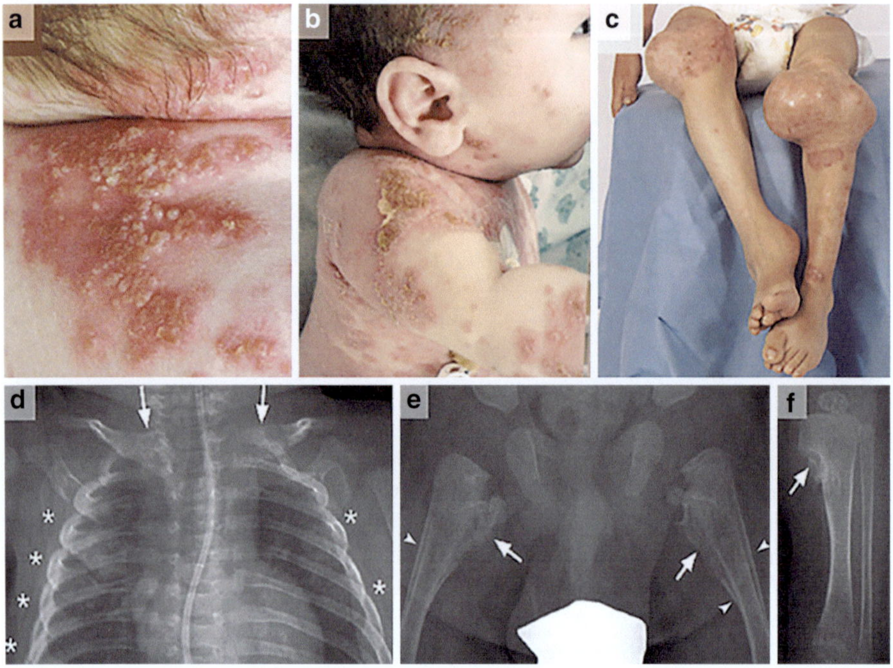

Fig. 6.1 Inflammatory skin and bone manifestations in patients with deficiency of IL-1Ra. The skin manifestations range from groupings of small pustules (Panel **a**) to a generalized pustulosis (Panel **b**). The bone manifestations include epiphyseal ballooning of multiple distal and proximal long bones in a patient from Puerto Rico (Panel **c**); the more typical radiographic manifestations include widening of multiple ribs (with affected ribs indicated with asterisks) and the clavicle (arrows) (Panel **d**), heterotopic ossification or periosteal cloaking of the proximal femoral metaphysis (arrows) and periosteal elevation of the diaphysis (arrowheads) (Panel **e**), and an osteolytic lesion with an sclerotic rim (Panel **f**, arrow). (From Aksentijevich et al. [3], with permission)

DIRA is a severe inflammatory disease that, if untreated, can evolve to systemic inflammatory response syndrome (SIRS) and death.

Dermatologic Manifestations The skin disease is characterized by a pustular dermatitis that can evolve from crops, to a generalized pustulosis or ichthyosiform lesions. Some patients present with nail changes, onychomadesis, anonychia, or pitting. Pathergy and mouth ulcers have been observed, and one case presented with pyoderma gangrenosum [3].

Skin biopsies have shown infiltration of the epidermis and dermis by neutrophils, formation of subcorneal pustules reminiscent of pustular psoriasis, infundibulofolliculitis, intracorneal and intraepidermal microabscesses, acanthosis, and hyperkeratosis. Neutrophilic eccrine hydradenitis, neutrophil-imbued parakeratosis with loss of granular cell layer have also been described. Immunofluorescence has been negative when tested [3, 4, 7].

Musculoskeletal Manifestations Patients present with severe joint pain on range of motion, joint swelling, sterile joint effusions, and prominent enlargement of joints (ballooning). Later changes include joint contractures, muscle atrophy, and growth retardation.

The most common radiographic features include diffuse osteopenia, epiphyseal ballooning of long bones, widening of anterior segments of ribs near the costochondral junctions, periostitis of long bones, and multifocal osteolytic lesions consistent with multifocal osteomyelitis affecting more frequently ribs, clavicles, and long bones. Less frequent features are heterotopic calcifications of proximal femurs, widening of the clavicles, metaphyseal erosions of long bones, osteolytic lesions in the skull, collapse of vertebral bodies with fusion, corner fractures on the distal femur and proximal tibia, odontoid nonfusion leading to atlantoaxial subluxation, and cervical vertebral fusion. The bone abnormalities including the osteolytic lesions can progress rapidly, and changes can be observed in a matter of few weeks.

The bone scintigraphy shows radiotracer uptake suggestive of osteomyelitis.

Bone biopsies have shown a non-specific inflammatory reaction, reactive woven bone, scattered osteoclasts, increased neutrophils, purulent osteomyelitis, fibrosis, and sclerosis. The cultures have been consistently negative for bacteria, fungi, and mycobacteria.

Other Manifestations Less commonly reported manifestations are:

Hepatosplenomegaly and interstitial lung disease [3].

Respiratory distress, with ground glass opacities and atelectasis on CT of the chest. The lung biopsy showed alveoli filled with macrophages and few neutrophils. This patient had also deep vein thrombosis on extremities, a screening for thrombophilic conditions (factor V of Leiden, protein C, protein S, and anti-thrombin III activity, lupus anticoagulant, and antiphospholipid antibodies), was all negative [4].

Dilated cardiomyopathy, corneal ulcerations, portal vein thrombosis with ascitis, and caput medusa [7].

DVT and internal jugular thrombosis after jugular catheterization [8, 9].

Two cases with CNS vasculitis, associated with the 175 Kb deletion [3, 4].

Episcleritis, conjunctivitis.

Systemic inflammatory response syndrome.

A fetus that died in utero at 27 weeks of gestation (with) had skin edema, ascites, short ribs, narrow thorax, polyhydramnios, necrotizing abscess in thymus, adrenal glands, and myocardium [6].

Laboratory

Laboratory testing reflects a severe inflammatory process with leukocytosis with neutrophilia, anemia, thrombocytosis, and highly elevated ESR up to 100 mmHg and CRP up to100 ng/ml. Cultures of skin lesions have shown contamination by staphylococcus, but no other bacteria has been recovered. Cultures of bone lesions have been negative for aerobic and anaerobic bacteria, fungi, and mycobacteria.

Screening for viral infections (CMV, HBV, HCV, rubella, HIV), syphilis, and toxoplasmosis, when tested, has been negative. Tests for rheumatoid factor (RF), antinuclear antibodies (ANA), antineutrophil cytoplasmic antibodies (ANCA), lymphocyte subsets, and immunoglobulin levels have been normal or negative. Tests for thrombophilic conditions have been negative.

Genetics

IL1RN, the mutated gene in DIRA, resides on the long arm of chromosome 2q13. Twenty patients have been reported so far who carry ten different loss of function germ line mutations. These mutations comprise four homozygous single point-nonsense mutations, five homozygous deletions (one in frame), and one compound heterozygous. All mutations except one result in either non-expressed or truncated proteins without biologic activity (Table 6.1). Heterozygous carrier relatives were asymptomatic conforming to a recessive pattern of inheritance (Table 6.1).

c229G>T is a nonsense mutation resulting in the amino acid mutation E77X. This mutation encodes for a truncated protein that is not secreted. The first five cases described were homozygous for the mutation and belonged to three Dutch unrelated families. The parents of the three families were carriers for the same mutation. Although no carriers were found among 351 Dutch controls (from a different area of the country), a founder effect is supported by the fact that the same mutation was found in 3 unrelated families [3].

c160C>T is a nonsense mutation resulting in the amino acid mutation Q54X. This mutation encodes a mutated protein that is not secreted. The mutation was found in two homozygous siblings from a consanguineous Lebanese family [3].

c355C>T is a nonsense mutation in exon four resulting in the amino acid mutation Q119X. This mutation creates a premature TAG stop codon that is expected to encode for a truncated protein. This mutation was found in the heterozygous parents of a Turkish consanguineous family. One pregnancy resulted in a fetal death at 27 weeks of gestation and the other on a premature infant born at 31 weeks of gestation who died at 4 months of age, both with features consistent with DIRA. No biological material was available for genetic analysis, but the prediction is that both were homozygous because both parents were heterozygous for the mutation. Modeling predicted a protein with defective binding to the receptor because the loss of amino acids A152, D153, Y172, and E175 that bind directly to the receptor; in addition the β-barrel is unable to fold properly because the β8, β9, and β12 strands are missing disrupting folding and impairing the ability of IL1Ra to bind to the receptor. Therefore, it predicts a nonfunctioning protein [6].

c76C>T is a nonsense mutation that results in the amino acid mutation R26X, reported in a single homozygous patient in a Turkish family [5].

64_1696del;p.IL1F9_IL1RNdel. This is a 175 Kb genomic deletion of the *IL1RN* locus encoding the IL-1Ra- and 5 IL-1-related genes: ILF9, ILF6, ILF8, IL 5, ILF10 (antagonist IL36RN, agonists IL36α, IL36β, and IL36γ of the IL36 receptor, and IL38), resulting in a non-expressed IL-1Ra. The deletion was reported in four homo-

Table 6.1 Summary of the published patients diagnosed with DIRA, their disease-causing mutations, and outcomes

Gender	Age at first symptoms (days)	Age of disease outcome at the time of report	Country of origin	Mutation	Reference
Male	0	Deceased	Netherlands	c.229G>T;p.Gly77*	[3]
Female	14	7.2 years	Netherlands	c.229G>T;p.Gly77*	[3]
Male	0	Deceased	Netherlands	c.229G>T;p.Gly77*	[3]
Female	2	Deceased	Netherlands	c.229G>T;p.Gly77*	[3]
Female	17	2 months	Netherlands	c.229G>T;p.Gly77*	[3]
Male	5	1.8 years	Lebanon	c.160C>T;p.Gln54*	[3]
Male	2	4 months	Lebanon	c.160C>T;p.Gln54*	[3]
Female	–	Aborted	Turkey	c355C>T;p.Gln119*	[6]
Male	7	Deceased	Turkey	c355C>T;p.Gln119*	[6]
Female	12 months	13 years	Turkey	c.76C>T;p.Arg26*	[5]
Male	8	9.5 years	Puerto Rico	-64_1696del;p.IL1F9 _IL1RNdel	[3]
Male	10	18 months	Puerto Rico	-64_1696del;p.IL1F9 _IL1RNdel	[4]
Male	14	15 years	Puerto Rico	-64_1696del;p.IL1F9 _IL1RNdel	[7]
Male	60	5 months	Puerto Rico	-64_1696del;p.IL1F9 _IL1RNdel	[10]
Female	7		Puerto Rican descent	-64_1696del;p.IL1F9 _IL1RNdel	[11]
Female	0	30 months	Brazil	c.213_227del;pAsp72_ Ile76del	[8]
Female	0	27 months	Brazil	c.213_227del;p.Asp72_ Ile76del	[8]
Male	14	13 months	Canada	c.156_157del;p. Asn52Lysfs*25	[3]
Female	21	17 months	Indian	Chr2_ hg19_113,865,011_ 113,887.227del	[12]
				C396delC;p. Thr133Profs*118	Berdeli, Infevers
Male	12	23 days	USA	c.229G>T;p.Gly*77 and c.140delC;p.T47TfsX4	[9]

*aminoacid position
Modified from Mendonca et al. [12]
Bardeli's mutation is registered in the Infevers database (http://fmf.igh.cnrs.fr/ISSAID/infevers/)

zygous patients from Puerto Rico. The mutation was found in 3 unrelated carriers in a panel of 119 controls from the same Northern part of Puerto Rico resulting in an allele frequency of 1.3% consistent with a founder effect. This frequency predicts an incidence of DIRA of 1 in 6300 births in Northern Puerto Rico [3]. A second patient with 175 Kb deletion (Reddy) [4] was the son of consanguineous parents who were heterozygous for the deletion and healthy [4] (Fig. 6.2). Three more cases have been

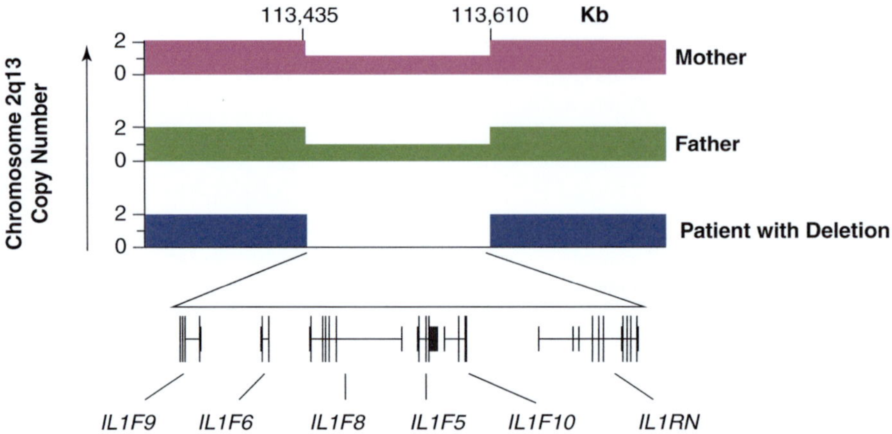

Fig. 6.2 Genetic characteristic of a patient with the 175 Kb deletion. Variation in genomic copy number in chromosome 2q13for the patient and his mother and father, showing a homozygous 175 Kb deletion in the patient and heterozygous in his parents. The deletion includes genes encoding sis members of the interleukin-1 family: the interleukin-1 receptor antagonist (*IL1RN*) and the interleukin-1 family members 5, 6, 8. 9, and 10. (From Reddy et al. [4], with permission)

reported from consanguineous and non-consanguineous parents [7, 10, 11]. All patients with the 175 Kb deletion are Puerto Rican or of Puerto Rican descent.

c.213_227del;pAsp72_Ile76del. This is a 15-bp in-frame deletion reported in two Brazilian unrelated patients, who were homozygous for the deletion suggesting a founder effect. The parents of both patients were heterozygous for the deletion. This mutation was not found in 200 ethnically matched and 200 not ethnically matched control chromosomes. This deletion encodes for a nonfunctional protein with no affinity for the IL-1R1. Ribbon modeling showed that the missing amino acids are in strand β4; loss of strand β4 can destabilize the other strands and disrupt formation of the β barrel and the binding to IL-1R1 [8].

c.156_157del;p.Asn52Lysfs*25. This mutation consists of a 2 bp deletion resulting in a frame shift, after which there is incorporation of 24 aberrant amino acids and a termination codon resulting in a truncated protein. This Newfoundland patient is homozygous and both parents heterozygous. Screening of 555 controls from the same country revealed 2 carriers of the mutation, resulting in an allele frequency 0.2% [3].

Chr2_hg19_113,865,011_113,887.227del. This is a 22.216 bp Kb deletion at the centromeric end of the *IL1RN* encompassing the first 4 exons (Fig. 6.3). It was described in an Indian patient who was homozygous for the deletion. The parents were non-consanguineous heterozygous for the deletion. The analysis of the patient's SNP array was suggestive of a "distant" relatedness o the parents and a founder effect [12].

c.229G>T;p.Gly*77/c.140delC;p.T47TfsX4. This is the first reported compound heterozygous for disease-causing mutations in DIRA. The c.229G>T;p.Gly*77 mutation is the same reported in families from the Netherlands. It is a nonsense mutation resulting in the amino acid mutation E77X that encodes for a truncated

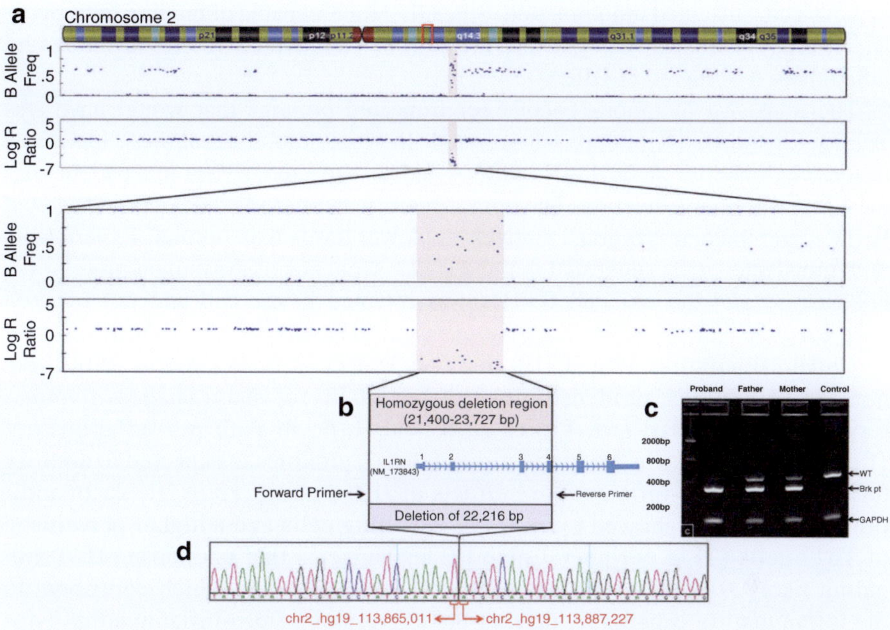

Fig. 6.3 Genetic analysis for the detection of the 22,216 bp *IL1RN* deletion. (**a**) SNP array data showing a homozygous deletion of IL1RN. The region deleted is indicated by a red box on the chromosome diagram. The B allele frequency (BAF) plot conveys the zygosity of a given SNP (blue dot), while the log R ratio (LRR) plot conveys the intensity or copy number. The homozygous deletion (shaded red) is indicated by the loss of intensity in the LRR plot and the absence of a coherent signal in the BAF plot. The deleted region includes the first four exons (two coding exons) of *IL1RN* (NM_173843). (**b**) Schematic representation of the deleted region of *IL1RN* gene predicted by SNP array. (**c**) Multiplex PCR products generated with three pairs of primers that amplify the wild-type allele, the breakpoint junction of the deletion or an internal control (GAPDH) were run in 2% agarose gel. Upper band indicates the presence of the wild-type (WT) allele, middle band indicates the presence of the deleted allele (Brk pt), and lower band serves as an internal control (GAPDH). (**d**) Sanger sequencing electropherogram depicting the breakpoint of the *IL1RN* deletion. (From Mendonca et al. [12] with permission)

protein that is not secreted. The second mutation c.140delC;p.T47TfsX4 is a one base pair deletion in exon 2 of the *IL1RN*. The deletion results in a frame shift and a premature e termination codon that encodes for a truncated protein. Both mutations were inherited in trans as the mother was carrier for the c.229G>T;p.Gly*77 and the father for the c.140delC;p.T47TfsX4 [9].

Functional Implications

Unlike other autoinflammatory diseases where elevated production of mature IL-1β drives the inflammatory process, in DIRA, the deficiency of the negative regulator IL-1Ra allows for unopposed signaling of IL-1 even at physiologic levels resulting in enhanced, sustained inflammation. Since IL-1Ra is capable of binding both IL-1α and IL-1β, it has been thought that the sum of their effects results in the severe inflammation observed in DIRA.

The nonsense mutations encode for truncated proteins that would have less affinity for the IL-1R but are not secreted. In whole blood cells, these mutations resulted in lower levels of IL-1Ra mRNA and, as expected, absent in a patient with the 175 Kb genomic deletion. The homozygous patients had no detectable secreted IL-1Ra, and the heterozygous relatives had lower levels than normal. Experiments with transfected cells suggested that the leader sequence of the mutant protein was not cleaved and the mutated IL-1Ra was retained in the cell and not secreted (Fig. 6.4).

Under stimulation with IL-1β, mononuclear cells from patients with these nonsense mutations, produced higher levels of IL-1α, macrophage inflammatory protein 1α (MIP-1α), TNFα, IL-8, and IL-6, all with pro-inflammatory effects. The increase in the production of these cytokines is expected to amplify the unopposed pro-inflammatory effects of IL-1α and IL1β in DIRA. In addition, skin biopsies showed more IL-17-secreting cells and a higher percentage of Th17 cells [3] in peripheral blood. This suggests that unopposed IL-1 signaling likely stimulates the differentiation of Th17 cells, which contribute to the inflammatory process by driving the expression of pro-inflammatory cytokines [3].

The transcriptome of unstimulated mononuclear cells from a patient with the 175 Kb deletion was more similar to that of a patient with neonatal-onset multisystemic inflammatory disease (NOMID/CINCA) but different from controls. However, the transcriptome of lipopolysaccharide (LPS)-stimulated mononuclear cells from this patient was more similar to that of the cells from a normal subject than to a NOMID/CINCA patient, with increase in the levels of transcripts for IL-1β, IL-1α, IL6, and IL-8 (Fig. 6.5). Measurement of cytokine levels in supernatants from LPS-stimulated monocytes confirmed a remarkable increase in the levels of IL-1β, IL-6, IL-8, IL-10, and TNFα in a control and the patient with the deletion, but not in a patient with NOMID/CINCA. Unstimulated mononuclear cells from the patient produced higher levels of IL-1β as compared to control cells and the parent's cells. These findings show that patients with DIRA maintain constant and chronic elevated levels of IL-1β. In addition, LPS-stimulated mononuclear cells from the parents of the patient with the deletion (both carriers) produced elevated levels of IL-1β, similar to those of the patient, and above the normal, demonstrating that haplo-insufficiency of the gene cluster on chromosome 2q13 results in an increase in IL-1β production [4]. The lower production of IL-1β in the patient with NOMID/CINCA may be the result of the rapid apoptosis of mononuclear cells in this condition triggered by LPS [14].

It has been hypothesized that the signaling of IL-1α may explain the different phenotypes of DIRA compared with NOMID/CINCA, which is driven by IL1β. The expression of IL-1α and IL-1β are different in the skin and bone [15]. IL-1α may play a role in the osteomyelitis in DIRA due to its ability to activate osteoclasts [16] and the development of neutrophilic pustulosis, as IL-1α and IL-1Ra are highly expressed in keratinocytes [17], stimulate their migration [18], and modulate anti-

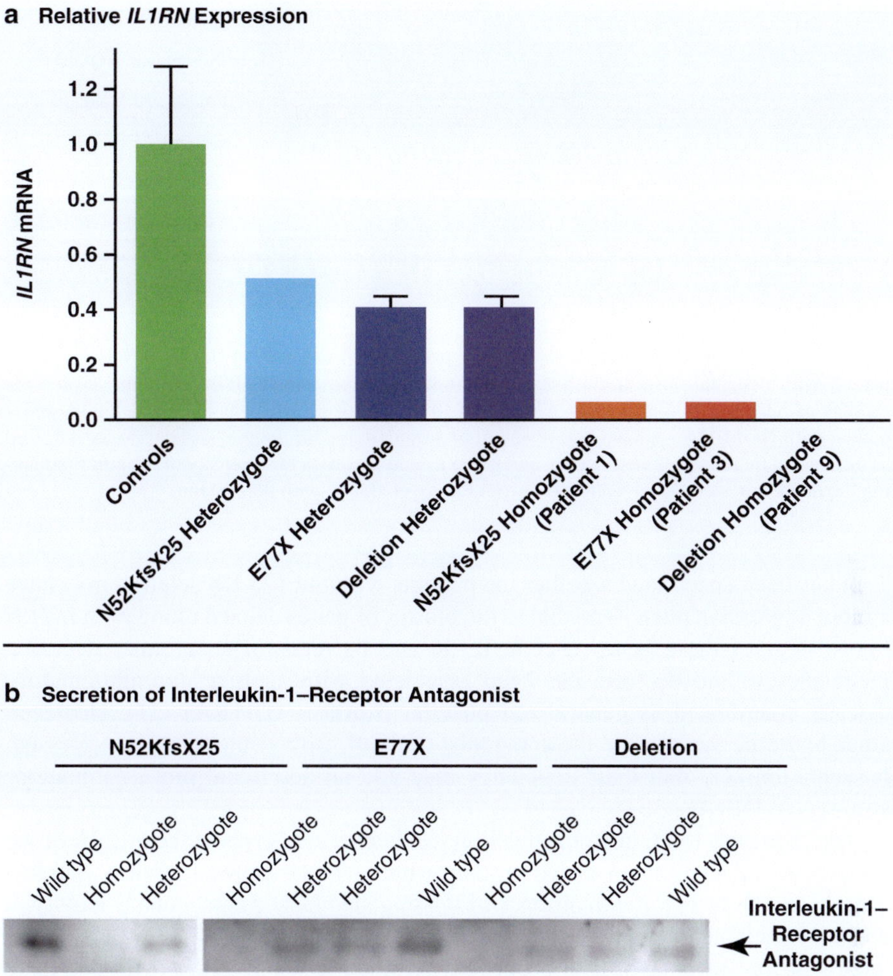

Fig. 6.4 Mechanism of disease caused by deficiency of interleukin-1 receptor antagonist. Relative messenger RNA (mRNA) levels of IL1RN, encoding the interleukin-1 receptor antagonist, in whole blood were determined by means of quantitative polymerase-chain-reaction assay (Panel **a**). Levels are shown for seven controls, one Newfoundland subject heterozygous for the N52KfsX25 mutation, three Dutch subjects heterozygous for the E77X mutation, two Puerto Rican subjects heterozygous for the 175 Kb genomic deletion, and one patient homozygous for each of these three mutations. T bars indicate the standard deviations, where applicable. In Panel **b** whole blood specimens from homozygotes and heterozygotes for each of these three mutations, as well as controls (with the wild-type sequence) were stimulated ex vivo with lipopolysaccharide to induce secretion of glycosylated interleukin-1-receptor antagonist by leukocytes. Resultant protein levels, detected by means of Western blot using an antibody specific for the N-terminal are shown. (From Aksentijevich et al. [3], with permission)

microbial responses [19]. In addition, IL-1-induced TNFα has been proposed as the driver of skin lesions, because treatment of the *IL1RN* knockout mouse with TNF inhibitors improved the skin lesions [20].

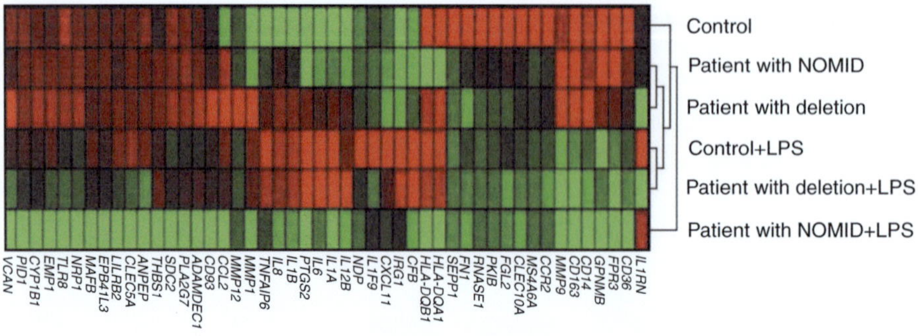

Fig. 6.5 Gene expression characteristics of a patient with deletion of the IL1RN locus and a patient with neonatal-onset multisystem inflammatory disease (NOMID). The gene expression profiles of peripheral-blood mononuclear cells from a control, a patient IL1RN deletion, and a patient with NOMID are shown before and after stimulation with lipopolysaccharide for 4 h. Red represents an increase in transcription, and green a decrease, with the intensity of the color indicating the degree of increase or decrease. (From Reddy et al. [4], with permission)

It has been speculated whether the patients with the 175 Kb deletion may have a more aggressive phenotype due to the cluster of genes deleted along with *IL1RN* locus. Four of these genes encode IL-36 and its receptor antagonist, IL-36Ra. Deficiency of the IL-36Ra has been associated with another autoinflammatory disease, manifested as generalized pustular psoriasis (DITRA) [21]. However, since both, the agonist and the antagonist of the IL-36 receptor are not expressed, it seems unlikely that their deficiency may add an additional pro-inflammatory stimulus in DIRA.

The Brazilian 15 bp in-frame deletion resulted in low levels of the mRNA of the mutated *IL-1RN* and the secreted protein, which when expressed in vitro, had low affinity for the receptor with absence of binding, and lacked antagonistic activity in an IL-1β mediated phospho-JNK nuclear translocation assay. Total WBCs stimulated with IL-1α, Il-1β or LPS produced increased levels of TNFα, MIP-1α, IL-6, IL-8, IL-1α and IL-1β. Both patients had severe disease [8].

In summary, the overall outcome of the deficiency of the IL1Ra is not only a positive feed-back in the production of IL-1α and IL-1β, but also an increase in the production of other pro-inflammatory cytokines such as IL-6, IL-8, TNFα, MIP-1α.

It has been remarkable the high frequency (30%) of preterm delivery in DIRA and the report of a case with likely onset of disease in utero. These facts suggest that increase in the IL-1 signaling must have a role in these outcomes. This possibility is supported by the previously documented association of elevated levels of IL-1β with preterm labor. It has been hypothesized that the high concentration of IL-1Ra in the amniotic fluid could be protective for the fetus. Both, the elevated IL-1 in the fetus and mother (an obligated heterozygous), and the deficiency of IL1Ra in amniotic fluid may play a role in the prematurity observed in DIRA [22–24].

Animal Models

The *IL1rn*-knockout murine models have failed to recapitulate the characteristic neutrophilic pustulosis and sterile osteomyelitis of DIRA.

The *IL1ra* knockout mouse model develops arthritis, psoriasis-like skin lesions and arteritis but not the bone abnormalities characteristic of DIRA. The mouse phenotype is influenced by its genetic background; it exhibits psoriatic-like skin lesions and arthritis in BALB/cA, and aortitis and small vessel vasculitis in BALBc/C57BL [25, 26].

In these models it appears that the enhanced IL-1 signaling with elevated levels of IL-8 and IL-6 drives the expansion of Th17 cells, which have an impact in the development of inflammation by inducing pro-inflammatory cytokines and neutrophil accumulation [27, 28]. From the animal models it appears that IL-17 plays a role in the inflammatory arthritis of the *IL1ra* knockout mice. The animal models and the finding of increased expression of IL-17 in the skin lesions of patients with DIRA support a role for IL-17 in the pathogenesis of inflammation in this condition.

The role of IL-1α in the pathogenesis of DIRA has not been resolved by the animal models. The *IL1rn* knockout mice does not develop the severe skin or bone inflammation characteristic of DIRA, suggesting that tissue expression of IL-1α and IL-1β may be different in humans and mice.

Diagnosis and Differential Diagnosis

The diagnosis of DIRA is established by the demonstration of mutations in the *IL1RN* locus.

The diagnosis of DIRA should be suspected in an infant presenting in the neonatal period with pustular lesions, osteitis, and systemic inflammation. Infectious and noninfectious diseases should be included in the differential diagnosis of DIRA.

From the dermatologic perspective, the cutaneous pustular lesions of DIRA can be incorporated in the group of diffuse infantile pustulosis [29]. Diffuse infantile pustulosis is the presentation of multiple dermatologic conditions including bullous impetigo, tinea, bacterial folliculitis, scabies, miliaria, pustular psoriasis, IgA pemphigus, acrodermatitis enteropathica, eosinophilic pustular folliculitis, erythema toxicum neonatorum, and transient neonatal pustular melanosis. These conditions should be considered in the differential diagnosis of the cutaneous component of DIRA and make a skin biopsy necessary.

A condition that presents with bone abnormalities similar to DIRA is infantile cortical hyperostosis. This is an autosomal dominant disease associated with mutations in *COL1A1*. Infantile cortical hyperostosis is a self-limiting disease that lacks the systemic inflammation and pustulosis of DIRA. Considering that the bone manifestation of DIRA could be by imaging indistinguishable from infectious osteomyelitis, a bone biopsy for microscopic analysis and cultures is recommended.

Among the autoinflammatory diseases, two present with skin and bone inflammation in the neonatal period: the NOMID/CINCA and Majeed syndromes. NOMID/

CINCA is associated with dominant gain of function mutations in NLRP3 that allow for spontaneous assembly of the NLRP3 inflammasome and overproduction of IL-1β. Patients with NOMID/CINCA have signs of systemic inflammation and a skin dermatosis at birth that is urticarial with perivascular inflammation on biopsy but no the pustulosis characteristic of DIRA. NOMID/CINCA patients lack the multifocal osteomyelitis, respiratory involvement, and thrombosis seen in DIRA. On the counterpart, DIRA lacks the hearing loss and aseptic meningitis of NOMID/CINCA.

Majeed syndrome presents with chronic recurrent multifocal osteomyelitis, neutrophilic dermatosis (from Sweet's syndrome to chronic pustulosis), periodic fever, and dyserythropoietic anemia, and is associated with mutations in *LPIN2*. The dyserythropoietic anemia is a characteristic and unique manifestation of Majeed's syndrome and differentiates it from DIRA. A third condition, although not frequently of neonatal onset, is synovitis, acne, pustulosis, hyperostosis, and osteitis syndrome (SAPHO); no mutations have been associated with this condition. Mevalonate kinase deficiency MVKD may present in infants, but unlike DIRA, patients have fever, prominent lymphadenopathy, abdominal pain, and a non-pustular exanthema. Finally, the differential diagnosis includes the deficiency in the interleukin-36 receptor antagonist (DITRA), a related condition characterized by generalized pustular psoriasis (Marrakchi) [21].

Prognosis

DIRA is a severe autoinflammatory disease. About 30% of these patients start life as small for gestational-age premature infants. Untreated patients not only suffer pain, prolonged hospitalizations, and organ damage but the progressive inflammation can evolve to respiratory distress, SIRS with multi-organ failure, and death. Of the 20 reported cases, 25% have died at variable ages. There are no patients reported that have survived to adulthood without amti-IL-1treatment. It has been observed that disease flares can be triggered by infections or stress.

Untreated bone lesions result in severe functional limitations due to bone deformities, joint contractures, vertebral collapse, and muscle atrophy. One child died in later life from pulmonary hemosiderosis with interstitial fibrosis. One case of intrauterine death possible related to in utero DIRA has been reported [6]. Because of the dire prognosis of untreated patients, early diagnosis is critical, and genetic testing should be done in suspected cases, especially in areas with known founder mutations, as is the case of Northern Puerto Rico.

Treatment

Attempts to treat with NSAIDs, steroids, and disease-modifying antirheumatic drugs such as methotrexate, azathioprine, cyclosporine, thalidomide, IVIG, and interferon gamma have resulted in partial or no response. Steroid treatment results in transient control of the inflammation with reduction of ESR and CRP. Some patients have required high doses of IV methylprednisolone up to 5 mg/Kg. None of these agents has induced long-term remission of the disease.

Treatment with anakinra, a recombinant human IL-1Ra, which replaces the deficient endogenous IL-1Ra, has resulted in a rapid and remarkable response sometimes within hours. The pustulosis improves within days and later fully resolves. The arthritis and musculoskeletal pain improves rapidly, and there is radiologic improvement of bone lesions within a few months. The inflammatory indices, WBC, ESR and CRP have normalized in all but one patient with the 175 Kb deletion. All treated patients have reached remission and discontinued steroids. The discontinuation of anakinra has resulted in a rapid relapse of the disease that has resolved with reinitiation of treatment. The patients treated early in infancy have developed normally while maintaining treatment with anakinra. The bone mineral density has improved reflecting the relevance of IL-1 in osteoclast activation and bone loss [16].

Two patients have developed an allergic reaction to anakinra, one of them expressing a truncated IL-1Ra and another expressing no IL-1Ra. Both patients were desensitized and able to continue treatment [12]. It is hypothesized that the lack of endogenous IL-1Ra may predispose these patients to develop an allergic reaction to a neo-antigen.

A single patient has been reported to respond to canakinumab, a monoclonal antibody to IL-1β [5]. There is no long-term follow-up available, or more extensive use of canakinumab to assess whether it would be as effective as the IL-1α and IL-1β blokade by anakinra.

Rilonacept is a long-acting soluble decoy receptor engineered as a dimeric fusion protein that contains of the ligand-binding domains of the extracellular portion of the human IL-1R linked to the Fc region of a human IgG1. It captures both IL-1α and IL-1β, blocking their binding to the cellular receptor [13], making it equivalent to the mechanism of action of anakinra and the native IL-1Ra. Because of its half-life of 8 days, it has been an attractive option for IL-1 blockade.

A recently study was conducted to assess the efficacy of rilonacept in maintaining remission of DIRA in children treated with anakinra, to determine necessary doses, and to evaluate safety [30]. Six mutation-positive children were enrolled in this open-label pilot study of weekly injections of rilonacept 2.2 mg/Kg with dose escalation to 4.4 mg/Kg. Five of six patients required dose escalation due to skin lesions. After dose escalation, all patients remained in remission for the 24 months of the study maintaining normal laboratory inflammatory indices (WBC, ESR, CRP, Platelets). All patients maintained normal growth as determined by height and weight. No serious adverse events were reported, and no patients discontinued treatment due to adverse events. This study demonstrates that capture of IL-1α and IL-1β by a monoclonal antibody, is an effective treatment for DIRA. The response to rilonacept was similar to that of anakinra, but patients and parents were inclined to prefer a weekly injection.

Given the severity of the disease and its potential lethality, treatment with IL-I-1inhibiton should be started as early as possible and maintained for life, because none of the untreated patients has survived to adult life.

References

1. Leung VC, Lee KE. Infantile cortical hyperostosis with intramedullary lesions. J Pediatr Orthop. 1985;5(3):354–7.
2. Ivker RA, Grin-Jorgensen CM, Vega VK, Hoss DM, Grant-Kels JM. Infantile generalized pustular psoriasis associated with lytic lesions of the bone. Pediatr Dermatol. 1993;10(3):277–82.
3. Aksentijevich I, Masters SL, Ferguson PJ, Dancey P, Frenkel J, van Royen-Kerkhoff A, et al. An autoinflammatory disease with deficiency of the interleukin-1-receptor antagonist. N Engl J Med. 2009;360(23):2426–37.
4. Reddy S, Jia S, Geoffrey R, Lorier R, Suchi M, Broeckel U, et al. An autoinflammatory disease due to homozygous deletion of the IL1RN locus. N Engl J Med. 2009;360(23):2438–44.
5. Ulusoy E, Karaca NE, El-Shanti H, Kilicoglu E, Aksu G, Kutukculer N. Interleukin-1 receptor antagonist deficiency with a novel mutation; late onset and successful treatment with canakinumab: a case report. J Med Case Rep. 2015;9:145.
6. Altiok E, Aksoy F, Perk Y, Taylan F, Kim PW, Ilikkan B, et al. A novel mutation in the interleukin-1 receptor antagonist associated with intrauterine disease onset. Clin Immunol. 2012;145(1):77–81.
7. Brau-Javier CN, Gonzales-Chavez J, Toro JR. Chronic cutaneous pustulosis due to a 175-kb deletion on chromosome 2q13: excellent response to anakinra. Arch Dermatol. 2012;148(3):301–4.
8. Jesus AA, Osman M, Silva CA, Kim PW, Pham TH, Gadina M, et al. A novel mutation of IL1RN in the deficiency of interleukin-1 receptor antagonist syndrome: description of two unrelated cases from Brazil. Arthritis Rheum. 2011;63(12):4007–17.
9. Stenerson M, Dufendach K, Aksentijevich I, Brady J, Austin J, Reed AM. The first reported case of compound heterozygous IL1RN mutations causing deficiency of the interleukin-1 receptor antagonist. Arthritis Rheum. 2011;63(12):4018–22.
10. Minkis K, Aksentijevich I, Goldbach-Mansky R, Magro C, Scott R, Davis JG, et al. Interleukin 1 receptor antagonist deficiency presenting as infantile pustulosis mimicking infantile pustular psoriasis. Arch Dermatol. 2012;148(6):747–52.
11. Schnellbacher C, Ciocca G, Menendez R, Aksentijevich I, Goldbach-Mansky R, Duarte AM, et al. Deficiency of interleukin-1 receptor antagonist responsive to anakinra. Pediatr Dermatol. 2013;30(6):758–60.
12. Mendonca LO, Malle L, Donovan FX, Chandrasekharappa SC, Montealegre Sanchez GA, Garg M, et al. Deficiency of Interleukin-1 receptor antagonist (DIRA): report of the first Indian patient and a novel deletion affecting IL1RN. J Clin Immunol. 2017;37(5):445–51.
13. Economides AN, Carpenter LR, Rudge JS, Wong V, Koehler-Stec EM, Hartnett C, et al. Cytokine traps: multi-component, high-affinity blockers of cytokine action. Nat Med. 2003;9(1):47–52.
14. Saito M, Nishikomori R, Kambe N, Fujisawa A, Tanizaki H, Takeichi K, et al. Disease-associated CIAS1 mutations induce monocyte death, revealing low-level mosaicism in mutation-negative cryopyrin-associated periodic syndrome patients. Blood. 2008;111(4):2132–41.
15. Hacham M, Argov S, White RM, Segal S, Apte RN. Distinct patterns of IL-1 alpha and IL-1 beta organ distribution--a possible basis for organ mechanisms of innate immunity. Adv Exp Med Biol. 2000;479:185–202.
16. Tani-Ishii N, Tsunoda A, Teranaka T, Umemoto T. Autocrine regulation of osteoclast formation and bone resorption by IL-1 alpha and TNF alpha. J Dent Res. 1999;78(10):1617–23.
17. Corradi A, Franzi AT, Rubartelli A. Synthesis and secretion of interleukin-1 alpha and interleukin-1 receptor antagonist during differentiation of cultured keratinocytes. Exp Cell Res. 1995;217(2):355–62.
18. Chen JD, Lapiere JC, Sauder DN, Peavey C, Woodley DT. Interleukin-1 alpha stimulates keratinocyte migration through an epidermal growth factor/transforming growth factor-alpha-independent pathway. J Invest Dermatol. 1995;104(5):729–33.

19. Bando M, Hiroshima Y, Kataoka M, Shinohara Y, Herzberg MC, Ross KF, et al. Interleukin-1alpha regulates antimicrobial peptide expression in human keratinocytes. Immunol Cell Biol. 2007;85(7):532–7.
20. Nakajima A, Matsuki T, Komine M, Asahina A, Horai R, Nakae S, et al. TNF, but not IL-6 and IL-17, is crucial for the development of T cell-independent psoriasis-like dermatitis in Il1rn−/− mice. J Immunol. 2010;185(3):1887–93.
21. Marrakchi S, Guigue P, Renshaw BR, Puel A, Pei XY, Fraitag S, et al. Interleukin-36-receptor antagonist deficiency and generalized pustular psoriasis. N Engl J Med. 2011;365(7):620–8.
22. Vitoratos N, Mastorakos G, Kountouris A, Papadias K, Creatsas G. Positive association of serum interleukin-1beta and CRH levels in women with pre-term labor. J Endocrinol Investig. 2007;30(1):35–40.
23. Romero R, Gotsch F, Pineles B, Kusanovic JP. Inflammation in pregnancy: its roles in reproductive physiology, obstetrical complications, and fetal injury. Nutr Rev. 2007;65(12 Pt 2):S194–202.
24. Chow SS, Craig ME, Jones CA, Hall B, Catteau J, Lloyd AR, et al. Differences in amniotic fluid and maternal serum cytokine levels in early midtrimester women without evidence of infection. Cytokine. 2008;44(1):78–84.
25. Horai R, Saijo S, Tanioka H, Nakae S, Sudo K, Okahara A, et al. Development of chronic inflammatory arthropathy resembling rheumatoid arthritis in interleukin 1 receptor antagonist-deficient mice. J Exp Med. 2000;191(2):313–20.
26. Nicklin MJ, Hughes DE, Barton JL, Ure JM, Duff GW. Arterial inflammation in mice lacking the interleukin 1 receptor antagonist gene. J Exp Med. 2000;191(2):303–12.
27. Nakae S, Saijo S, Horai R, Sudo K, Mori S, Iwakura Y. IL-17 production from activated T cells is required for the spontaneous development of destructive arthritis in mice deficient in IL-1 receptor antagonist. Proc Natl Acad Sci U S A. 2003;100(10):5986–90.
28. Koenders MI, Devesa I, Marijnissen RJ, Abdollahi-Roodsaz S, Boots AM, Walgreen B, et al. Interleukin-1 drives pathogenic Th17 cells during spontaneous arthritis in interleukin-1 receptor antagonist-deficient mice. Arthritis Rheum. 2008;58(11):3461–70.
29. Mengesha YM, Bennett ML. Pustular skin disorders: diagnosis and treatment. Am J Clin Dermatol. 2002;3(6):389–400.
30. Garg M, de Jesus AA, Chapelle D, Dancey P, Herzog R, Rivas-Chacon R, et al. Rilonacept maintains long-term inflammatory remission in patients with deficiency of the IL-1 receptor antagonist. JCI Insight. 2017;2(16).

Chapter 7
Deficiency of the Interleukin-36 Receptor Antagonist (DITRA) and Generalized Pustular Psoriasis

Arturo Diaz

Interleukin-36 receptor antagonist deficiency, DITRA MIM:614204, and generalized pustular psoriasis are life-threatening diseases characterized by a disseminated dermatitis, pustular psoriasis, and fever. The link of DITRA to loss-of-function recessive mutations in the interleukin-36 receptor antagonist *IL23RN* locus was first described by Marrakchi et al. in 2011 [1]. The mutations encode for an unstable protein with poor interaction with its receptor allowing for an unopposed effect of IL-36 that results in enhanced production of pro-inflammatory cytokines and systemic inflammation.

Epidemiology

Psoriasis is a relatively common disease affecting up to 8.5% of individuals in some populations, being more frequent in populations living more distant from the equator [2]. There are several forms of psoriasis; the most common is chronic plaque psoriasis (vulgaris) present in approximately 80% of the patients with psoriasis. Psoriasis vulgaris may present with extracutaneous manifestations such as psoriatic arthritis, a spondyloarthropathy affecting axial and peripheral joints, enthesitis, and iritis.

Pustular psoriasis is a rare disease that has been classified in generalized and localized forms. The generalized forms include acute generalized pustular psoriasis (GPP), also known as generalized pustular psoriasis of von Zumbusch, and annular pustular psoriasis (subacute). Localized forms of pustular psoriasis include acrodermatitis continua of Hallopeau that affects mostly the fingers, and palmoplantar pustulosis.

A. Diaz
Division of Rheumatology, Beth Israel Deaconess Medical Center,
Harvard Medical School, Boston, MA, USA
e-mail: adiaz3@bidmc.harvard.edu

P. Efthimiou (ed.), *Auto-Inflammatory Syndromes*,
https://doi.org/10.1007/978-3-319-96929-9_7

Generalized pustular psoriasis (GPP) is a multisystemic life-threatening inflammatory disease characterized by recurrent episodes of sudden onset, although subacute and chronic courses have been described [3]. It affects mostly adults in the middle age (40–60 years) and infrequently affects children. However in patients with DITRA, GPP occurs at earlier age and even in childhood; in the initial report, 12 of 19 patients had disease onset in childhood [1]. While there is no sex predominance [4, 5], a form of GPP called impetigo herpetiformis has been observed to occur in pregnancy, suggesting a hormonal influence in the disease [6]. Several series have reported history of previous plaque psoriasis from 30% to 78%, but it appears that the subgroup of patients with *IL36RN* mutations have less frequent history of plaque psoriasis [7].

Several precipitating factors have been identified; the most common is the withdrawal of systemic or potent topical steroids as well as other agents such as cyclosporine [3]. Triggering of GPP by other agents such as treatment with ustekinumab, TNF inhibitors, and pegylated interferon-alpha-2b have been reported sporadically [8–11]. Infections, particularly respiratory streptococcal infections, have been reported as a trigger in 15% of cases [3, 5]. Menstruation and pregnancy have been also identified as triggers.

Mucocutaneous Manifestations

The typical presentation of GPP is characterized by the sudden onset of a diffuse and painful erythema, followed by the formation of minuscule pustules that eventually coalesce to form large sterile purulent collections. The purulent lesions resolve in about 1 week leaving a residual erythema with scaling. As is typical of the disease, recurrence of pustular lesions in other areas occurs. The annular form has similar course but the erythema is surrounded by a ring of pustules. Patients with GPP may present with mucocutaneous involvement that may include oral pustules, cheilitis, geographic tongue, and nail changes. Mucosal involvement appears to be more frequent in patients with *IL36RN* mutations [12].

Extracutaneous Manifestations

Patients with GPP and DITRA present with manifestations of systemic inflammation such as high-grade fever up to 42 °C, chills, and malaise, joint pain. Liver dysfunction occurring in about 50% of patients is a prominent complication with jaundice, elevated transaminases and bilirubin, and histologic features of neutrophilic or sclerosing cholangitis [13, 14]. The spectrum of ocular inflammation includes uveitis, iritis, and conjunctivitis. Renal dysfunction with oliguric renal failure has been reported as well as neutrophilic pneumonitis, acute respiratory distress syndrome, and sepsis. Frequently, patients require management in the ICU to treat fluid and electrolyte imbalances, and deaths secondary to sepsis have been reported.

Laboratory

Laboratory abnormalities include elevation of acute phase reactants such as leukocytosis that can be highly elevated, elevated ESR, and CRP. There is elevation of liver function tests and hypoalbuminemia in 50% of patients that tends to correlate with the level of leukocytosis. Fluid and electrolyte imbalances are present in patients with extensive areas of skin involved [13]. Elevated antistreptolysins have been reported in patients with history of an upper respiratory infection as the trigger. There are no serologic markers for DITRA.

Pathology

Skin biopsies show psoriasiform changes, spongiform pustules of Kogoj (aggregates of neutrophils between degenerated keratinocytes within the upper Malpighian layer of the epidermis, forming a subcorneal macropustule), acanthosis with elongation of rete ridges, and parakeratosis in the stratum corneum. Immunostaining shows infiltration of the skin with CD8 T cells, CD3 T cells, and macrophages [1]. Acute generalized exanthematous pustulosis (AGEP) is in the differential and is suggested by the presence of eosinophils and necrotic keratinocytes.

Genetics

The *IL36RN* gene resides on chromosome 2q13-q14.1. In 2011, Marrakchi et al. communicated the linkage of a recessive missense mutation in the *IL36RN* locus in 16 affected members from 9 Tunisian families with GPP. *IL36RN* encodes for the IL36Ra; the mutation predicted the substitution of a proline for leucine at position 27 (L27P). Initial studies were consistent with a reduction of function of the mutated protein; therefore, the term "deficiency of the interleukin-36 receptor antagonist" (DITRA) was proposed to refer to this disease. All the families had a disease with an autosomal recessive pattern of inheritance, and all but one (family 6), had some degree of consanguinity. Co-segregation of the disease and a common 1.2 Mb haplotype suggested a founder effect. It was estimated that the most recent common ancestor carrying the mutation lived 13 generations ago [1].

Twenty variants in the *IL36RN* locus have been registered in the Infevers database (http://fmf.igh.cnrs.fr/ISSAID/infevers/). The gene contains five exons. Nineteen variants consist of a substitution and one of a deletion localized on exons 2, 3, and 4.

One variant is localized in intron 3. The countries of origin of the registered cases are Algeria China, Germany, Iraq, Japan, Pakistan, Spain, Tunisia, and the UK; *IL36RN* mutations have been reported in more than 70 cases worldwide.

Three important questions are whether patients with non-familial GPP carry *IL36RN* mutations, whether patients with other forms of psoriasis carry mutations, and whether patients with *IL36RN* mutations form a homogeneous group/disease.

Regarding the first question, it has been found that some patients with non-familial sporadic GPP carry *IL36RN* mutations. In a study in unrelated patients with sporadic GPP, 7/84 (8%) were homozygous or compound heterozygous *IL36RN* mutations [15], while another smaller study found more frequent mutations in 7/19 patients (39%) [16]. These studies demonstrate that most patients with non-familial sporadic GPP do not harbor *IL36RN* mutations and should not be classified as DITRA.

Patients with other forms of psoriasis such as acrodermatitis chronica of Hallopeau, and palmoplantar pustulosis [15, 17, 18], and even in drug reactions manifested as acute generalized exanthematous pustulosis [19, 20] have been found although rarely to carry *IL36RN* mutations; therefore, these mutations are not exclusive of GPP.

It has been suggested that patients that present with GPP without having before other forms of psoriasis are more likely to harbor *IL36RN* mutations [21]. A Japanese study of patients with GPP found *IL36RN* mutations in only 2/20 (10%) patients with a history of plaque psoriasis compared with 9/11 (81%) patients without history of plaque psoriasis [7] supporting this impression. Overall it appears that *IL36RN* mutations underline a spectrum of psoriatic phenotypes [15], which suggests that the IL-36 pathway may direct the predisposition to several forms of psoriasis.

Other factors, genetic, epigenetic, and environmental, may contribute to the phenotype in DITRA. Gain-of-function mutations and polymorphisms in caspase recruitment domain family member 14 (CARD14), an epidermal regulator of NF-kB, have been reported in plaque psoriasis as well as in GPP [22, 23]. The mutations appear to be associated with cases of GPP with plaque psoriasis, but not with GPP alone, which is more associated with *IL36RN* mutations. These data suggested that GPP alone is genetically different from GPP with plaque psoriasis, at least in the Japanese population.

Loss-of-function mutations in the adaptor protein complex 1 (AP-1) subunit σ1C (AP1S3) have been linked to GPP. AP-1 is a heterotetramer that promotes vesicular trafficking between the trans-Golgi network and the endosomes. AP1S3 silencing in keratinocytes disrupted the endosomal translocation of the innate pattern recognition receptor TLR-3 (Toll-like receptor 3), resulting in inhibition of downstream signaling [24].

Functional Studies

The region surrounding amino acid 27 (the first reported mutated) is highly conserved across species, and the leucine at this position is conserved on mammalian species, suggesting that is functionally important. *IL36RN* shares a 44% analogy with the *IL1RN*, the mutated gene in DITRA.

The L27P mutation did not affect the stability or rate of degradation of the IL-36Ra mRNA. However, structural modeling suggested that the mutation affects the stability of the protein and the interaction with its receptor (interleukin-1 receptor-related protein 2). The mutated protein had a very low expression and was less effective than the wild-type protein at inhibiting an IL-36γ-induced response in an IL-8 reporter assay. This impaired function resulted in increased production of pro-inflammatory cytokines specially IL-8 by the patient's keratinocytes homozygous for the mutation stimulated with IL-1β, IL-36α, IL-36β, and IL-36γ. In addition IL-36γ was overproduced in keratinocytes stimulated with IL-1β. This enhanced inflammatory response was confirmed by measuring cytokines in serum of patients during a flare; patients had 25-fold increase in IL-8 production as compared to controls. In full correlation, biopsies of skin lesions from patients showed an increase in staining for IL-36α, Il-36β, and more robustly IL-36γ [1].

The three IL-36 agonists signal through the IL36R which recruits the IL-1R accessory protein IL-1RAcP, triggering downstream activation of the pro-inflammatory nuclear factor-kB (NF-kB) and mitogen-activated protein kinase (MAPK) pathways [25, 26], leading to enhanced transcription and release of pro-inflammatory cytokines. The IL-36 cytokines and their receptor are highly expressed in skin [27] and other epithelial tissues and likely to play a role in innate immunity (Fig. 7.1).

Keratinocytes from patients with the L27P mutations produced higher amounts of IL-8 in response to stimulation with polyinosinic-polycytidylic acid (poly[L-C]), a synthetic ligand for Toll-like receptor 3, involved in response to infections; it is speculated that this may explain the frequent triggering of flares of GPP by common infections [1]. The role of IL-36 in GPP has been supported by a mouse model overexpressing IL-36α which develops pustular lesions; these lesions exacerbate by simultaneous deficiency of IL-36Ra [28, 29], recapitulating the human disease.

Based on the evidence that homozygous and compound heterozygous for *IL-36RN* mutations are associated with different forms of pustular psoriasis (GPP, palmoplantar pustular psoriasis, acrodermatitis continua of Hallopeau, and acute generalized exanthematous pustular eruption), Tauber et al. [30] investigated the outcome of different mutations in the function of the protein and their correlation with the various phenotypes, to establish genotype-phenotype correlations. They used site-directed mutagenesis to generate the mutants and expression in HEK293T cells. They found three groups:

1. Null mutations with complete absence of IL-36Ra protein expression
2. Mutations with decreased protein expression
3. Mutations with unchanged protein expression

In a functional assay measuring the ability to repress the IL-36-dependent activation of NF-kB, it was found complete functional impairment in null mutations, and partial or no impairment was observed in other mutations, then considered hypomorphic.

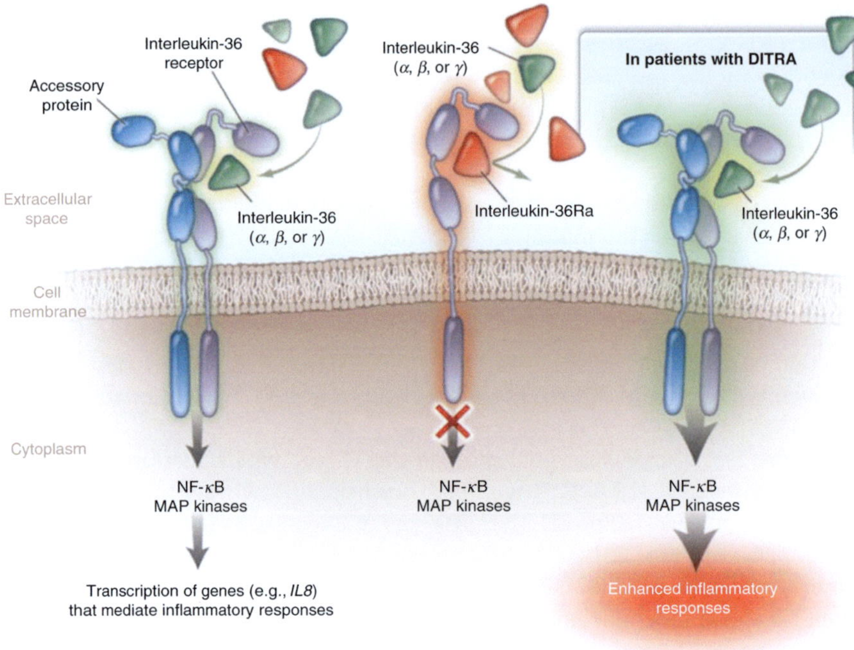

Fig. 7.1 Disinhibition of the signaling pathway activated by interleukin-1 family proteins in generalized pustular psoriasis. Interleukin-36α, interleukin-36β, and interleukin-36γ exert their actions by binding to the interleukin-36 receptor, interleukin-1 receptor-like 2. Ligand binding to this receptor enables the recruitment of the interleukin-1 receptor accessory protein, leading to signal transduction involving activation of nuclear factor-kB (NF-kB) and mitogen-activated protein (MAP) kinases. The interleukin-36 receptor antagonist (interleukin-36Ra) also binds to the interleukin-36 receptor, which blocks binding by the agonist ligands but fails to recruit accessory protein and therefore does not lead to biologic activity. Interleukin-36Ra antagonizes their action and inhibits downstream inflammatory signaling (NF-kB and MAP kinases) avoiding exacerbated inflammatory responses. DITRA denotes deficiency on interleukin-36 receptor antagonist

Null mutations were associated with severe clinical phenotype GPP and AGEPE, while the hypomorphic mutations were associated with localized disease (PPP ACH) and generalized variants. The detection of the same mutations in generalized and localized pustular phenotypes implies that other factors may play a role in determining the phenotype, such as disease-modifying genes, environmental factors, or epigenetic events. In addition, it was proposed that long-term follow-up is necessary to assess the true expression of the disease in each individual.

It was found that there was a lack of altered protein expression or function for Lys35Arg and Arg102Trp, suggesting that these are indeed polymorphisms. The fact that no mutations were found on two GPP families and ten patients with sporadic disease suggested a genetic heterogeneity of the disease.

Diagnosis

The diagnosis of DITRA is established by the presence of GPP in any of its varieties and the demonstration of mutations in the *IL36RN* locus. Skin biopsies are necessary to rule out other pustular diseases.

Prognosis

DITRA is a life-threatening multisystemic inflammatory disease marked by lifelong relapses. The severity of the disease is reflected by its high mortality; in the initial report by Marrakchi, there were 5 deaths from septicemia among 16 affected individuals. Infections, drugs, and other factors trigger relapses.

Treatment

There are no trials assessing the treatment of DITRA. Current treatment is based on the experience and recommendations for GPP and small series and case reports of treatment of patients with DITRA.

Treatment of GPP has included topical and systemic therapies. Topical treatments have a limited efficacy and practicality in GPP. The first-line systemic therapy recommended by the 2012 consensus statement from the task force of the National Psoriasis Foundation Medical Board [31] includes acitretin, methotrexate, the TNF inhibitor infliximab, and cyclosporine. Acitretin and methotrexate are used for stable non-severe disease. Methotrexate appears to be effective in about 70% of patients [32]. For severe disease, infliximab and cyclosporine tend to induce a faster response. However, the experience with infliximab is limited to a small retrospective report showing fast and excellent response in 8 of 10 patients [33]. Case reports have communicated the efficacy of the TNF inhibitors etanercept and adalimumab. Combination therapy of a TNF inhibitor with a non-biologic agent has been reported as effective.

Second-line therapy includes inhibitors of the Th17 pathway, photochemotherapy, and combination therapy. The IL-17 inhibitor monoclonal antibody secukinumab has been proved effective in plaque psoriasis, but there is limited experience in GPP. In a 52-week analysis from a phase III open-label multicenter Japanese study that included 12 patients, according to a clinical global impression, 10 patients (83%) had a rating of "very much improved," and one patient showed no improvement. Although small, this trial shows efficacy of this agent.

A case report has shown efficacy of secukinumab, in a patient with DITRA whose flow cytometry of cells from affected skin showed 25-fold more IL-17A-producing

CD4+ T cells [34]. It has been reported a correlation between elevated IL-36 levels in psoriatic lesions and increased levels of IL-17, but the relationship between IL-36 and Th17 differentiation remains unknown [35].

Two pediatric cases of DITRA unresponsive to multiple treatments responded to high dose ustekinumab, a monoclonal antibody to the p40 subunit of IL-12 and IL-23 [36], suggesting that blockade of the IL-23/Th17 axis is effective in DITRA. IL-12/IL-23 inhibition appears to be effective in pustular psoriasis regardless of the presence of *IL36RN* mutations [37]. The role of IL-17 is supported from an animal model in which psoriasiform lesions were induced by imiquimod via Toll-like receptor 7; in this model, IL-36-deficient mice were protected from the disease in an IL-1 independent manner. This in turn suggests a cross talk between IL-36 and the IL-23/Th17 axis [38].

The unopposed effect of IL-36 in DITRA upregulates the NF-kB and MAPK pathways resulting in enhanced production of IL-1 and other pro-inflammatory cytokines. Case reports have shown the efficacy of anakinra an IL-1 receptor antagonist [39, 40] in patients with DITRA. It is unclear at present time whether blocking the IL-23/Th17 axis or the IL-1 or TNFa pathways would be more effective or safer for DITRA.

Two cases of late-onset DITRA were successfully treated with granulocyte and monocyte apheresis using an adsorbent column of cellulose acetate beds. The mechanism of action is unclear, although immunoglobulins and complement are also removed [41].

Based on the observation that TLR4 activators such as bacterial infections trigger relapses of GPP and activate the NF-kB and MAPK pathways resulting in production of pro-inflammatory cytokines, Shibata et al. developed an animal model in which *IL36rn −/−* mice were treated with the TLR4 agonist LPS [42]. The mice developed pustulosis, liver inflammation with sterile abscesses, and hind paw enthesitis, highly resembling GPP. Treatment of these animals with the TLR4 antagonist TAK-242 (resatorvid) which binds the intracellular domain of the TLR4 and inhibits the production of LPS-induced inflammatory mediators, resulted in improvement of all symptoms related to GPP. Treatment with intraperitoneal anti-IL-17 antibodies had minimal effect. Although the role of TLR4 in the development of GPP has not been elucidated, blocking the TLR4 pathway appears an attractive therapeutic option to explore.

References

1. Marrakchi S, Guigue P, Renshaw BR, Puel A, Pei XY, Fraitag S, et al. Interleukin-36-receptor antagonist deficiency and generalized pustular psoriasis. N Engl J Med. 2011;365(7):620–8.
2. Parisi R, Symmons DP, Griffiths CE, Ashcroft DM, Identification, Management of P, et al. Global epidemiology of psoriasis: a systematic review of incidence and prevalence. J Invest Dermatol. 2013;133(2):377–85.
3. Choon SE, Lai NM, Mohammad NA, Nanu NM, Tey KE, Chew SF. Clinical profile, morbidity, and outcome of adult-onset generalized pustular psoriasis: analysis of 102 cases seen in a tertiary hospital in Johor, Malaysia. Int J Dermatol. 2014;53(6):676–84.

4. de Oliveira ST, Maragno L, Arnone M, Fonseca Takahashi MD, Romiti R. Generalized pustular psoriasis in childhood. Pediatr Dermatol. 2010;27(4):349–54.
5. Zelickson BD, Muller SA. Generalized pustular psoriasis. A review of 63 cases. Arch Dermatol. 1991;127(9):1339–45.
6. Oumeish OY, Parish JL. Impetigo herpetiformis. Clin Dermatol. 2006;24(2):101–4.
7. Sugiura K, Takemoto A, Yamaguchi M, Takahashi H, Shoda Y, Mitsuma T, et al. The majority of generalized pustular psoriasis without psoriasis vulgaris is caused by deficiency of interleukin-36 receptor antagonist. J Invest Dermatol. 2013;133(11):2514–21.
8. Shmidt E, Wetter DA, Ferguson SB, Pittelkow MR. Psoriasis and palmoplantar pustulosis associated with tumor necrosis factor-alpha inhibitors: the Mayo Clinic experience, 1998 to 2010. J Am Acad Dermatol. 2012;67(5):e179–85.
9. Koizumi H, Tokuriki A, Oyama N, Ido H, Sugiura K, Akiyama M, et al. Certolizumab pegol, a pegylated anti-TNF-alpha antagonist, caused de novo-onset palmoplantar pustulosis followed by generalized pustular psoriasis in a patient with rheumatoid arthritis. J Dermatol. 2017;44(6):723–4.
10. Wenk KS, Claros JM, Ehrlich A. Flare of pustular psoriasis after initiating ustekinumab therapy. J Dermatolog Treat. 2012;23(3):212–4.
11. Gregoriou S, Kazakos C, Christofidou E, Kontochristopoulos G, Vakis G, Rigopoulos D. Pustular psoriasis development after initial ustekinumab administration in chronic plaque psoriasis. Eur J Dermatol. 2011;21(1):104–5.
12. Navarini AA, Simpson MA, Borradori L, Yawalkar N, Schlapbach C. Homozygous missense mutation in IL36RN in generalized pustular dermatosis with intraoral involvement compatible with both AGEP and generalized pustular psoriasis. JAMA Dermatol. 2015;151(4):452–3.
13. Borges-Costa J, Silva R, Goncalves L, Filipe P, Soares de Almeida L, Marques Gomes M. Clinical and laboratory features in acute generalized pustular psoriasis: a retrospective study of 34 patients. Am J Clin Dermatol. 2011;12(4):271–6.
14. Viguier M, Allez M, Zagdanski AM, Bertheau P, de Kerviler E, Rybojad M, et al. High frequency of cholestasis in generalized pustular psoriasis: Evidence for neutrophilic involvement of the biliary tract. Hepatology. 2004;40(2):452–8.
15. Setta-Kaffetzi N, Navarini AA, Patel VM, Pullabhatla V, Pink AE, Choon SE, et al. Rare pathogenic variants in IL36RN underlie a spectrum of psoriasis-associated pustular phenotypes. J Invest Dermatol. 2013;133(5):1366–9.
16. Korber A, Mossner R, Renner R, Sticht H, Wilsmann-Theis D, Schulz P, et al. Mutations in IL36RN in patients with generalized pustular psoriasis. J Invest Dermatol. 2013;133(11):2634–7.
17. Abbas O, Itani S, Ghosn S, Kibbi AG, Fidawi G, Farooq M, et al. Acrodermatitis continua of Hallopeau is a clinical phenotype of DITRA: evidence that it is a variant of pustular psoriasis. Dermatology. 2013;226(1):28–31.
18. Takahashi T, Fujimoto N, Kabuto M, Nakanishi T, Tanaka T. Mutation analysis of IL36RN gene in Japanese patients with palmoplantar pustulosis. J Dermatol. 2017;44(1):80–3.
19. Sugiura K, Shoda Y, Akiyama M. Generalized pustular psoriasis triggered by amoxicillin in monozygotic twins with compound heterozygous IL36RN mutations: comment on the article by Navarini et al. J Invest Dermatol. 2014;134(2):578–9.
20. Navarini AA, Valeyrie-Allanore L, Setta-Kaffetzi N, Barker JN, Capon F, Creamer D, et al. Rare variations in IL36RN in severe adverse drug reactions manifesting as acute generalized exanthematous pustulosis. J Invest Dermatol. 2013;133(7):1904–7.
21. Capon F. IL36RN mutations in generalized pustular psoriasis: just the tip of the iceberg? J Invest Dermatol. 2013;133(11):2503–4.
22. Jordan CT, Cao L, Roberson ED, Duan S, Helms CA, Nair RP, et al. Rare and common variants in CARD14, encoding an epidermal regulator of NF-kappaB, in psoriasis. Am J Hum Genet. 2012;90(5):796–808.
23. Ammar M, Jordan CT, Cao L, Lim E, Bouchlaka Souissi C, Jrad A, et al. CARD14 alterations in Tunisian patients with psoriasis and further characterization in European cohorts. Br J Dermatol. 2016;174(2):330–7.

24. Setta-Kaffetzi N, Simpson MA, Navarini AA, Patel VM, Lu HC, Allen MH, et al. AP1S3 mutations are associated with pustular psoriasis and impaired Toll-like receptor 3 trafficking. Am J Hum Genet. 2014;94(5):790–7.
25. Debets R, Timans JC, Homey B, Zurawski S, Sana TR, Lo S, et al. Two novel IL-1 family members, IL-1 delta and IL-1 epsilon, function as an antagonist and agonist of NF-kappa B activation through the orphan IL-1 receptor-related protein 2. J Immunol. 2001;167(3):1440–6.
26. Towne JE, Garka KE, Renshaw BR, Virca GD, Sims JE. Interleukin (IL)-1F6, IL-1F8, and IL-1F9 signal through IL-1Rrp2 and IL-1RAcP to activate the pathway leading to NF-kappaB and MAPKs. J Biol Chem. 2004;279(14):13677–88.
27. Kumar S, McDonnell PC, Lehr R, Tierney L, Tzimas MN, Griswold DE, et al. Identification and initial characterization of four novel members of the interleukin-1 family. J Biol Chem. 2000;275(14):10308–14.
28. Blumberg H, Dinh H, Dean C Jr, Trueblood ES, Bailey K, Shows D, et al. IL-1RL2 and its ligands contribute to the cytokine network in psoriasis. J Immunol. 2010;185(7):4354–62.
29. Blumberg H, Dinh H, Trueblood ES, Pretorius J, Kugler D, Weng N, et al. Opposing activities of two novel members of the IL-1 ligand family regulate skin inflammation. J Exp Med. 2007;204(11):2603–14.
30. Tauber M, Bal E, Pei XY, Madrange M, Khelil A, Sahel H, et al. IL36RN mutations affect protein expression and function: a basis for genotype-phenotype correlation in pustular diseases. J Invest Dermatol. 2016;136(9):1811–9.
31. Robinson A, Van Voorhees AS, Hsu S, Korman NJ, Lebwohl MG, Bebo BF Jr, et al. Treatment of pustular psoriasis: from the Medical Board of the National Psoriasis Foundation. J Am Acad Dermatol. 2012;67(2):279–88.
32. Ozawa A, Ohkido M, Haruki Y, Kobayashi H, Ohkawara A, Ohno Y, et al. Treatments of generalized pustular psoriasis: a multicenter study in Japan. J Dermatol. 1999;26(3):141–9.
33. Viguier M, Aubin F, Delaporte E, Pages C, Paul C, Beylot-Barry M, et al. Efficacy and safety of tumor necrosis factor inhibitors in acute generalized pustular psoriasis. Arch Dermatol. 2012;148(12):1423–5.
34. Cordoro KM, Ucmak D, Hitraya-Low M, Rosenblum MD, Liao W. Response to Interleukin (IL)-17 Inhibition in an Adolescent With Severe Manifestations of IL-36 Receptor Antagonist Deficiency (DITRA). JAMA Dermatol. 2017;153(1):106–8.
35. Carrier Y, Ma HL, Ramon HE, Napierata L, Small C, O'Toole M, et al. Inter-regulation of Th17 cytokines and the IL-36 cytokines in vitro and in vivo: implications in psoriasis pathogenesis. J Invest Dermatol. 2011;131(12):2428–37.
36. Bonekamp N, Caorsi R, Viglizzo GM, Graaf M, Minoia F, Grossi A, et al. High-dose ustekinumab for severe childhood deficiency of interleukin-36 receptor antagonist (DITRA). Ann Rheum Dis. 2018;77:1241–3.
37. Arakawa A, Ruzicka T, Prinz JC. Therapeutic efficacy of interleukin 12/interleukin 23 blockade in generalized pustular psoriasis regardless of IL36RN mutation status. JAMA Dermatol. 2016;152(7):825–8.
38. Tortola L, Rosenwald E, Abel B, Blumberg H, Schafer M, Coyle AJ, et al. Psoriasiform dermatitis is driven by IL-36-mediated DC-keratinocyte crosstalk. J Clin Invest. 2012;122(11):3965–76.
39. Huffmeier U, Watzold M, Mohr J, Schon MP, Mossner R. Successful therapy with anakinra in a patient with generalized pustular psoriasis carrying IL36RN mutations. Br J Dermatol. 2014;170(1):202–4.
40. Rossi-Semerano L, Piram M, Chiaverini C, De Ricaud D, Smahi A, Kone-Paut I. First clinical description of an infant with interleukin-36-receptor antagonist deficiency successfully treated with anakinra. Pediatrics. 2013;132(4):e1043–7.
41. Tominaga C, Yamamoto M, Imai Y, Yamanishi K. A case of old age-onset generalized pustular psoriasis with a deficiency of IL-36RN (DITRA) treated by granulocyte and monocyte apheresis. Case Rep Dermatol. 2015;7(1):29–35.
42. Shibata A, Sugiura K, Furuta Y, Mukumoto Y, Kaminuma O, Akiyama M. Toll-like receptor 4 antagonist TAK-242 inhibits autoinflammatory symptoms in DITRA. J Autoimmun. 2017;80:28–38.

Chapter 8
Cryopyrin-Associated Periodic Syndromes (CAPS)

Marinka Twilt and Susanne M. Benseler

Introduction

Cryopyrin-associated periodic syndrome (CAPS) is an autoinflammatory disease spectrum characterized by chronic systemic and organ inflammation due to an abnormal regulation of the innate immune system. Goldbach-Mansky characterized autoinflammatory diseases in general as disorders of amplified danger sensing and cytokine dysregulation [1]. CAPS has most commonly an autosomal dominant inheritance and is caused by single germline or somatic gain-of-function mutations in the *NLRP3* (nucleotide-binding domain, leucine-rich repeat family, pyrin domain containing 3) gene formerly known as *CIAS1* (cold-induced autoinflammatory syndrome 1) gene encoding the protein cryopyrin on chromosome 1q44 [2]. The discovery of this gene linked three different phenotypes, which were initially described as independent disease entities: familial cold autoinflammatory syndrome (FCAS) [3], Muckle-Wells syndrome (MWS) [4, 5], and neonatal-onset multisystem inflammatory disorder (NOMID), initially described as chronic infantile neurologic, cutaneous and articular (CINCA) syndrome [6, 7]. In addition, patients can present with overlapping symptoms of the identified CAPS severity phenotypes. Therefore, CAPS is now considered as a clinical continuum rather than three distinct clinical phenotypes [5, 8].

M. Twilt (✉)
Alberta Children's Hospital, Calgary, AB, Canada
e-mail: marinka.twilt@ahs.ca

S. M. Benseler
Department of Paediatrics, Alberta Children's Hospital, Calgary, AB, Canada

Cumming School of Medicine, University of Calgary, Calgary, AB, Canada
e-mail: susanne.benseler@albertahealthservices.ca

P. Efthimiou (ed.), *Auto-Inflammatory Syndromes*,
https://doi.org/10.1007/978-3-319-96929-9_8

Epidemiology

CAPS is a rare disease. In 2010, German study estimated the prevalence of CAPS at 1 per million [9], while a year later a French publication reported an estimated prevalence of 1 in 360,000 [10]. In 2016, Mehr et al. reported Australian data confirming an estimated population prevalence of 1 per million persons [11]. Toplak et al. documented that the availability of genetic testing has resulted in increased recognition and significantly reduced delay to diagnosis of all autoinflammatory diseases since the identification of the MEFV gene, the first gene associated with autoinflammation in 1997 [12].

Genetics and Pathophysiology

In 2001, Hoffman et al. first reported gain-of-function mutations in the *NRLP3* gene (CIAS1) encoding the "putative pyrin-like protein" – subsequently labeled as cryopyrin – in FCAS and MWS patients [2]. Initial cases were based on multiplex families; however sporadic cases due to de novo mutations have also been described, in particular for the severe phenotype CINCA/NOMID. Gain-of-function mutations in the *NLRP3* gene result in the loss of an important gatekeeper of the IL-1 inflammasome. Increase in cryopyrin function, which regulates the activation and cleavage of caspase-1, causes increased cleavage of the pro-inflammatory cytokines, IL-1β and IL-18 [13, 14]. Other functions attributed to the NLRP3 inflammasome include NF-κB activation and pyroptotic cell death [15]. In NOMID/CINCA about 60% of patients were found to have missense mutations in the *NLPR3* gene [16].

To date, 205 heterozygous non-synonymous variants in NLRP3 have been reported in patients with clinical features of CAPS (Infevers database: http://fmf.igh.cnrs.fr/ISSAD/infevers/). Some mutations associated with clinical phenotypes of CAPS have been confirmed to be caspase-1 activating in vitro, but the majority has not been tested. Large pedigrees with pathogenic *NLPR3* variants have been report. In 2016, Sobolewska et al. described the predominant phenotype of skin rash and ocular involvement in a five-generation family with the AV439V mutation, which is associated with a heterogeneous clinical spectrum of FCAS/MWS-overlap syndrome [17]. Many authors including Kuemmerle-Deschner emphasized the poor genotype-phenotype correlation and high degree of variability in the phenotype within families [18]. However, distinct risk alleles have been identified for severe, early organ manifestations such a sensorineural hearing loss and early deafness [19].

Patients with low-penetrance variants of autoinflammatory genes remain a clinical challenge [20]. Recently, Kuemmerle-Deschner et al. described the clinical phenotype and in vitro functional impact of the low-penetrance variants of *NLPR3*, Q703K, R488K, and V198 M in patients with a clinical phenotype of autoinflammation [21]. Patients had an atypical clinical phenotype with prominent fevers and gastrointestinal symptoms, less hearing loss, eye disease, and renal involvement.

Anti-IL-1 treatment appeared to be less effective, with complete resolution of symptoms occurring in only 50% of patients [21]. Notably, patients were found to have an intermediate biologic phenotype, including IL-1β- and non-IL-1β-mediated inflammatory pathway activation. To confuse matters even further, recent reports have identified pathogenic and low-penetrance *NLRP3* variants in animal models and patients with distinct inflammatory organ diseases such as inflammatory brain diseases and multiple sclerosis in the absence of CAPS typical symptoms [22, 23].

A significant proportion of patients have a defined CAPS phenotype, but no confirmed mutation when assessed in routine fever panels. In some patients, disease causing somatic mutations can be found. In fact, in 33% of NOMID/CINCA mutation-negative patients and 12% of patients with a clinical diagnosis of MWS in the absence of a NLRP3 mutation, next-generation sequencing techniques identified somatic mutations [24]. This approach is commonly limited to research setting and not routine clinical care environments. It is also important to note that access to genetic testing varies between countries and healthcare systems.

Clinical Phenotypes

CAPS is a systemic inflammatory disease with characteristic organ inflammation and dysfunction [25]. Systemic features include fatigue, fever, and irritability. Historically, autoinflammatory diseases were termed periodic fever syndromes, a terminology that was often difficult to reconcile in CAPS, since distinct episodes followed by symptom-free intervals are often missing and fever may be absent, especially in adult patients [26]. Systemic inflammation, while constitutively present in CAPS patients, dramatically worsens with endogenous and exogenous triggers such as cold and infections. Organ disease varies in severity across the disease spectrum and includes predominant skin, eye, renal, musculoskeletal, and CNS involvement. Skin disease is characterized by an urticaria-like rash, which is commonly triggered by cold temperature, stress, or infections [27]. The rash is typically not itchy and does not respond to antihistamine therapy. Histologically a predominantly neutrophilic dermatitis is seen [2, 28]. Eye involvement is common in patients with CAPS including the highly prevalent non-purulent conjunctivitis, uveitis, and less frequently papilledema due to CNS inflammation, which is a hallmark of CINCA/NOMID [29, 30]. Mucous membranes can be involved in CAPS including oral and nasal hyperemia and ulcers. Chest symptoms can be seen; in particular CAPS-associated pericarditis have been reported [31]. Abdominal symptoms including stomach pains and vomiting or diarrhea are seen particular in children with CAPS and in patients with low-penetrance variants [21]. The spectrum of renal manifestations includes proteinuria and impaired renal function due to amyloidosis ultimately requiring renal replacement, if untreated [32, 33]. Musculoskeletal manifestations range from arthralgia, myalgia, and arthritis to severe bone inflammation resulting in skeletal deformities due to disruption of directional growth and marrow expansion due to inflammation. Typical clinical findings are patellar overgrowth and frontal bossing as seen in CINCA/NOMID patients [34]. Short stature is commonly seen in children with severe CAPS; its etiology is multifactorial including severe systemic inflammation, failure to thrive, and growth disturbances due to inflammation. CNS manifestations are seen primarily in the moderate to severe phenotypes including typically headaches, aseptic meningitis, raised intracranial pressure and secondary papilledema, hydrocephalus, focal deficits due to focal inflammatory lesions, and impaired cognition [35].

Sensorineural hearing loss due to inner ear inflammation is the hallmark of CAPS [36]. Hearing loss typically first affects the higher frequencies above 4KHz (see Fig. 8.1). Over time, the hearing threshold increases across all frequencies. Untreated it results in irreversible deafness. The mechanism is not completely understood. Nakanishi et al. recently explored CAPS syndromic and non-syndromic families with *NLRP3* missense mutations and confirmed that resident macrophage-/monocyte-like cells within the cochlea can mediate local autoinflammation via activation of the NLRP3 inflammasome resulting in secretion of IL-1beta, even in the absence of systemic features of CAPS [37].

Diagnosis and Classification

Characteristic clinical features are the cornerstone of diagnosing and classifying CAPS [38]. Classification criteria were recently proposed aiming to identify patients with CAPS within cohorts of patients with autoinflammation for

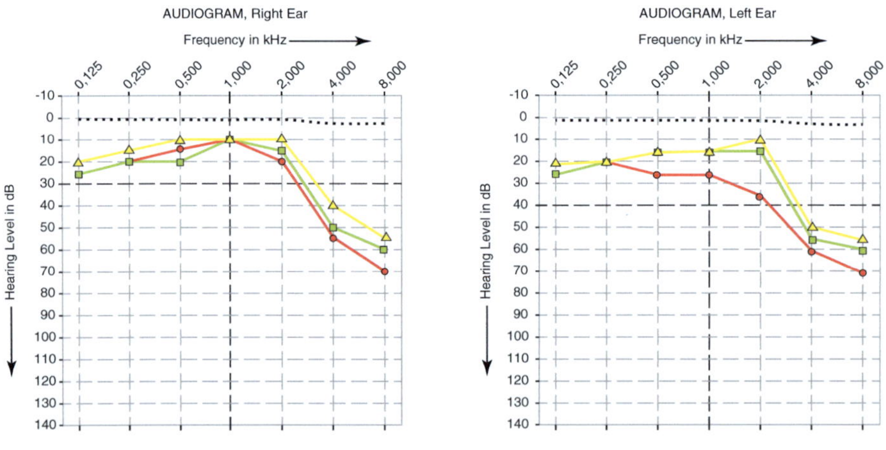

Fig. 8.1 Natural history of early high-frequency hearing loss in a 13-year-old boy with moderate CAPS. Bilateral progression of high-frequency sensorineural hearing loss over a 12-month period in an untreated adolescent patient with CAPS. Each line represents the hearing threshold measurement documented in 6-month intervals. The dotted line represents the normal hearing threshold

Table 8.1 CAPS diagnostic criteria[a]

Raised inflammatory markers (CRP/SAA)
Coupled with ≥2 of 6 CAPS typical signs or symptoms
Urticarial-like rash
Cold-/stress-triggered episodes
Sensorineural hearing loss
Musculoskeletal symptoms including arthralgia/arthritis/myalgia
Chronic aseptic meningitis
Skeletal abnormalities including epiphyseal overgrowth/frontal bossing

[a]Adapted from Kuemmerle-Deschner et al. [39]

participation in research studies [38]. In 2017, diagnostic criteria for CAPS were proposed. The most important aspect of these criteria is the coupling of characteristic clinical features with raised CAPS-typical inflammatory markers, which helps distinguishing CAPS from CAPS-mimics even when the genetic testing is negative or unavailable (Table 8.1). Criteria with low specificity such as urticaria-like rash may in doubt require additional histological confirmation of perivascular and/or periadnexal neutrophilic infiltration. These criteria performed well for all CAPS patients independent of *NLPR3* mutation presence or absence [39].

Inflammatory Markers

C-reactive protein (CRP) and serum amyloid A (SAA) are the most widely available inflammatory markers relevant for monogenic diseases of the innate immunity such as CAPS [40, 41]. In active CAPS, inflammatory makers are coupled with clinical features. During the seemingly symptom-free interval, they may be close to normal in patients on the mild end of the severity spectrum, yet continuously elevated in patients with the severe phenotype. In trials, both CRP and SAA were found to correlate well with disease activity and treatment response [42–44].

The neutrophil-derived protein S100A12 and its homologues MRP8/14 (S100A8/9) may provide additional precision to detecting inflammation in autoinflammatory diseases such as CAPS [45, 46] and may increase the ability to detect subclinical inflammation over CRP and SAA [46]. Pro-inflammatory cytokine profiles have been measured in patients with CAPS [44, 46]; their clinical utility is currently limited. Rodriguez-Smith et al. demonstrated that CSF cytokines correlate well with aseptic meningitis and blood-brain barrier dysfunction in CINCA/NOMID and may serve as biomarkers of inflammation [47]. Equally, microarray-based gene expression profiling that has been reported to define a CAPS disease-related signature and predict treatment responsiveness is currently primarily utilized in the research context [48].

In everyday practice, CRP and in many places SAA remain the key accessible biomarkers of CAPS. In addition, complete blood counts and differential commonly demonstrate raised neutrophils and platelets in active CAPS. The sedimentation rates are raised, while autoantibodies are typically negative and complement levels are normal or mildly raised. Spinal taps reveal raised opening pressures and raised white blood counts and protein levels in children with CNS involvement [49].

Additional Testing

Beyond serial inflammatory markers, patients with CAPS required routine monitoring of organ inflammation and function [50]. Screening for early, high-frequency hearing loss is critically important to detect sensorineural hearing loss at an early, potentially reversible stage [51]. Modified audiograms including higher frequencies beyond the routine so-called 4-pure tone averages (4-PTA) of 0.5-4KHz are important to request [36]. Early sensorineural hearing loss in CAPS first occurs at frequencies of 6–10KHz and is best detected when conducting a so-called high-frequency pure tone averages (HF-PTA) [51]. Ophthalmological assessments are required to detect inflammatory manifestations of CAPS in the eye and inflammatory sequelae. Urine analysis should screen for proteinuria; frequently protein/creatinine ratios are determined. CNS manifestations should be explored using magnetic resonance imaging, spinal taps including opening pressures and cell counts, and formal cognitive assessments, when indicated [50]. Different strategies are available to monitor amyloidosis including biopsies and amyloid scans; these are required in advanced disease states [50].

Monitoring of Children and Adults with CAPS

In 2015, the international community of pediatric rheumatologists unified in the European Union-funded SHARE initiative published evidence-based recommendations for the management of children and adults with CAPS [50, 52]. Overarching principles include the need for patient- and family-centered care models provided by multidisciplinary teams in a tertiary center with expertise in CAPS, where available. Access to genetic counseling and attention to completion of attenuated vaccines as appropriate was mandated. Of note, vaccination against *Streptococcus pneumoniae* has been shown to result in severe, life-threatening systemic inflammation due to CAPS reactivation in some patients [53]. Clinicians are therefore required to balance potential benefits of pneumococcal immunization against safety concerns. In CAPS, the 13-valent pneumococcal conjugate vaccine might be favorable over the polysaccharide vaccine [54]. The SHARE experts emphasized the need for standardized monitoring of disease activity and damage. Disease activity is commonly monitored by patient diary-based approaches such as the autoinflammatory diseases activity index (AIDAI) and its score [55]. A disease damage instrument for all autoinflammatory diseases, the autoinflammatory diseases damage index (ADDI), has been developed [56].

Regular monitoring visits of children and adults with CAPS are required. General assessments including review of children's growth and development, disease activity, and damage instruments should be partnered with inflammatory markers and CAPS-specific testing of hearing, eye, and renal involvement. Patient with severe disease phenotypes require monitoring of CNS and bone involvement. A strong emphasis should be given to disease burden and impact on well-being, functioning, and social participation [56]. Psychosocial support for patients and families is commonly needed [57].

Treatment

The treatment of CAPS aims to control the IL-1-driven inflammation, prevent organ dysfunction and damage, and improve the overall health-related quality of life. In 2003 Hawkins et al. were the first to treat CAPS patients (MWS) with anti-IL-1 therapy [58]. The group reported rapid improvement of clinical signs and symptoms and improved inflammatory markers within days of starting treatment with anakinra [58]. Ever since, a composite measure is used to determine disease activity control in CAPS. Treatment studies typically define complete response as (1) the absence of CAPS typical symptoms, (2) the normalization of CRP and/or SAA levels, and (3) low/normal disease activity estimated on a 10 cm visual analog scale [43].

To date, anti-IL-1 therapy options for CAPS include (1) canakinumab, the monoclonal, human anti-IL-1β antibody; (2) anakinra, the recombinant human anti-IL-1 receptor antibody; and (3) rilonacept, the soluble IL-1 decoy receptor [59]. Access to the different anti-IL-1 treatment options varies dramatically across healthcare systems and countries.

All three anti-IL-1 regimens have been studied and found to be effective in patients with CAPS [27, 43, 60–62]. The European Medicines Agency (EMA) approved canakinumab for CAPS patients ≥2 years of age and ≥7.5 kg body weight including all CINCA/NOMID, MWS, and severe FCAS. EMA also approved anakinra for all CAPS patients ages ≥8 months and ≥10 kg. Rilonacept has no EMA approval. The US Food and Drug Administration (FDA) approved all three anti-IL-1 therapies, canakinumab for CAPS patients ≥4 years of age, anakinra for CINCA/NOMID, and rilonacept for FCAS and MWS in patients ≥12 years of age. It remains uncertain if a preference should be given to one specific anti-IL-1 regimen based on the CAPS severity or specific organ disease. For the mild phenotypes of FCAS, the initial studies confirm the effectiveness of rilonacept [27, 63–65]; subsequently both anakinra and canakinumab have been shown to be effective. For MWS and the moderate spectrum of CAPS, first anakinra [44, 58, 66–69] and then canakinumab [44] have been used more commonly to control disease activity. Interestingly, there are case reports documenting reversibility of what is thought to be CAPS-related damage following treatment with anti-IL-1 therapy such as hearing loss [19, 36] and renal amyloidosis [70]. Finally for the severe phenotype of CINCA/NOMID, anakinra was first shown to be effective [34, 62, 71–73]; subsequently Sibley et al. demonstrated effectiveness of canakinumab [61]. There remain concerns about the ability of all anti-IL-1 therapies to cross the blood-brain barrier effectively. Studies in nonhuman primate models without meningitis revealed that anakinra drug levels in the CSF were only a third of serum levels; however declines were slower in the CSF compared to serum providing a rationale for increased anakinra doses in patients with ongoing CNS inflammation [30].

Recent studies have highlighted the effectiveness of anti-IL-1 therapy in real-life settings and suggested a "treat-to-target" approach including an iterative assessment of disease activity and anti-IL-1 dose adjustments being the most effective approach to achieve control of inflammation and prevent organ damage (see Fig. 8.2) [74, 75]. It was documents that younger patients consistently *needed higher* doses of anti-IL-1 therapy to achieve disease activity control [74]. Beyond the often access-option-driven selection of the anti-IL-1 regimen, considerations should be given to continuous versus interval treatment, dose and interval adjustments, intolerance and patient preferences, as well as specific circumstances such as pregnancy and breastfeeding [76].

The 2015 SHARE recommendations specify that IL-1 inhibition is indicated for the whole spectrum of CAPS and at any age [50]. Furthermore, IL-1 inhibition

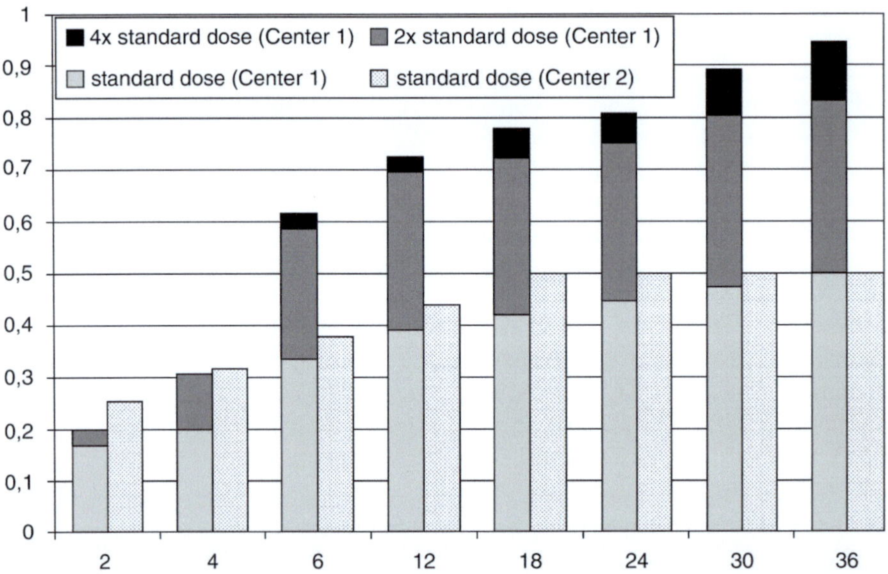

Fig. 8.2 Treat-to-target in CAPS: Canakinumab dosing in complete responders comparing two high-volume autoinflammatory disease centers in Germany. The study assessed the real-life effectiveness of canakinumab in CAPS comparing centers with different treatment strategies. Center 1 adopted a treat-to-target strategy resulting in significantly higher rates of complete response compared to Center 2, where CAPS patients were kept on the recommended standard dose. (Modified from Kuemmerle-Deschner [74])

should be started as early as possible in CAPS patients with active disease to prevent organ damage. The recommendations state that there is no evidence for the efficacy of disease-modifying antirheumatic drugs (DMARDs) or biological therapy other than anti-IL-1 therapy for children and adults with CAPS. However, for symptomatic adjunctive therapy, short courses of NSAIDs and corticosteroids may be used. Importantly adjunctive therapy such as physiotherapy, orthotic devices, and hearing aids is recommended as appropriate. Access to psychosocial support for school, workplace, and family are essential for patients with rare diseases including CAPS.

Outcome

The long-term outcome of patients with CAPS has dramatically improved with increased awareness and subsequent clinical diagnosis, access to genetic testing, and effective and safe anti-IL-1 therapies [77]. A rapid diagnosis and early start of therapy remains critically important, since CAPS patients accrual organ damage over time, if inflammation remains uncontrolled. Control of inflammation typically results in resolution of CAPS-associated clinical signs and symptoms, normalization of inflammatory markers, and halt of damage progression.

Trial-based long-term efficacy and safety of canakinumab in CAPS was reported at 24 months [78]. Complete remission was achieved in 78% (85/109) canakinumab-naive patients, of whom 93% were already asymptomatic within 8 days of therapy. The relapse rate of all responders was 10%, and dose adjustments were required in 24%, primarily children and patients with severe CAPS. Adverse events were mild to moderate, commonly infections noted in 66%, while 10% had severe infections all response to standard therapies. Increased dosing did not correlate with a higher risk of adverse events. A total of 92% of patient reported no injection side reactions (79). Real-life-based treatment effectiveness was found to be significantly lower in a recent multicenter study across Germany [74]. Overall complete remission was attained in only 53% of CAPS patients ranging from 14% in severe and 79% in mild CAPS phenotypes. Centers with "treat-to-target" approaches and treatment dose adjustment strategies had dramatically higher rates of complete remission (90 versus 50%) [74]. These and other studies made several important points: (1) IL-1 inhibition in CAPS is effective; however younger patients and those with more severe phenotypes need higher treatment doses to achieve control of disease activity; (2) treatment responses are sustained in 90% of patients; and (3) infections are the main adverse event to watch for in patients with CAPS treated with IL-1 inhibition.

Limited data is available for disease- and treatment-related long-term damage in CAPS. Only recently an instrument was developed to systematically capture damage, the autoinflammatory diseases damage index (ADDI) [56]. Long-term outcome appears to be strongly correlated to the severity of the phenotype and the delay to starting effective treatment.

Children with CINCA/NOMID are commonly symptomatic in the first year of life with fevers, rashes, and CNS manifestations. In 2015, Levy et al. reported the characteristics of 136 CAPS patients from the cross-sectional Eurofever Registry of contemporary outcomes and documented neurological manifestations in 54 patients (40%) including headaches in 70%, papilledema in 52%, meningitis in 26%, hydrocephalus in 18%, and mental retardation in 16% [79]. Mamoudjy et al. reported the contemporary neurological outcome of 24 patients of 9 children and 15 adults with CAPS followed for a median time of 10 years. The vast majority had an onset of symptoms within the first year of life, however was diagnosed between 0 and 53 years of age. A total 71% had neurological involvement. The most common findings were learning difficulties requiring educational support in 58% [80]. Neven et al. documented the contemporary outcome of 10 patients with CINCA/NOMID ages 3 months to 19.8 years at start of anakinra therapy and followed for 26–42 months [62]. At the last follow-up, 50% had residual aseptic meningitis. In the vast majority, dose adjustments were made due to ongoing CNS inflammation. Deficits were strongly associated with delay to effective therapy. Growth parameters were only assessed in five of the eight older children, in whom anakinra was started before completion of puberty; a dramatic increase in median growth which improved from 3 (0.5–4.5) to 7 (7–7.5) cm/year was documented [62]. Amyloidosis was present in two patients at baseline and did not change; however proteinuria improved in all affected patients and no new renal damage occurred [62]. These studies suggest several important points when caring for CINCA/NOMID patients: (1) early start of therapy may prevent neurological deficits, (2) CNS inflammation requires higher anti-IL-1 treatment doses, (3) effective IL-1 inhibition can result in growth in patients with growth potential, and (4) effective treatment improves early renal damage and prevents amyloidosis.

Historically, children and adults with moderate CAPS/MWS have suffered from debilitating fatigue, rashes, sensorineural hearing loss, and renal failure [4]. Contemporary, treated outcomes of moderate CAPS are dramatically better. Similar to other autoinflammatory diseases, moderate CAPS has two phases, systemic and organ inflammation and organ damage (see Fig. 8.3). Treatment started in the first

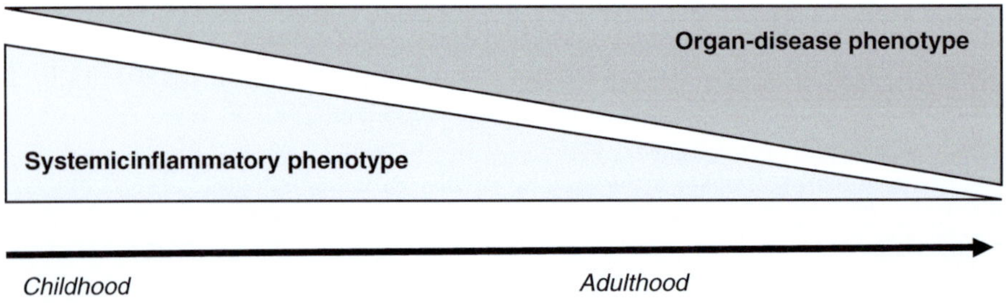

Fig. 8.3 The clinical phenotype changes across the age spectrum: the example of moderate CAPS/ Muckle-Wells syndrome. The clinical presentation of patients with autoinflammatory syndromes may vary depending on the age of the patient. While children commonly present with clinical and laboratory features of systemic inflammation including fever, older patients may have organ dysfunction and damage as the leading clinical phenotype. (*Modified from Kuemmerle-Deschner [26])

phase has been shown to effectively prevent organ damage such as deafness and renal amyloidosis [26]. Anti-IL-1 therapy was also found to dramatically improve fatigue and result in better health-related quality of life [81]. There appear to remain several unmet needs in CAPS that need to be addressed in order to improve participation and achieve the best possible outcomes.

References

1. Sanchez GA, de Jesus AA, Goldbach-Mansky R. Monogenic autoinflammatory diseases: disorders of amplified danger sensing and cytokine dysregulation. Rheum Dis Clin N Am. 2013;39(4):701–34.
2. Hoffman HM, Mueller JL, Broide DH, Wanderer AA, Kolodner RD. Mutation of a new gene encoding a putative pyrin-like protein causes familial cold autoinflammatory syndrome and Muckle-Wells syndrome. Nat Genet. 2001;29(3):301–5.
3. Kile R, Rusk H. A case of cold urticaria with an unusual family history. JAMA. 1940;114:1067–8.
4. Muckle TJ, Wells M. Urticaria, deafness, and amyloidosis: a new heredo-familial syndrome. Q J Med. 1962;31:235–48.
5. Dode C, Le Du N, Cuisset L, Letourneur F, Berthelot JM, Vaudour G, et al. New mutations of CIAS1 that are responsible for Muckle-Wells syndrome and familial cold urticaria: a novel mutation underlies both syndromes. Am J Hum Genet. 2002;70(6):1498–506.
6. Feldmann J, Prieur AM, Quartier P, Berquin P, Certain S, Cortis E, et al. Chronic infantile neurological cutaneous and articular syndrome is caused by mutations in CIAS1, a gene highly expressed in polymorphonuclear cells and chondrocytes. Am J Hum Genet. 2002;71(1):198–203.
7. Prieur AM, Griscelli C, Lampert F, Truckenbrodt H, Guggenheim MA, Lovell DJ, et al. A chronic, infantile, neurological, cutaneous and articular (CINCA) syndrome. A specific entity analysed in 30 patients. Scand J Rheumatol Suppl. 1987;66:57–68.
8. Granel B, Philip N, Serratrice J, Ene N, Grateau G, Dode C, et al. CIAS1 mutation in a patient with overlap between Muckle-Wells and chronic infantile neurological cutaneous and articular syndromes. Dermatology. 2003;206(3):257–9.
9. Lainka E, Neudorf U, Lohse P, Timmann C, Bielak M, Stojanov S, et al. Analysis of cryopyrin-associated periodic syndromes (CAPS) in German children: epidemiological, clinical and genetic characteristics. Klin Padiatr. 2010;222(6):356–61.
10. Cuisset L, Jeru I, Dumont B, Fabre A, Cochet E, Le Bozec J, et al. Mutations in the autoinflammatory cryopyrin-associated periodic syndrome gene: epidemiological study and lessons from eight years of genetic analysis in France. Ann Rheum Dis. 2011;70(3):495–9.
11. Mehr S, Allen R, Boros C, Adib N, Kakakios A, Turner PJ, et al. Cryopyrin-associated periodic syndrome in Australian children and adults: epidemiological, clinical and treatment characteristics. J Paediatr Child Health. 2016;52(9):889–95.
12. Balow JE Jr, Shelton DA, Orsborn A, Mangelsdorf M, Aksentijevich I, Blake T, et al. A high-resolution genetic map of the familial Mediterranean fever candidate region allows identification of haplotype-sharing among ethnic groups. Genomics. 1997;44(3):280–91.
13. Hoffman HM, Patel DD. Genomic-based therapy: targeting interleukin-1 for autoinflammatory diseases. Arthritis Rheum. 2004;50(2):345–9.
14. Lachmann HJ, Lowe P, Felix SD, Rordorf C, Leslie K, Madhoo S, et al. In vivo regulation of interleukin 1beta in patients with cryopyrin-associated periodic syndromes. J Exp Med. 2009;206(5):1029–36.
15. de Jesus AA, Canna SW, Liu Y, Goldbach-Mansky R. Molecular mechanisms in genetically defined autoinflammatory diseases: disorders of amplified danger signaling. Annu Rev Immunol. 2015;33:823–74.

16. Goldbach-Mansky R, Dailey NJ, Canna SW, Gelabert A, Jones J, Rubin BI, et al. Neonatal-onset multisystem inflammatory disease responsive to interleukin-1beta inhibition. N Engl J Med. 2006;355(6):581–92.
17. Sobolewska B, Angermair E, Deuter C, Doycheva D, Kuemmerle-Deschner J, Zierhut M. NLRP3 A439V mutation in a large family with cryopyrin-associated periodic syndrome: description of ophthalmologic symptoms in correlation with other organ symptoms. J Rheumatol. 2016;43(6):1101–6.
18. Kuemmerle-Deschner JB, Koetter I, Dannecker GE, Bialkowski A, Tzaribachev N, Koch S, et al. New CIAS1 E311K mutation and cytokine profile in a family of 3 generations with the clinical picture of muckle-wells syndrome. Clin Exp Rheumatol. 2004;22:531.
19. Kuemmerle-Deschner JB, Koitschev A, Ummenhofer K, Hansmann S, Plontke SK, Koitschev C, et al. Hearing loss in muckle-wells syndrome. Arthritis Rheum. 2013;65(3):824–31.
20. Pelagatti MA, Meini A, Caorsi R, Cattalini M, Federici S, Zulian F, et al. Long-term clinical profile of children with the low-penetrance R92Q mutation of the TNFRSF1A gene. Arthritis Rheum. 2011;63(4):1141–50.
21. Kuemmerle-Deschner JB, Verma D, Endres T, Broderick L, de Jesus AA, Hofer F, et al. Clinical and molecular phenotypes of low-penetrance variants of NLRP3: diagnostic and therapeutic challenges. Arthritis Rheumatol. 2017;69(11):2233–40.
22. Schuh E, Lohse P, Ertl-Wagner B, Witt M, Krumbholz M, Frankenberger M, et al. Expanding spectrum of neurologic manifestations in patients with NLRP3 low-penetrance mutations. Neurol Neuroimmunol Neuroinflamm. 2015;2(4):e109.
23. Barclay W, Shinohara ML. Inflammasome activation in multiple sclerosis and experimental autoimmune encephalomyelitis (EAE). Brain Pathol. 2017;27(2):213–9.
24. Kummerle-Deschner JB, Lohse P. Genetics of cryopyrin-associated periodic syndrome. Z Rheumatol. 2017;76(4):313–21.
25. Kuemmerle-Deschner JB. CAPS--pathogenesis, presentation and treatment of an autoinflammatory disease. Semin Immunopathol. 2015;37(4):377–85.
26. Kuemmerle-Deschner JB, Dembi Samba S, Tyrrell PN, Kone-Paut I, Marie I, Deschner N, et al. Challenges in diagnosing Muckle-Wells syndrome: identifying two distinct phenotypes. Arthritis Care Res (Hoboken). 2014;66(5):765–72.
27. Hoffman HM, Rosengren S, Boyle DL, Cho JY, Nayar J, Mueller JL, et al. Prevention of cold-associated acute inflammation in familial cold autoinflammatory syndrome by interleukin-1 receptor antagonist. Lancet. 2004;364(9447):1779–85.
28. Arostegui JI, Aldea A, Modesto C, Rua MJ, Arguelles F, Gonzalez-Ensenat MA, et al. Clinical and genetic heterogeneity among Spanish patients with recurrent autoinflammatory syndromes associated with the CIAS1/PYPAF1/NALP3 gene. Arthritis Rheum. 2004;50(12):4045–50.
29. Tarabishy AB, Hise AG, Traboulsi EI. Ocular manifestations of the autoinflammatory syndromes. Ophthalmic Genet. 2012;33(4):179–86.
30. Goldbach-Mansky R. Current status of understanding the pathogenesis and management of patients with NOMID/CINCA. Curr Rheumatol Rep. 2011;13(2):123–31.
31. Insalaco A, Prencipe G, Buonuomo PS, Ceccherini I, Bracaglia C, Pardeo M, et al. A novel mutation in the CIAS1/NLRP3 gene associated with an unexpected phenotype of cryopyrin-associated periodic syndromes. Clin Exp Rheumatol. 2014;32(1):123–5.
32. Bilginer Y, Akpolat T, Ozen S. Renal amyloidosis in children. Pediatr Nephrol. 2011;26(8):1215–27.
33. Lachmann HJ, Goodman HJ, Gilbertson JA, Gallimore JR, Sabin CA, Gillmore JD, et al. Natural history and outcome in systemic AA amyloidosis. N Engl J Med. 2007;356(23):2361–71.
34. Sibley CH, Plass N, Snow J, Wiggs EA, Brewer CC, King KA, et al. Sustained response and prevention of damage progression in patients with neonatal-onset multisystem inflammatory disease treated with anakinra: a cohort study to determine three- and five-year outcomes. Arthritis Rheum. 2012;64(7):2375–86.
35. Parker T, Keddie S, Kidd D, Lane T, Maviki M, Hawkins PN, et al. Neurology of the cryopyrin-associated periodic fever syndrome. Eur J Neurol. 2016;23(7):1145–51.
36. Koitschev A, Gramlich K, Hansmann S, Benseler S, Plontke SK, Koitschev C, et al. Progressive familial hearing loss in Muckle-Wells syndrome. Acta Otolaryngol. 2012;132(7):756–62.

37. Nakanishi H, Kawashima Y, Kurima K, Chae JJ, Ross AM, Pinto-Patarroyo G, et al. NLRP3 mutation and cochlear autoinflammation cause syndromic and nonsyndromic hearing loss DFNA34 responsive to anakinra therapy. Proc Natl Acad Sci U S A. 2017;114(37):E7766–E75.
38. Federici S, Sormani MP, Ozen S, Lachmann HJ, Amaryan G, Woo P, et al. Evidence-based provisional clinical classification criteria for autoinflammatory periodic fevers. Ann Rheum Dis. 2015;74(5):799–805.
39. Kuemmerle-Deschner JB, Ozen S, Tyrrell PN, Kone-Paut I, Goldbach-Mansky R, Lachmann H, et al. Diagnostic criteria for cryopyrin-associated periodic syndrome (CAPS). Ann Rheum Dis. 2017;76(6):942–7.
40. van der Hilst JC, Simon A, Drenth JP. Hereditary periodic fever and reactive amyloidosis. Clin Exp Med. 2005;5(3):87–98.
41. Pastore S, Paloni G, Caorsi R, Ronfani L, Taddio A, Lepore L, et al. Serum amyloid protein A concentration in cryopyrin-associated periodic syndromes patients treated with interleukin-1 beta antagonist. Clin Exp Rheumatol. 2014;32(4 Suppl 84):S63–6.
42. Gillespie J, Mathews R, McDermott MF. Rilonacept in the management of cryopyrin-associated periodic syndromes (CAPS). J Inflamm Res. 2010;3:1–8.
43. Lachmann HJ, Kone-Paut I, Kuemmerle-Deschner JB, Leslie KS, Hachulla E, Quartier P, et al. Use of canakinumab in the cryopyrin-associated periodic syndrome. N Engl J Med. 2009;360(23):2416–25.
44. Kuemmerle-Deschner JB, Wittkowski H, Tyrrell PN, Koetter I, Lohse P, Ummenhofer K, et al. Treatment of Muckle-Wells syndrome: analysis of two IL-1-blocking regimens. Arthritis Res Ther. 2013;15(3):R64.
45. Wittkowski H, Frosch M, Wulffraat N, Goldbach-Mansky R, Kallinich T, Kuemmerle-Deschner J, et al. S100A12 is a novel molecular marker differentiating systemic-onset juvenile idiopathic arthritis from other causes of fever of unknown origin. Arthritis Rheum. 2008;58(12):3924–31.
46. Wittkowski H, Kuemmerle-Deschner JB, Austermann J, Holzinger D, Goldbach-Mansky R, Gramlich K, et al. MRP8 and MRP14, phagocyte-specific danger signals, are sensitive biomarkers of disease activity in cryopyrin-associated periodic syndromes. Ann Rheum Dis. 2011;70(12):2075–81.
47. Rodriguez-Smith J, Lin YC, Tsai WL, Kim H, Montealegre-Sanchez G, Chapelle D, et al. Cerebrospinal fluid cytokines correlate with aseptic meningitis and blood-brain barrier function in neonatal-onset multisystem inflammatory disease: central nervous system biomarkers in neonatal-onset multisystem inflammatory disease correlate with central nervous system inflammation. Arthritis Rheumatol. 2017;69(6):1325–36.
48. Balow JE Jr, Ryan JG, Chae JJ, Booty MG, Bulua A, Stone D, et al. Microarray-based gene expression profiling in patients with cryopyrin-associated periodic syndromes defines a disease-related signature and IL-1-responsive transcripts. Ann Rheum Dis. 2013;72(6):1064–70.
49. Finetti M, Omenetti A, Federici S, Caorsi R, Gattorno M. Chronic infantile neurological cutaneous and articular (CINCA) syndrome: a review. Orphanet J Rare Dis. 2016;11(1):167.
50. ter Haar NM, Oswald M, Jeyaratnam J, Anton J, Barron KS, Brogan PA, et al. Recommendations for the management of autoinflammatory diseases. Ann Rheum Dis. 2015;74(9):1636–44.
51. Kuemmerle-Deschner JB, Koitschev A, Tyrrell PN, Plontke SK, Deschner N, Hansmann S, et al. Early detection of sensorineural hearing loss in Muckle-Wells-syndrome. Pediatr Rheumatol Online J. 2015;13(1):43.
52. Wulffraat NM, Vastert B, Consortium S. Time to share. Pediatr Rheumatol Online J. 2013;11(1):5.
53. Walker UA, Hoffman HM, Williams R, Kuemmerle-Deschner J, Hawkins PN. Brief report: severe inflammation following vaccination against Streptococcus pneumoniae in patients with cryopyrin-associated periodic syndromes. Arthritis Rheumatol. 2016;68(2):516–20.
54. Jaeger VK, Hoffman HM, van der Poll T, Tilson H, Seibert J, Speziale A, et al. Safety of vaccinations in patients with cryopyrin-associated periodic syndromes: a prospective registry based study. Rheumatology (Oxford). 2017;56(9):1484–91.

55. Piram M, Kone-Paut I, Lachmann HJ, Frenkel J, Ozen S, Kuemmerle-Deschner J, et al. Validation of the auto-inflammatory diseases activity index (AIDAI) for hereditary recurrent fever syndromes. Ann Rheum Dis. 2014;73(12):2168–73.
56. Ter Haar NM, Annink KV, Al-Mayouf SM, Amaryan G, Anton J, Barron KS, et al. Development of the autoinflammatory disease damage index (ADDI). Ann Rheum Dis. 2017;76(5):821–30.
57. Lepore L, Paloni G, Caorsi R, Alessio M, Rigante D, Ruperto N, et al. Follow-up and quality of life of patients with cryopyrin-associated periodic syndromes treated with Anakinra. J Pediatr. 2010;157(2):310–5. e1
58. Hawkins PN, Lachmann HJ, McDermott MF. Interleukin-1-receptor antagonist in the Muckle-Wells syndrome. N Engl J Med. 2003;348(25):2583–4.
59. Dinarello CA, Simon A, van der Meer JW. Treating inflammation by blocking interleukin-1 in a broad spectrum of diseases. Nat Rev Drug Discov. 2012;11(8):633–52.
60. Hoffman HM, Throne ML, Amar NJ, Sebai M, Kivitz AJ, Kavanaugh A, et al. Efficacy and safety of rilonacept (interleukin-1 trap) in patients with cryopyrin-associated periodic syndromes: results from two sequential placebo-controlled studies. Arthritis Rheum. 2008;58(8):2443–52.
61. Sibley CH, Chioato A, Felix S, Colin L, Chakraborty A, Plass N, et al. A 24-month open-label study of canakinumab in neonatal-onset multisystem inflammatory disease. Ann Rheum Dis. 2015;74(9):1714–9.
62. Neven B, Marvillet I, Terrada C, Ferster A, Boddaert N, Couloignier V, et al. Long-term efficacy of the interleukin-1 receptor antagonist anakinra in ten patients with neonatal-onset multisystem inflammatory disease/chronic infantile neurologic, cutaneous, articular syndrome. Arthritis Rheum. 2010;62(1):258–67.
63. Church LD, Savic S, McDermott MF. Long term management of patients with cryopyrin-associated periodic syndromes (CAPS): focus on rilonacept (IL-1 trap). Biologics. 2008;2(4):733–42.
64. Goldbach-Mansky R, Shroff SD, Wilson M, Snyder C, Plehn S, Barham B, et al. A pilot study to evaluate the safety and efficacy of the long-acting interleukin-1 inhibitor rilonacept (interleukin-1 trap) in patients with familial cold autoinflammatory syndrome. Arthritis Rheum. 2008;58(8):2432–42.
65. Hoffman HM, Throne ML, Amar NJ, Cartwright RC, Kivitz AJ, Soo Y, Weinstein SP. Long-term efficacy and safety profile of rilonacept in the treatment of cryopryin-associated periodic syndromes: results of a 72-week open-label extension study. Clin Ther. 2012;34(10):2091–103.
66. Hawkins PN, Lachmann HJ, Aganna E, McDermott MF. Spectrum of clinical features in Muckle-Wells syndrome and response to anakinra. Arthritis Rheum. 2004;50(2):607–12.
67. Kuemmerle-Deschner JB, Tyrrell PN, Koetter I, Wittkowski H, Bialkowski A, Tzaribachev N, et al. Efficacy and safety of anakinra therapy in pediatric and adult patients with the autoinflammatory Muckle-Wells syndrome. Arthritis Rheum. 2011;63(3):840–9.
68. Mirault T, Launay D, Cuisset L, Hachulla E, Lambert M, Queyrel V, et al. Recovery from deafness in a patient with Muckle-Wells syndrome treated with anakinra. Arthritis Rheum. 2006;54(5):1697–700.
69. Rynne M, Maclean C, Bybee A, McDermott MF, Emery P. Hearing improvement in a patient with variant Muckle-Wells syndrome in response to interleukin 1 receptor antagonism. Ann Rheum Dis. 2006;65(4):533–4.
70. Scarpioni R, Rigante D, Cantarini L, Ricardi M, Albertazzi V, Melfa L, et al. Renal involvement in secondary amyloidosis of Muckle-Wells syndrome: marked improvement of renal function and reduction of proteinuria after therapy with human anti-interleukin-1beta monoclonal antibody canakinumab. Clin Rheumatol. 2015;34(7):1311–6.
71. Boschan C, Witt O, Lohse P, Foeldvari I, Zappel H, Schweigerer L. Neonatal-onset multisystem inflammatory disease (NOMID) due to a novel S331R mutation of the CIAS1 gene and response to interleukin-1 receptor antagonist treatment. Am J Med Genet A. 2006;140(8):883–6.
72. Lovell DJ, Bowyer SL, Solinger AM. Interleukin-1 blockade by anakinra improves clinical symptoms in patients with neonatal-onset multisystem inflammatory disease. Arthritis Rheum. 2005;52(4):1283–6.

73. Miyamae T, Inaba Y, Nishimura G, Kikuchi M, Kishi T, Hara R, et al. Effect of anakinra on arthropathy in CINCA/NOMID syndrome. Pediatr Rheumatol Online J. 2010;8:9.
74. Kuemmerle-Deschner JB, Hofer F, Endres T, Kortus-Goetze B, Blank N, Weissbarth-Riedel E, et al. Real-life effectiveness of canakinumab in cryopyrin-associated periodic syndrome. Rheumatology (Oxford). 2016;55(4):689–96.
75. Russo RA, Melo-Gomes S, Lachmann HJ, Wynne K, Rajput K, Eleftheriou D, et al. Efficacy and safety of canakinumab therapy in paediatric patients with cryopyrin-associated periodic syndrome: a single-centre, real-world experience. Rheumatology (Oxford). 2014;53(4):665–70.
76. Youngstein T, Hoffmann P, Gul A, Lane T, Williams R, Rowczenio DM, et al. International multi-centre study of pregnancy outcomes with interleukin-1 inhibitors. Rheumatology (Oxford). 2017;56(12):2102–8.
77. Toplak N, Frenkel J, Ozen S, Lachmann HJ, Woo P, Kone-Paut I, et al. An international registry on autoinflammatory diseases: the Eurofever experience. Ann Rheum Dis. 2012;71(7):1177–82.
78. Kuemmerle-Deschner JB, Hachulla E, Cartwright R, Hawkins PN, Tran TA, Bader-Meunier B, et al. Two-year results from an open-label, multicentre, phase III study evaluating the safety and efficacy of canakinumab in patients with cryopyrin-associated periodic syndrome across different severity phenotypes. Ann Rheum Dis. 2011;70(12):2095–102.
79. Levy R, Gerard L, Kuemmerle-Deschner J, Lachmann HJ, Kone-Paut I, Cantarini L, et al. Phenotypic and genotypic characteristics of cryopyrin-associated periodic syndrome: a series of 136 patients from the Eurofever registry. Ann Rheum Dis. 2015;74(11):2043–9.
80. Mamoudjy N, Maurey H, Marie I, Kone-Paut I, Deiva K. Neurological outcome of patients with cryopyrin-associated periodic syndrome (CAPS). Orphanet J Rare Dis. 2017;12(1):33.
81. Marsaud C, Marie I, Kone-Paut I. Longterm followup of quality of life in patients with cryopyrin-associated periodic syndrome treated with canakinumab, an anti-interleukin 1beta monoclonal antibody. J Rheumatol. 2014;41(8):1721–2.

Chapter 9
Familial Mediterranean Fever

Selcan Demir, İlkin Elif Günel, and Seza Özen

Familial Mediterranean fever is the most common autoinflammatory disease (AID) over the world. FMF affects primarily the ethnic groups from the eastern Mediterranean basin such as Turks, Armenians, Arabs, and non-Ashkenazi Jews [1]. FMF is associated with mutations of the *MEFV* gene on chromosome 16p, which codes for the pyrin protein [2, 3]. Mutated pyrin causes an excessive inflammatory response via uncontrolled production of interleukin (IL)-1 [4]. Although the responsible gene for FMF has been identified, the molecular and genetic studies showed that the pathogenesis, inheritance, and penetrance of FMF are more complicated. It has been 20 years since the gene associated with FMF has been defined. However, the past 20 years have taught us that the chapter is not closed and that there is still much to be investigated.

Clinically FMF is characterized by recurrent and self-limited attacks of fever and polyserositis. The most significant complication of the chronic inflammation in FMF is secondary amyloidosis.

Colchicine is still the mainstay of FMF treatment. The regular use of colchicine can reduce the severity and frequency of inflammatory attacks and suppress chronic subclinical inflammation and prevent complications [5–8]. Recent advances in molecular studies have led new therapeutic options in FMF. If colchicine fails, anti-IL-1 therapy is a promising second-line therapy.

S. Demir · S. Özen (✉)
Department of Pediatrics, Division of Rheumatology, Hacettepe University Faculty of Medicine, Ankara, Turkey
e-mail: sezaozen@hacettepe.edu.tr

İ. E. Günel
Department of Pediatrics, Hacettepe University Faculty of Medicine, Ankara, Turkey

P. Efthimiou (ed.), *Auto-Inflammatory Syndromes*,
https://doi.org/10.1007/978-3-319-96929-9_9

Genetics

The mutations in the *MEFV* gene, which are composed of 10 exons, were first described in 1997. The *MEFV* gene is located on chromosome 16 (16p 13.3) and encodes a protein consisting of 781 amino acids termed pyrin or marenostrin [2, 3, 9], which is a part of the NLRP3 inflammasome complex. Mutant pyrin causes an exaggerated inflammation with excessive production of IL-1 [4]. To date, there are about 300 known sequence variants of *MEFV*, and all reported mutations and the associated phenotypes are recorded in the INFEVERS database (http://fmf.igh.cnrs.fr/ISSAID/infevers/) [10]. However, some of them are not associated with the FMF phenotype and their significance is not clear. The most common pathogenic mutations worldwide are the p.M694V, M694I, M680I, and V726A. In 2009, Booty et al. showed that screening for the set of most common mutations appears sufficient to diagnose FMF in presence of clinical symptoms [11]. In 2012, Shinar et al. proposed recommendations for interpretation of genetic testing for FMF [12]. The consensus was set to test for 14 variants (the first 9 are defined as clearly pathogenic, and the other 5 are variants of uncertain significance): M694V, M694I, M680I, V726A, R761H, A744S, E167D, T267I, I692del, K695R, E148Q, P369S, F479L, and I591T. In 2015, the SHARE (Single Hub and Access point for pediatric Rheumatology in Europe) initiative has established evidence-based recommendations for genetic diagnosis of FMF [10]. These recommendations are presented in Table 9.1.

Table 9.1 Recommendations for familial Mediterranean fever (FMF) genetic diagnosis

Recommendation	Strength of evidence
1. FMF is a clinical diagnosis, which can be supported but not excluded by genetic testing	B
2. Consider patients homozygous for M694V at risk of developing, with very high probability, a severe phenotype	B
3. FMF patients carrying two of the common mutated alleles (homozygotes or compound heterozygotes), especially for M694V mutation or mutations at position 680–694 on exon 10, must be considered at risk of having a more severe disease	B
4. The E148Q variant is common, of unknown pathogenic significance, and as the only MEFV variant does not support the diagnosis of FMF	B
5. Patients homozygous for M694V mutation are at risk of early-onset disease	C
6. Individuals homozygous for M694V who are not reporting symptoms should be evaluated and followed closely in order to consider therapy	A
7. For individuals with two pathogenic mutations for FMF who do not report symptoms, if there are risk factors for AA amyloidosis (such as the country, family history, and persistently elevated inflammatory markers, particularly serum amyloid A protein), close follow-up should be started and treatment considered	B
8. Consultation with an autoinflammatory disease specialist may be helpful in order to aid in the indication and interpretation of the genetic testing and diagnosis	C

Adapted from Ref. [10]

The *MEFV* gene mutations in exon 10 are associated with the most severe form of disease, and genetic variants on exon 2 and on exon 3 are associated with milder form of disease. M694V is the most common mutation, which has been associated with severe disease, early onset, and a higher risk of AA amyloidosis [10, 13]. According to the SHARE recommendations, the patients carrying two mutated alleles in position 680–694 on exon 10 must be considered at risk of having more severe disease [10]. The second most frequent mutation after M694V is the E148Q on exon 2, and its pathogenic role is still controversial. E148Q is a common variant in the general population. Ben-Chetrit et al. showed a similar frequency for E148Q mutation in patients and healthy controls [14]. Tchernitchko et al. demonstrated that E148Q allele frequency was comparable among patients and asymptomatic relatives, and they concluded E148Q as a benign polymorphism [15]. However, some reports suggest that patients with homozygous E148Q might have FMF phenotype [16, 17]. In 2012, Shinar et al. has defined E148Q as a variant of unknown significance in a consensus conference [12], and according to the SHARE recommendations, this fact is also highlighted [10].

The inheritance of FMF is autosomal recessive inheritance. However, a substantial number of clinically FMF patients have only one MEVF mutation. Furthermore, 10–20% of patients who meet the diagnostic criteria for FMF have no demonstrable *MEFV* mutations [11, 13]. Because of the incomplete penetrance and the varying expression of FMF phenotype, it has been suggested that there are additional factors like modifier genes, epigenetics, or environmental factors affecting the expression of the disease. Marek et al. studied the clinical and genetic features of heterozygous FMF patients and performed haplotype studies. They showed that the heterozygous patients tend to have milder disease, but the disease could not be practically distinguished clinically from that in homozygous patients [18]. Federici et al. suggested a "dose effect" associated with the *MEFV* gene mutations. They demonstrated an increasing symptom frequency from patients carrying a single low-penetrance mutation to patients with high-penetrance mutations [19]. Lachmann et al. demonstrated that both basal and peak acute phase protein concentrations were higher in *MEFV* heterozygotes than in wild-type controls, demonstrating a "pro-inflammatory" condition among FMF carriers [20]. In addition, Kalyoncu et al. showed that acute rheumatic fever, arthralgia, and febrile episodes of more than four times per year were more frequent in asymptomatic heterozygous parents of children with FMF [21]. It has been shown that serum amyloid could increase the severity of the symptoms of FMF by activating NLRP3 inflammasome, resulting in excessive IL-1B secretion [22]. Supporting this observation, the presence of SAA1 allele was strongly associated with renal amyloidosis in FMF patients [23, 24].

The first study showing the effect of environment on FMF was in 1974. Schwabe et al. reported that the Armenian FMF patients who lived in the USA did not develop renal amyloidosis [25]. In the same line, Touitou et al. analyzed the features of 2482 FMF patients from 14 different countries, and they concluded that the country recruitment, rather than *MEFV* genotype, was the most important risk factor for renal amyloidosis in FMF [26]. Our group has shown that Turkish FMF children who live in Germany have a milder disease phenotype compared with the ones living in Turkey [16]. This observation was subsequently confirmed in the Eurofever registry [16].

Pathogenesis

The *MEFV* gene encodes pyrin, 781 amino acid protein, expressed mainly in cells polymorph nuclear neutrophils, eosinophils, and monocyte series [27]. Pyrin is essential to form inflammasomes, multiprotein complexes playing a major role in both innate and adaptive immune systems [28]. Pyrin consists of three fundamental domains: N-terminal RING domain, B-box domain, and C-terminal coiled-coil domain. It has an additional C-terminal. B30.2/rfp/PRY/SPRY domain is where most of the major disease associated mutations are clustered [29]. Pyrin interacts with the inflammasome adaptor protein (ASC) and modulates caspase-1 and IL-1 activation [30]. Mutation of pyrin causes an exaggerated inflammation via excessive IL-1 production [4]. Until recently there were conflicting results on whether the mutations on *MEFV* gene were gain-of-function mutations [11, 31] or loss-of-function [32, 33] mutations. In 2011, with the generation of knock-in mice harboring the mouse pyrin protein fused to the human B30.2 domain containing FMF-associated mutations, large amounts of IL-1β secretion have been shown in an ASC and caspase-1-dependent, NLRP3-independent manner [34]. These data [34] and several later studies [35, 36] supported that FMF-associated mutations are gain of function and pyrin itself promotes ASC oligomerization and forms a caspase-1-activating complex.

Twenty years after the identification of the gene, we recently have understood the function of pyrin. Xu et al. have also demonstrated that the modification and inactivation of Rho GTPases by different pathogenic bacteria toxins induce the activation of the pyrin inflammasome [36]. They suggested that pyrin senses a downstream event in the actin cytoskeleton pathway rather than directly recognizing Rho modification [36]. Park et al. has enlightened these mechanisms further. They demonstrated that pyrin is phosphorylated by RhoA-activated serine-threonine kinases (PKN1 and PKN2) and binds to regulatory 14-3-3 protein leading to inactivation of the pyrin inflammasome formation. In the presence of several bacterial toxins and FMF causing *MEFV* mutations, RhoA is inactivated resulting in a lowered threshold for activation of the pyrin inflammasome [37]. Gao et al. have observed that site-specific dephosphorylation and microtubule dynamics influenced activation of pyrin inflammasome. Targeting drugs, including colchicine, blocked activation of the pyrin inflammasome by inhibiting oligomerization of pyrin with ASC. It did not affect pyrin dephosphorylation and 14-3-3 dissociation [38]. Moreover, Gorp et al. have showed that pyrin inflammasome activation led by microtubules formation is not effective in FMF patients that harbor mutations in B30.2/SPRY domain [39]. Although recent studies have elucidated more about the mechanism of pyrin, there are still many questions that we need to answer about the pathogenesis of FMF.

Clinical Manifestations

Clinical episode usually starts during childhood or adolescence, 90% of them having had an onset of the disease by age 20 [1, 40, 41]. FMF attacks can last for 12–72 h. Attacks are characterized by fever and serositis along with an increase in acute phase reactants. The serositis may manifest as peritoneal, pleural, joint, or skin inflammation, sometimes in combination. Abdominal pain with fever is the most frequent presentation. Pain can be generalized or focused in a quadrant, sometimes mimicking acute appendicitis, and the range is from mild to severe [1, 41, 42]. Pleural pain is generally unilateral. Rarely, a small effusion, friction rub, or atelectasis may be present [42]. Joint manifestations, especially arthralgia which is more common than arthritis, can sometimes be the first sign of the disease in children [43]. FMF arthritis is usually monoarticular; however in children, it may have involvement of several joints symmetrically or asymmetrically, with pain and large effusions [41, 44, 45]. The aspirate will be sterile but may have leukocyte counts as high as 100,000/mm^3. Three clinical phenotypes have been suggested for FMF: type 1, which is usually associated with recurrent short episodes of inflammation and serositis; type 2, characterized by the evidence of reactive amyloid-associated (AA) amyloidosis, the most common complication of FMF, as the first clinical manifestation of the disease in an otherwise asymptomatic individual; and type 3, known as the "silent" homozygous or compound heterozygote state, in which two *MEFV* mutations are found without signs or symptoms of FMF nor of AA amyloidosis [46]. Twenty percent of patients have the so-called exertional leg pain, muscle pain in the lower extremities after physical exercise [47]. Colchicine-induced myopathy is a very rare side effect [47, 48]. The only cutaneous finding in FMF is the erysipeloid erythematous rash on the dorsum of the foot, ankle, or lower leg [41, 44, 49, 50].

Pericarditis is a rare condition [51]. In prepubescent boys, unilateral acute scrotal pain episodes may rarely occur [41, 52]. In patients with FMF, certain rheumatic diseases such as Behçet disease [53, 54], polyarteritis nodosa [53, 55], microscopic polyarteritis [56], and glomerulonephritis [57, 58] are more frequent as compared to the healthy population. The increase in these rheumatic diseases has been suggested to be due to the inflammatory milieu [21]. Neurological symptoms are rare; however headache may rarely occur in pediatric patients.

Laboratory Investigations

Acute phase reactants such as ESR, C-reactive protein, and serum amyloid A (SAA) increase during FMF attacks [44]. Elevation of acute phase serum proteins in between attacks is accepted to reflect ongoing inflammation and susceptibility to develop systemic amyloidosis, which is the most serious sequela of FMF [59–61]. Systemic amyloidosis presents with SAA deposition mainly in the kidney but also in many organs such as the gastrointestinal tract, spleen, kidneys, adrenals, thyroid, and lungs [1]. There are some predisposing risk factors for amyloidosis such as a positive family history of this complication, male sex, the α/α genotype at the SAA1 locus, and poor compliance with colchicine therapy. Many studies confirm that M694V mutation is more common in patients with amyloidosis, arthritis, and erysipeloid erythema [43, 62–65]. Microalbuminuria is an early indicator of impaired renal function. It is recommended to do periodic urinalysis which is an important part of continuing care for FMF patients. Amyloidosis can be confirmed by biopsy of the kidney or rectum, if proteinuria is detected [66].

Diagnosis

Since FMF usually requires lifelong treatment, it is crucial to establish a timely, correct diagnosis. The diagnosis of FMF relies mainly on clinical findings, and molecular analysis of the *MEFV* gene provides genetic confirmation [46]. The presence of short (12–72 h), recurrent (three or more) febrile episodes and abdominal, chest, joint, or skin manifestations with no discernible infectious cause suggest a clinical diagnosis of FMF [67, 68]. The supportive factors can be positive family history, onset before the age of 20, ethnicity, and favorable response to colchicine therapy. There are some sets of classification and diagnostic criteria for FMF. The first set of criteria was created for adults by the experts in Tel Hashomer Hospital [1]. Livneh et al. [67] revised the criteria in 1997, excluding some manifestations of the Tel Hashomer criteria especially amyloidosis. However, there were clear differences between adult and pediatric FMF cases such as the fever-only attacks in some children and inability of some pediatric patients to express the severity and exact location of the pain. Although the Tel Hashomer criteria were very successful in diagnosing the patients, the specificity was low (54.6%) in children [69] In 2009, Turkish pediatricians [69] defined criteria for children with FMF as well (Table 9.2) [68]. Among Turkish children, the criteria (two out of five criteria for diagnosis) reached a sensitivity and specificity of 88.8% and 92.2%, respectively [68]. There are more than 50 mutations described in *MEFV* [70]; however a number of sequence variants are not pathogenic. The exchange of valine or isoleucine for methionine at position 694 (M694V and M694I), the substitution of alanine for valine at position 726 (V726A) and the substitution of isoleucine for methionine at residue 680 (M680I) are the most common mutations among patients. Exon 2 of *MEFV* includes a number of missense substitutions, most of which are variants of unknown significance; the most well

Table 9.2 Turkish FMF pediatric criteria

Fever (axillary, >38 °C, ≥ 3 attacks of 6–72-h duration)
Abdominal pain (≥3 attacks of 6–72-h duration)
Chest pain (≥3 attacks of 6–72-h duration)
Arthritis (oligoarthritis, ≥3 attacks of 6–72-h duration)
Family history of FMF

Adapted from Ref. [68]
Diagnosis: 2 out of 5 criteria

known is the substitution of glutamine for glutamic acid at residue 148 (E148Q). Despite complete sequencing of the coding region of *MEFV*, it is more likely 30 % of patients with clinical signs of FMF just have one demonstrable mutation [11, 18, 71]. Recently mutations in exon 2 of *MEFV* (S242R and E244K) have been associated with neutrophilic dermatoses, inherited in a dominant fashion [72].

Treatment

An international group of experts published recommendations for the management of FMF in 2016 [73]. These recommendations are presented in Table 9.3. According to these recommendations, the main goal of treatment should be complete control of unprovoked attacks and minimizing subclinical inflammation between attacks. Colchicine has been the mainstay of FMF treatment since 1972 [74]. Colchicine can reduce the frequency and severity of attacks and suppress subclinical inflammation between attacks and improve quality of life [5–7]. Furthermore, it prevents the development of secondary amyloidosis in patients with FMF [8]. Colchicine is generally safe and well tolerated in children [75]. Colchicine is known to prevent microtubule elongation by binding to tubulin monomers and inhibit polymer formation, which is necessary for pyrin inflammasome assembly [76]. It is recommended that colchicine should be started as soon as the patient is clinically diagnosed. Physicians should follow up these asymptomatic individuals regularly [73]. If the asymptomatic patient has M694V homozygous mutations, which is more commonly associated with the secondary amyloidosis, the physician may start colchicine treatment, especially in countries where amyloidosis is frequent [12]. Colchicine treatment is generally started at the subtherapeutic dose of 0.5 mg/day (or 0.6 mg/day depending on the available drug formulation) and monitored according to disease activity and the patient's tolerance. Higher doses up to 2 mg/day can be used to control ongoing disease activity and amyloidosis [73]. The major side effects of colchicine are gastrointestinal, diarrhea, and transient elevation of transaminases.

A minority group of FMF patients do not respond to colchicine or are intolerant to the drug because of its side effects. Since the mutation in the pyrin protein has been clearly associated with increased IL-1 production, anti-IL-1 treatment has emerged as a promising second-line therapy in patients with resistant disease [30, 77]. Several studies have reported successful results in colchicine-resistant patients with IL-1-blocking agents [78–80]. IL-1 blockade can also reverse proteinuria in patients with secondary amyloidosis [77, 79, 80]. However, there is no evidence for using anti-IL-1 treatment without colchicine to prevent amyloidosis. Thus, a maximal tolerated dose of colchicine is recommended with anti-IL-1 treatment [73]. Anti-TNF treatment can be successful, especially in patients with FMF and chronic arthritis and sacroiliitis [81].

The Autoinflammatory Disease Activity Index (AIDAI), which is a patient-based symptom diary, is used to monitor disease activity in FMF and other autoinflammatory diseases. AIDAI contains 13 symptoms, and it should be scored daily by

Table 9.3 The European League Against Rheumatism recommendations for the management of FMF with grade of recommendation

Recommendation	Grade
1. Ideally, FMF should be diagnosed and initially treated by a physician with experience in FMF	D
2. The ultimate goal of treatment in FMF is to reach complete control of unprovoked attacks and minimizing subclinical inflammation in between attacks	C
3. Treatment with colchicine should start as soon as a clinical diagnosis is made	A
4. Dosing can be in single or divided doses, depending on tolerance and compliance	D
5. The persistence of attacks or of subclinical inflammation represents an indication to increase the colchicine dose	C
6. Compliant patients not responding to the maximum tolerated dose of colchicine can be considered nonrespondent or resistant; alternative biological treatments are indicated in these patients	B
7. FMF treatment needs to be intensified in AA amyloidosis using the maximal tolerated dose of colchicine and supplemented with biologics as required	C
8. Periods of physical or emotional stress can trigger FMF attacks, and it may be appropriate to increase the dose of colchicine temporarily	D
9. Response, toxicity, and compliance should be monitored every 6 months	D
10. Liver enzymes should be monitored regularly in patients with FMF treated with colchicine; if liver enzymes are elevated greater than twofold the upper limit of normal, colchicine should be reduced and the cause further investigated	D
11. In patients with decreased renal function, the risk of toxicity is very high, and therefore signs of colchicine toxicity, as well as CPK, should be carefully monitored and colchicine dose reduced accordingly	C
12. Colchicine toxicity is a serious complication and should be adequately suspected and prevented	C
13. When suspecting an attack, always consider other possible causes. During the attacks, continue the usual dose of colchicine and use NSAID	C
14. Colchicine should not be discontinued during conception, pregnancy, or lactation; current evidence does not justify amniocentesis	C
15. In general, men do not need to stop colchicine prior to conception; in the rare case of azoospermia or oligospermia proven to be related to colchicine, temporary dose reduction or discontinuation may be needed	C
16. Chronic arthritis in a patient with FMF might need additional medications, such as DMARDs, intra-articular steroid injections, or biologics	C
17. In protracted febrile myalgia, glucocorticoids lead to the resolution of symptoms; NSAID and IL-1-blockade might also be a treatment option; NSAIDs are suggested for the treatment of exertional leg pain	C
18. If a patient is stable with no attacks for more than 5 years and no elevated APR, dose reduction could be considered after expert consultation and with continued monitoring	D

Adapted from Ref. [73]

APR acute phase reactants, *CPK* creatinine phosphokinase, *DMARDs* disease-modifying antirheumatic drugs, *FMF* familial Mediterranean fever, *IL-1* interleukin-1, *NSAID* nonsteroidal anti-inflammatory drugs

Grades of recommendation: *A* high, *B* moderate, *C* low, *D* very low

Name:				**Age:**				Month:			Year:		
Symptoms associated with autoinflammatory syndrome today													
Day	Fever ≥38°C (100.4°F)	Overall Symtomps	Abdominal pain	Nausea/ vomitting	Diarrhea	Head aches	Chest pain	Painful nodes	Arthralgia or myalgia	Swelling of the joints	Eye manifestations	Skin rash	Pain relief drug taken
score	0 or 1	0 or 1	0 or 1	0 or 1	0 or 1	0 or 1	0 or 1	0 or 1	0 or 1	0 or 1	0 or 1	0 or 1	
1													
2													
3													
…													
31													

Fig. 9.1 Autoinflammatory Diseases Activity Index diary. Notes: each line refers to a day in a month (Adapted from Ref. [82])

patients or by parents as yes or no (Fig. 9.1). AIDAI score is very easy to use, and it provides to assess disease activity and response to therapy [82].

The research in the past 20 years has taught us a lot about the clinical and pathogenic characteristics of FMF. However much remains to be investigated. Why do some patients have more severe disease? Why do some heterozygotes display the phenotype? What is the phenotype-genotype correlation in regard to the many variants that have been identified? Are all pyrin mutations associated with a FMF phenotype? What is the effect of environment? These are questions that will keep us working on the field in the years to come.

References

1. Sohar E, Gafni J, Pras M, Heller H. Familial Mediterranean fever. A survey of 470 cases and review of the literature. Am J Med. 1967;43(2):227–53.
2. The International FMF Consortium. Ancient missense mutations in a new member of the RoRet gene family are likely to cause familial Mediterranean fever. Cell. 1997;90(4):797–807.
3. French FMFC. A candidate gene for familial Mediterranean fever. Nat Genet. 1997;17(1):25–31.
4. Berkun Y, Ben-Chetrit E. Pyrin and cryopyrin--similar domain sequence but opposite inflammatory consequence. Clin Exp Rheumatol. 2007;25(4 Suppl 45):S6–8.
5. Livneh A, Langevitz P. Diagnostic and treatment concerns in familial Mediterranean fever. Baillieres Best Pract Res Clin Rheumatol. 2000;14(3):477–98.
6. Majeed HA, Rawashdeh M, el-Shanti H, Qubain H, Khuri-Bulos N, Shahin HM. Familial Mediterranean fever in children: the expanded clinical profile. QJM. 1999;92(6):309–18.
7. Zemer D, Livneh A, Danon YL, Pras M, Sohar E. Long-term colchicine treatment in children with familial Mediterranean fever. Arthritis Rheum. 1991;34(8):973–7.
8. Zemer D, Pras M, Sohar E, Modan M, Cabili S, Gafni J. Colchicine in the prevention and treatment of the amyloidosis of familial Mediterranean fever. N Engl J Med. 1986;314(16):1001–5.
9. Stoffels M, Szperl A, Simon A, Netea MG, Plantinga TS, van Deuren M, et al. MEFV mutations affecting pyrin amino acid 577 cause autosomal dominant autoinflammatory disease. Ann Rheum Dis. 2014;73(2):455–61.
10. Giancane G, Ter Haar NM, Wulffraat N, Vastert SJ, Barron K, Hentgen V, et al. Evidence-based recommendations for genetic diagnosis of familial Mediterranean fever. Ann Rheum Dis. 2015;74(4):635–41.

11. Booty MG, Chae JJ, Masters SL, Remmers EF, Barham B, Le JM, et al. Familial Mediterranean fever with a single MEFV mutation: where is the second hit? Arthritis Rheum. 2009;60(6):1851–61.
12. Shinar Y, Obici L, Aksentijevich I, Bennetts B, Austrup F, Ceccherini I, et al. Guidelines for the genetic diagnosis of hereditary recurrent fevers. Ann Rheum Dis. 2012;71(10):1599–605.
13. Touitou I. The spectrum of Familial Mediterranean Fever (FMF) mutations. Eur J Hum Genet. 2001;9(7):473–83.
14. Ben-Chetrit E, Lerer I, Malamud E, Domingo C, Abeliovich D. The E148Q mutation in the MEFV gene: is it a disease-causing mutation or a sequence variant? Hum Mutat. 2000;15(4):385–6.
15. Tchernitchko D, Legendre M, Cazeneuve C, Delahaye A, Niel F, Amselem S. The E148Q MEFV allele is not implicated in the development of familial Mediterranean fever. Hum Mutat. 2003;22(4):339–40.
16. Ozen S, Demirkaya E, Amaryan G, Kone-Paut I, Polat A, Woo P, et al. Results from a multicentre international registry of familial Mediterranean fever: impact of environment on the expression of a monogenic disease in children. Ann Rheum Dis. 2014;73(4):662–7.
17. Yilmaz E, Ozen S, Balci B, Duzova A, Topaloglu R, Besbas N, et al. Mutation frequency of Familial Mediterranean Fever and evidence for a high carrier rate in the Turkish population. Eur J Hum Genet. 2001;9(7):553–5.
18. Marek-Yagel D, Berkun Y, Padeh S, Abu A, Reznik-Wolf H, Livneh A, et al. Clinical disease among patients heterozygous for familial Mediterranean fever. Arthritis Rheum. 2009;60(6):1862–6.
19. Federici S, Calcagno G, Finetti M, Gallizzi R, Meini A, Vitale A, et al. Clinical impact of MEFV mutations in children with periodic fever in a prevalent western European Caucasian population. Ann Rheum Dis. 2012;71(12):1961–5.
20. Lachmann HJ, Sengul B, Yavuzsen TU, Booth DR, Booth SE, Bybee A, et al. Clinical and subclinical inflammation in patients with familial Mediterranean fever and in heterozygous carriers of MEFV mutations. Rheumatology (Oxford). 2006;45(6):746–50.
21. Kalyoncu M, Acar BC, Cakar N, Bakkaloglu A, Ozturk S, Dereli E, et al. Are carriers for MEFV mutations "healthy"? Clin Exp Rheumatol. 2006;24(5 Suppl 42):S120–2.
22. Niemi K, Teirila L, Lappalainen J, Rajamaki K, Baumann MH, Oorni K, et al. Serum amyloid A activates the NLRP3 inflammasome via P2X7 receptor and a cathepsin B-sensitive pathway. J Immunol. 2011;186(11):6119–28.
23. Atoyan S, Hayrapetyan H, Sarkisian T, Ben-Chetrit E. MEFV and SAA1 genotype associations with clinical features of familial Mediterranean fever and amyloidosis in Armenia. Clin Exp Rheumatol. 2016;34(6 Suppl 102):72–6.
24. Cazeneuve C, Ajrapetyan H, Papin S, Roudot-Thoraval F, Genevieve D, Mndjoyan E, et al. Identification of MEFV-independent modifying genetic factors for familial Mediterranean fever. Am J Hum Genet. 2000;67(5):1136–43.
25. Schwabe AD, Peters RS. Familial Mediterranean Fever in Armenians. Analysis of 100 cases. Medicine (Baltimore). 1974;53(6):453–62.
26. Touitou I, Sarkisian T, Medlej-Hashim M, Tunca M, Livneh A, Cattan D, et al. Country as the primary risk factor for renal amyloidosis in familial Mediterranean fever. Arthritis Rheum. 2007;56(5):1706–12.
27. Centola M, Wood G, Frucht DM, Galon J, Aringer M, Farrell C, et al. The gene for familial Mediterranean fever, MEFV, is expressed in early leukocyte development and is regulated in response to inflammatory mediators. Blood. 2000;95(10):3223–31.
28. de Torre-Minguela C, Mesa Del Castillo P, Pelegrin P. The NLRP3 and pyrin inflammasomes: implications in the pathophysiology of autoinflammatory diseases. Front Immunol. 2017;8:43.
29. Weinert C, Morger D, Djekic A, Grutter MG, Mittl PR. Crystal structure of TRIM20 C-terminal coiled-coil/B30.2 fragment: implications for the recognition of higher order oligomers. Sci Rep. 2015;5:10819.
30. Park H, Bourla AB, Kastner DL, Colbert RA, Siegel RM. Lighting the fires within: the cell biology of autoinflammatory diseases. Nat Rev Immunol. 2012;12(8):570–80.

31. Yu JW, Fernandes-Alnemri T, Datta P, Wu J, Juliana C, Solorzano L, et al. Pyrin activates the ASC pyroptosome in response to engagement by autoinflammatory PSTPIP1 mutants. Mol Cell. 2007;28(2):214–27.
32. Papin S, Cuenin S, Agostini L, Martinon F, Werner S, Beer HD, et al. The SPRY domain of Pyrin, mutated in familial Mediterranean fever patients, interacts with inflammasome components and inhibits proIL-1beta processing. Cell Death Differ. 2007;14(8):1457–66.
33. Hesker PR, Nguyen M, Kovarova M, Ting JP, Koller BH. Genetic loss of murine pyrin, the Familial Mediterranean Fever protein, increases interleukin-1beta levels. PLoS One. 2012;7(11):e51105.
34. Chae JJ, Cho YH, Lee GS, Cheng J, Liu PP, Feigenbaum L, et al. Gain-of-function Pyrin mutations induce NLRP3 protein-independent interleukin-1beta activation and severe autoinflammation in mice. Immunity. 2011;34(5):755–68.
35. Gavrilin MA, Abdelaziz DH, Mostafa M, Abdulrahman BA, Grandhi J, Akhter A, et al. Activation of the pyrin inflammasome by intracellular Burkholderia cenocepacia. J Immunol. 2012;188(7):3469–77.
36. Xu H, Yang J, Gao W, Li L, Li P, Zhang L, et al. Innate immune sensing of bacterial modifications of Rho GTPases by the Pyrin inflammasome. Nature. 2014;513(7517):237–41.
37. Park YH, Wood G, Kastner DL, Chae JJ. Pyrin inflammasome activation and RhoA signaling in the autoinflammatory diseases FMF and HIDS. Nat Immunol. 2016;17(8):914–21.
38. Gao W, Yang J, Liu W, Wang Y, Shao F. Site-specific phosphorylation and microtubule dynamics control Pyrin inflammasome activation. Proc Natl Acad Sci U S A. 2016;113(33):E4857–66.
39. Van Gorp H, Saavedra PH, de Vasconcelos NM, Van Opdenbosch N, Vande Walle L, Matusiak M, et al. Familial Mediterranean fever mutations lift the obligatory requirement for microtubules in Pyrin inflammasome activation. Proc Natl Acad Sci U S A. 2016;113(50):14384–9.
40. Ben-Chetrit E, Levy M. Familial Mediterranean fever. Lancet. 1998;351(9103):659–64.
41. Gedalia A, Adar A, Gorodischer R. Familial Mediterranean fever in children. J Rheumatol Suppl. 1992;35:1–9.
42. Brauman A, Gilboa Y. Recurrent pulmonary atelectasis as a manifestation of familial Mediterranean fever. Arch Intern Med. 1987;147(2):378–9.
43. Brik R, Shinawi M, Kasinetz L, Gershoni-Baruch R. The musculoskeletal manifestations of familial Mediterranean fever in children genetically diagnosed with the disease. Arthritis Rheum. 2001;44(6):1416–9.
44. Samuels J, Aksentijevich I, Torosyan Y, Centola M, Deng Z, Sood R, et al. Familial Mediterranean fever at the millennium. Clinical spectrum, ancient mutations, and a survey of 100 American referrals to the National Institutes of Health. Medicine. 1998;77(4):268–97.
45. Ince E, Cakar N, Tekin M, Kendirli T, Ozkaya N, Akar N, et al. Arthritis in children with familial Mediterranean fever. Rheumatol Int. 2002;21(6):213–7.
46. Soriano A, Manna R. Familial Mediterranean fever: new phenotypes. Autoimmun Rev. 2012;12(1):31–7.
47. Langevitz P, Zemer D, Livneh A, Shemer J, Pras M. Protracted febrile myalgia in patients with familial Mediterranean fever. J Rheumatol. 1994;21(9):1708–9.
48. Majeed HA, Al-Qudah AK, Qubain H, Shahin HM. The clinical patterns of myalgia in children with familial Mediterranean fever. Semin Arthritis Rheum. 2000;30(2):138–43.
49. Azizi E, Fisher BK. Cutaneous manifestations of familial Mediterranean fever. Arch Dermatol. 1976;112(3):364–6.
50. Barzilai A, Langevitz P, Goldberg I, Kopolovic J, Livneh A, Pras M, et al. Erysipelas-like erythema of familial Mediterranean fever: clinicopathologic correlation. J Am Acad Dermatol. 2000;42(5 Pt 1):791–5.
51. Kees S, Langevitz P, Zemer D, Padeh S, Pras M, Livneh A. Attacks of pericarditis as a manifestation of familial Mediterranean fever (FMF). QJM. 1997;90(10):643–7.
52. Eshel G, Vinograd I, Barr J, Zemer D. Acute scrotal pain complicating familial Mediterranean fever in children. Br J Surg. 1994;81(6):894–6.
53. Ben-Chetrit E, Cohen R, Chajek-Shaul T. Familial mediterranean fever and Behcet's disease--are they associated? J Rheumatol. 2002;29(3):530–4.

54. Schwartz T, Langevitz P, Zemer D, Gazit E, Pras M, Livneh A. Behcet's disease in Familial Mediterranean fever: characterization of the association between the two diseases. Semin Arthritis Rheum. 2000;29(5):286–95.
55. Ozdogan H, Arisoy N, Kasapcapur O, Sever L, Caliskan S, Tuzuner N, et al. Vasculitis in familial Mediterranean fever. J Rheumatol. 1997;24(2):323–7.
56. Ozen S, Ben-Chetrit E, Bakkaloglu A, Gur H, Tinaztepe K, Calguneri M, et al. Polyarteritis nodosa in patients with Familial Mediterranean Fever (FMF): a concomitant disease or a feature of FMF? Semin Arthritis Rheum. 2001;30(4):281–7.
57. Akpolat T, Akpolat I, Karagoz F, Yilmaz E, Kandemir B, Ozen S. Familial Mediterranean fever and glomerulonephritis and review of the literature. Rheumatol Int. 2004;24(1):43–5.
58. Said R, Hamzeh Y, Said S, Tarawneh M, al-Khateeb M. Spectrum of renal involvement in familial Mediterranean fever. Kidney Int. 1992;41(2):414–9.
59. Duzova A, Bakkaloglu A, Besbas N, Topaloglu R, Ozen S, Ozaltin F, et al. Role of A-SAA in monitoring subclinical inflammation and in colchicine dosage in familial Mediterranean fever. Clin Exp Rheumatol. 2003;21(4):509–14.
60. Korkmaz C, Ozdogan H, Kasapcopur O, Yazici H. Acute phase response in familial Mediterranean fever. Ann Rheum Dis. 2002;61(1):79–81.
61. Tunca M, Kirkali G, Soyturk M, Akar S, Pepys MB, Hawkins PN. Acute phase response and evolution of familial Mediterranean fever. Lancet. 1999;353(9162):1415.
62. Cazeneuve C, Sarkisian T, Pecheux C, Dervichian M, Nedelec B, Reinert P, et al. MEFV-gene analysis in armenian patients with Familial Mediterranean fever: diagnostic value and unfavorable renal prognosis of the M694V homozygous genotype-genetic and therapeutic implications. Am J Hum Genet. 1999;65(1):88–97.
63. Gershoni-Baruch R, Brik R, Zacks N, Shinawi M, Lidar M, Livneh A. The contribution of genotypes at the MEFV and SAA1 loci to amyloidosis and disease severity in patients with familial Mediterranean fever. Arthritis Rheum. 2003;48(4):1149–55.
64. Kone Paut I, Dubuc M, Sportouch J, Minodier P, Garnier JM, Touitou I. Phenotype-genotype correlation in 91 patients with familial Mediterranean fever reveals a high frequency of cutaneomucous features. Rheumatology. 2000;39(11):1275–9.
65. Shinar Y, Livneh A, Langevitz P, Zaks N, Aksentijevich I, Koziol DE, et al. Genotype-phenotype assessment of common genotypes among patients with familial Mediterranean fever. J Rheumatol. 2000;27(7):1703–7.
66. Blum A, Sohar E. The diagnosis of amyloidosis. Ancillary procedures. Lancet. 1962;1(7232):721–4.
67. Livneh A, Langevitz P, Zemer D, Zaks N, Kees S, Lidar T, et al. Criteria for the diagnosis of familial Mediterranean fever. Arthritis Rheum. 1997;40(10):1879–85.
68. Yalcinkaya F, Ozen S, Ozcakar ZB, Aktay N, Cakar N, Duzova A, et al. A new set of criteria for the diagnosis of familial Mediterranean fever in childhood. Rheumatology. 2009;48(4):395–8.
69. Sonmez HE, Batu ED, Ozen S. Familial Mediterranean fever: current perspectives. J Inflamm Res. 2016;9:13–20.
70. Touitou I, Lesage S, McDermott M, Cuisset L, Hoffman H, Dode C, et al. Infevers: an evolving mutation database for auto-inflammatory syndromes. Hum Mutat. 2004;24(3):194–8.
71. Ozen S. Changing concepts in familial Mediterranean fever: is it possible to have an autosomal-recessive disease with only one mutation? Arthritis Rheum. 2009;60(6):1575–7.
72. Moghaddas F, Llamas R, De Nardo D, Martinez-Banaclocha H, Martinez-Garcia JJ, Mesa-Del-Castillo P, et al. A novel Pyrin-Associated Autoinflammation with Neutrophilic Dermatosis mutation further defines 14-3-3 binding of pyrin and distinction to Familial Mediterranean Fever. Ann Rheum Dis. 2017;76:2085.
73. Ozen S, Demirkaya E, Erer B, Livneh A, Ben-Chetrit E, Giancane G, et al. EULAR recommendations for the management of familial Mediterranean fever. Ann Rheum Dis. 2016;75(4):644–51.
74. Goldfinger SE. Colchicine for familial Mediterranean fever. N Engl J Med. 1972;287(25):1302.
75. Padeh S, Gerstein M, Berkun Y. Colchicine is a safe drug in children with familial Mediterranean fever. J Pediatr. 2012;161(6):1142–6.

76. Ravelli RB, Gigant B, Curmi PA, Jourdain I, Lachkar S, Sobel A, et al. Insight into tubulin regulation from a complex with colchicine and a stathmin-like domain. Nature. 2004;428(6979):198–202.
77. Ozen S, Bilginer Y, Aktay Ayaz N, Calguneri M. Anti-interleukin 1 treatment for patients with familial Mediterranean fever resistant to colchicine. J Rheumatol. 2011;38(3):516–8.
78. Grattagliano I, Bonfrate L, Ruggiero V, Scaccianoce G, Palasciano G, Portincasa P. Novel therapeutics for the treatment of familial Mediterranean fever: from colchicine to biologics. Clin Pharmacol Ther. 2014;95(1):89–97.
79. van der Hilst J, Moutschen M, Messiaen PE, Lauwerys BR, Vanderschueren S. Efficacy of anti-IL-1 treatment in familial Mediterranean fever: a systematic review of the literature. Biologics. 2016;10:75–80.
80. Hashkes PJ, Spalding SJ, Giannini EH, Huang B, Johnson A, Park G, et al. Rilonacept for colchicine-resistant or -intolerant familial Mediterranean fever: a randomized trial. Ann Intern Med. 2012;157(8):533–41.
81. Bilgen SA, Kilic L, Akdogan A, Kiraz S, Kalyoncu U, Karadag O, et al. Effects of anti-tumor necrosis factor agents for familial mediterranean fever patients with chronic arthritis and/or sacroiliitis who were resistant to colchicine treatment. J Clin Rheumatol. 2011;17(7):358–62.
82. Piram M, Kone-Paut I, Lachmann HJ, Frenkel J, Ozen S, Kuemmerle-Deschner J, et al. Validation of the auto-inflammatory diseases activity index (AIDAI) for hereditary recurrent fever syndromes. Ann Rheum Dis. 2014;73(12):2168–73.

Chapter 10
Type I Interferonopathies: From Pathophysiology to Clinical Expression

Christina Maria Flessa, Evangelia Argiriou, and Clio P. Mavragani

Introduction

Type I interferonopathies are a heterogeneous group of autoinflammatory and autoimmune diseases characterized by distinct genetic and phenotypic features and hallmarked by activation of type I interferon (IFN) pathway [1]. IFNs have been first described in 1957 by Isaacs and Lindenmann as soluble factors that "interfere" with viral replication in host cells [2, 3]. IFNs are classified into three subgroups, known as types I, II, and III, based on their structure, chromosomal location, and receptor specificity. In particular, type I interferons consist of 13 functional α-genes and single genes for interferon-β, interferon-ε, interferon-κ, and interferon-ω [4].

In 1979, it has been first reported that circulating IFN levels are increased in patients with several autoimmune diseases including systemic lupus erythematosus (SLE), Sjogren's syndrome and systemic sclerosis [5], a finding extensively replicated during the last decades [6–9]. An interesting early observation reported by Gresser et al. on experimental models implied a putatively harmful role of type I IFNs in developing embryos, which resulted in growth retardation, several organ damage, and necrosis [10]. Subsequently, it has been recognized a subset of patients presenting with progressive neurological problems resembling transplacental infections in the absence of an infectious agent. These abnormalities were transmitted following an autosomal recessive Mendelian pattern [11]. Of interest, serum and cerebrospinal fluid (CSF) of these patients suffering from the so-called Aicardi-Goutieres syndrome (AGS) demonstrated increased IFNα activity [12]. In 2003, the shared phenotypes between AGS, SLE and the utero-human immunodeficiency virus (HIV) infection, led Crow and colleagues to support type I IFN upregulation

Authors Christina Maria Flessa and Evangelia Argiriou are equally contributed to this work.

C. M. Flessa · E. Argiriou · C. P. Mavragani (✉)
Department of Physiology, School of Medicine, National and Kapodistrian University of Athens, Athens, Greece

P. Efthimiou (ed.), *Auto-Inflammatory Syndromes*,
https://doi.org/10.1007/978-3-319-96929-9_10

as a common denominator in these distinct clinical entities [13]. However, whether deregulation of type I IFN system is directly related to clinical manifestations remains to be further explored. Nevertheless, experimental and clinical evidence supports neurotoxic effects of IFNs in mice models and associations with thrombotic microangiopathy [14–16].

Over the past decade, it has been increasingly appreciated that certain clinical entities occurring early in life were characterized by a constellation of clinical features including chilblain-like skin lesions, lung inflammation, and intracranial calcifications together with overexpression of IFN-related genes. The latter has been shown to occur as a result of genetic aberrations of key molecules of the type I IFN pathway. Despite the fact that type I IFN activation is a common denominator in these disorders – the so-called interferonopathies – several differences in both clinical expression and underlying genetic background have been recognized. It seems that the observed variability relates to the presence of multiple biological effects of the type I IFN pathway molecules, the timing of IFN-related effects, as well as the impact of environmental stressors, such as cold or infections [1].

As mentioned above, interferonopathies are characterized by a mixture of autoinflammatory and autoimmune characteristics. Upregulation of type I IFNs results not only in the mobilization of innate immunity mechanisms, but also in chemokine expression and loss of self-tolerance, which ultimately leads to activation of autoreactive B and T cells and autoantibody production. Thus according to Crow and colleagues, type I interferonopathies can be considered "as autoinflammatory in origin with spill over into autoimmunity" [1], especially when there is a phenotypic overlap to SLE.

Nowadays, the current understanding of the mechanism contributing to the activation of innate immunity system against viral invasion, along with the identification of specific genetic aberrations leading to type I IFN activation, highlights the pivotal contribution of nucleic acid metabolism and signaling to type I IFN overexpression.

Type I IFN Pathway Signaling

Type I IFNs activate intracellular antimicrobial programs and influence the development of both innate and adaptive immune responses [17]. They are polypeptides that are secreted by infected cells, and their role can be summarized in three basic functions:

1. Limitation of the spread of microbial insults and especially viral pathogens by inducing an "antiviral state" in infected and neighboring cells.
2. Modulation of innate immune responses such as enhancement of antigen presentation and natural killer cell function together with restraining pro-inflammatory pathways.
3. Activation of the adaptive immune system, thus promoting the development of high-affinity antigen-specific T- and B-cell responses and immunological memory [17].

Canonical type I IFN signaling activates the Janus kinase (JAK)-signal transducer and activator of transcription (STAT) pathway, leading to transcription of IFN-stimulated genes (ISGs) [17]. More specifically, IFN acts as a ligand and binds a heterodimeric transmembrane protein receptor called IFNα/β receptor (IFNAR) which is composed of IFNAR1 and IFNAR2 subunits [17]. Recent data indicate that the signal can be transmitted through IFNAR1 alone, through specific binding of IFNβ to IFNAR1, which is independent of IFNAR2 [18]. In the canonical type I IFN pathway, IFN binding to its receptor activates the receptor-associated protein tyrosine kinases JAK1 and tyrosine kinase 2 (TYK2), which in turn phosphorylate the cytoplasmic transcription factors signal transducer and activator of transcription 1 (STAT1) and STAT2. The latter subsequently dimerize and translocate to the nucleus, where they associate with IFN-regulatory factor 9 (IRF9). As a result, they form a complex called IFN-stimulated gene factor 3 (ISGF3), which binds to its cognate DNA sequences, the IFN-stimulated response elements (ISREs), part of the IFN-stimulated genes (ISGs), and directs transcription of ISGs [19–22] (Fig. 10.1).

Recent evidence point toward the presence of a STAT2-/IRF9-dependent IFNα but STAT1-independent signaling pathway [23]. In this case, STAT2 is capable of forming stable homodimers, when phosphorylated in response to IFNα, and these homodimers interact with IRF9 and can activate transcription of ISGs that carry ISRE sequences [23, 24]. Beyond the canonical pathway, IFN stimulates other pathways as well, such as STAT3 (especially in the absence of STAT1), p38 and ERK, PI-3K cascades, as well as the mTOR-Akt-S6K axis [19, 25].

Activation of Type I IFN Pathway: Role of Toll-Like Receptors (TLRs) and Cytosolic Nucleic Acid Sensors

Activation of type I IFN system has been shown to occur either by sensing of exogenous or endogenous nucleic acids that can be recognized by two distinct categories of sensors: a. endosomal Toll-like receptors (TLRs) and b. cytosolic nucleic acid sensors. It is important that the immune system can distinguish between exogenous and self-nucleic acids in order to avoid unnecessary reactions against self.

Toll-Like Receptors (TLRs)

The main TLRs identifying nucleic acids include TLR3 which recognizes dsRNA, TLR7, and TLR8 triggered by ssRNA and TLR9 that senses unmethylated CpG DNA sequences. It is of note that mutations of these molecules have not been so far associated with type I interferonopathies [26–28].

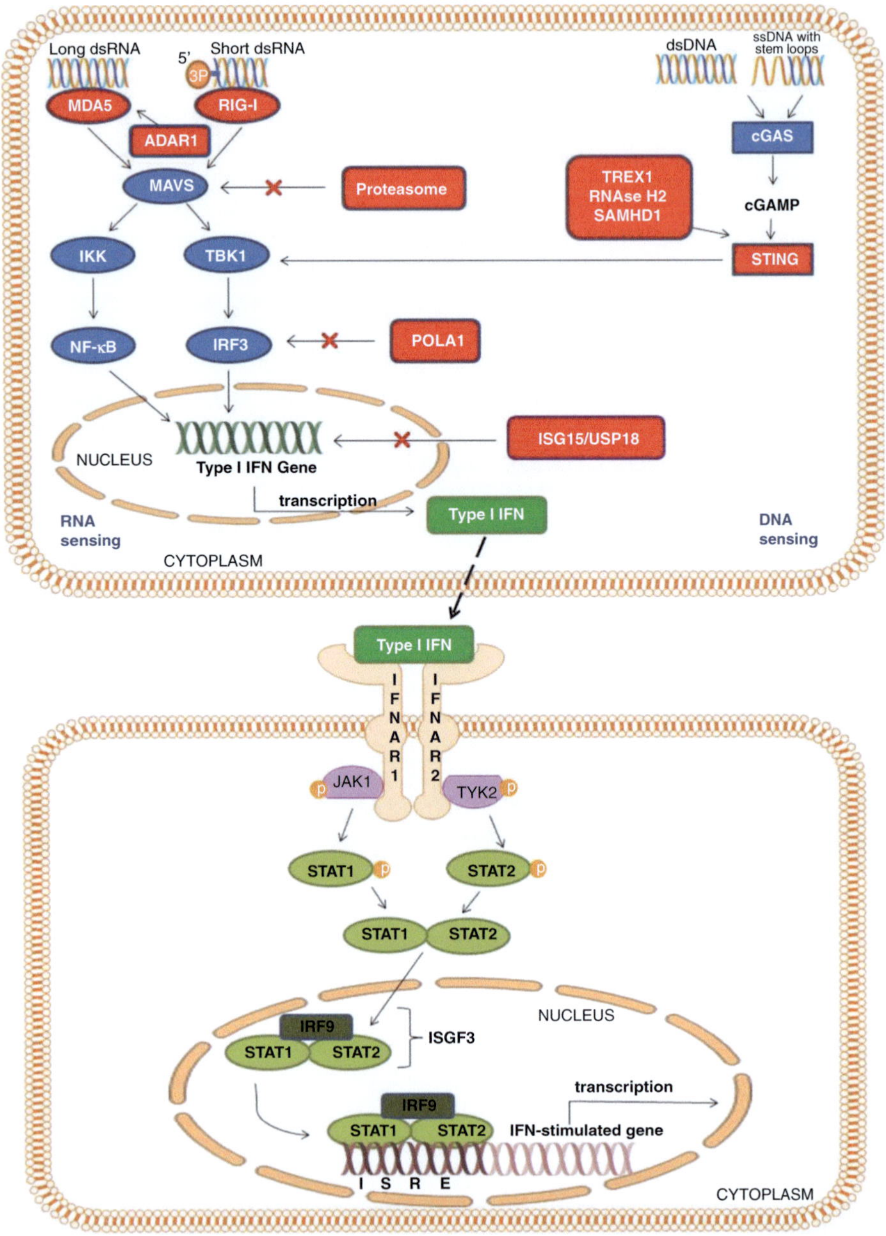

Fig. 10.1 Cytosolic nucleic acid sensing machinery resulting in type I IFN production (upper panel). Molecules implicated in the pathogenesis of type I interferonopathies are depicted in red. Lower panel: type I IFN signaling pathway following ligation of the type I IFN receptor leading to transcription of IFN-stimulated genes through the JAK/STAT pathway. *ADAR1* adenosine deaminase acting on RNA 1; *cGAMP* cyclic GMP-AMP; *cGAS* cyclic GMP-AMP synthase; *IFN* interferon; *IFNAR* IFNα receptor; *IKK* IκB kinase; *IRF3* IFN-regulatory factor 3; *IRF9* IFN-regulatory

(continued)

RNA Sensors

Three Toll-like receptors function in the endosomes to recognize pathogen-derived RNA: TLR3, TLR7, and TLR8 [29, 30]. TLR3 activates TIR-domain-containing adapter-inducing IFNβ (TRIF), whereas TLR7 and TLR8 activate MyD88. Both adaptor proteins lead to the activation of nuclear factor kappa-light-chain-enhancer of activated B cells (NF-κB), whereas IFN-regulatory factor 3 (IRF3) is activated by the TRIF pathway and IRF7 by the MyD88 pathway [31].

DNA Sensors

CpG DNA was initially found to be able to induce type I IFNs through TLR9 ligation in plasmacytoid dendritic cells (pDCs) [30]. TLR9 activates MyD88, which in turn leads to the activation of NF-κB and IRF7 in pDCs [31]. Nevertheless, cytoplasmic DNA of many other cell types that do not express TLR9 can also robustly produce type I IFNs [30] and will be discussed below.

Cytosolic Sensors

RNA Sensors

Cytosolic viral RNA is identified by retinoic acid-inducible gene I (RIG-I) and its homolog melanoma differentiation-associated gene 5 (MDA5) [30]. RIG-I is the founding member of the RIG-I-like receptor (RLR) family of cytosolic RNA sensors. The other two members are MDA5 and laboratory of genetics and physiology 2 (LGP2) [32]. Downstream of RIG-1, the adaptor protein mitochondrial antiviral signaling (MAVS) induces the cytosolic kinases IκB kinase (IKK) and TANK-binding kinase 1 (TBK1) which, in turn, activate the NF-κB, IRF3, and IRF7 pathways to induce type I IFNs [33]. Before the discovery of RLRs, two other proteins were implicated in the recognition of viral RNA: a. the IFN-inducible 2′–5′-oligoadenylate synthetase (OAS), an activator of the ribonuclease RNAse L [34] which degrades viral RNA inducing type I IFN production through the RIG-I pathway [30]

factor 9; *ISG* IFN-stimulated gene; *ISG15* interferon-stimulated gene 15; *ISGF3* IFN-stimulated gene factor 3; *ISRE* IFN-stimulated response element; *JAK* Janus kinase; *MAVS* mitochondrial antiviral signaling; *MDA5* melanoma differentiation-associated gene 5; *NF-κB* nuclear factor kappa-light-chain-enhancer of activated B cells; *POLA1* polymerase-α1; *RIG-I* retinoic acid-inducible gene I; *RNAse H2, RNase H2A, RNase H2B, and RNase H2C* ribonuclease H2 subunits A, B, and C; *SAMHD1* deoxynucleoside triphosphate triphosphohydrolase and ribonuclease SAM domain and HD domain 1;*STAT* signal transducer and activator of transcription; *STING* stimulator of IFN genes; *TBK1* TANK-binding kinase 1; *TREX1* three prime (3′) repair exonuclease 1; *TYK2* tyrosine kinase 2; *USP18* ubiquitin-specific peptidase 18 and b. the dsRNA-dependent protein kinase R (PKR) which suppresses translation initiation and also induces type I IFN production as a response to dsRNA in some cell types [35].

DNA Sensors

The mechanisms through which the immune system *senses DNA* were not elucidated until recent years. The activated pathway in this case is the RNA polymerase III/RIG-I pathway. More specifically, double-stranded poly(dA-dT) DNA is converted by the DNA-dependent enzyme RNA polymerase III (Pol III) to an RNA species in the cytosol that bears 5′-triphosphate and forms a double-stranded RNA [36]. This form of RNA acts as a ligand for RIG-I which triggers type I IFN production through MAVS [30, 36]. The strict dependence of Pol III on AT-rich sequence as well as the DNA-induced IFN production in a sequence-independent manner pointed toward the presence of another more general cytoplasmic DNA-sensing pathway [30]. In 2008, a molecule was identified as a crucial signaling adaptor for type I IFN induction and was named stimulator of IFN genes (STING) [37]. STING [also known as transmembrane protein 173 (TMEM173)] is a predominantly endoplasmic reticulum-localized protein which when stimulated with dsDNA relocalizes to Golgi apparatus and assembles into punctate structures that contain the kinase TBK1 [38]. Subsequently, the C-terminal tail (CTT) of the carboxy-terminal domain of STING provides a scaffold to bring IRF3 in close proximity to TBK1, leading to TBK1-dependent phosphorylation and activation of IRF3, which can subsequently induce the expression of type I IFN genes [28, 38]. Upstream activators of STING include pathogen-derived nucleotides [cyclic (3′–5′) diguanylate (c-di-GMP) and cyclic (3′–5′) diadenylate (c-di-AMP)] [39, 40] as well as second messengers (cyclic GMP-AMP or cGAMP) produced by the enzyme cyclic GMP-AMP synthase (cGAS) through an enzymatic degradation of cytosolic DNA [30, 41–43]. Additionally, genetic variants of DNAse II – an endonuclease located in lysosomes and expressed in a variety of cells – and three prime (3′) repair exonuclease 1 (TREX1), the most abundant 3′➔5′ DNA exonuclease in cells, have been both shown to promote autoimmune responses by inability of degrading cytoplasmic DNA [30, 44, 45]. TREX1 specifically targets and digests DNA reverse-transcribed from endogenous retroelements or replication debris [30, 44]. If not degraded, these endogenous DNA substrates further activate the STING-dependent cytosolic DNA-sensing pathway, triggering type I IFN-dependent autoimmune diseases [30].

Finally, the presence of DNA in the cytosol of macrophages can activate the inflammasome, a multiprotein complex that activates the proteolytic enzyme caspase-1 and leads to the maturation of IL-1β [30]. The receptor for cytosolic DNA in the inflammasome pathway is the protein absent in melanoma 2 (AIM2) [46].

Type I Interferonopathies: Genetic Defects and Clinical Phenotypes

A growing body of evidence points toward an activated type I IFN pathway in several autoimmune diseases, possibly as a result of inappropriate immune reactions against endogenous nucleic acids. Overproduction of type I IFN can be attributed to three main events [47] including (a) increased availability of endogenous nucleic acids as a result of defective clearance or impaired silencing mechanisms, (b) enhanced activation or sensitivity of an innate immune sensor or adaptive molecule, and (c) dysregulation of type I IFN response negative feedback loops. Inappropriate expression of endogenous nucleic acids as a result of defective epigenetic silencing such as methylation has been shown to be able to induce type I IFNs in both SLE and Sjogren's syndrome [48, 49] through TLR-dependent and TLR-independent pathways. More specifically, it has been suggested that L1 RNA can transduce the signal through both endosomal TLRs and the RIG-I and MDA5 pathways [49].

Next, we wished to present genetic, clinical, and laboratory characteristics of the main type I interferonopathies. Mutations in genes mainly affecting the recognition of DNA and RNA by cytosolic sensors as well as deregulation of type I IFN production seem to be causally linked with the so far recognized type I interferonopathies (Table 10.1, Figs. 10.1 and 10.2).

Phenotypes Related to Aberrant Nucleic Acid Sensing

DNA Sensors

STING-Associated Vasculopathy, Infantile Onset (SAVI)

STING-associated vasculopathy with onset in infancy (SAVI) is a monogenic autoinflammatory disorder with an autosomal dominant type of inheritance, due to de novo, heterozygous gain-of-function mutations in *TMEM173* gene. Of note, newly recognized mutations in exons 6 and 7 of *TMEM173* have recently been reported [50]. As a result, activation of type I IFN pathway occurs, through cGAS-STING-TBK1-IRF3 pathway. In a recent experimental model, it was shown that upregulation of IFN-related genes in the context of SAVI occurs independently of IRF3 stimulation [51].

Similarly to other interferonopathies such as AGS, TREX1-related familial chilblain lupus, and CANDLE syndrome, the main clinical manifestations – which occur in early childhood – include vasculitic skin manifestations. These are mainly manifested as ulcerating acral skin lesions in fingers, toes, ears, and nose following cold exposure. SAVI patients frequently present with pulmonary involvement as

Table 10.1 Classification of type I interferonopathies according to the underlying genetic abnormality and pathophysiology

Responsible gene/protein	Protein function	Phenotypes	Pathway activation	Type of inheritance
Nucleic acid sensors				
DNA				
TREX1 (TREX1)	Cytosolic DNAse	AGS, RVCL, FCL, SLE	cGAS-STING-TBK1-IRF3	Autosomal dominant or recessive
RNA				
RIG-1 (RIG-1)	dsRNA sensor	Atypical SMS	MAVS	Autosomal dominant (gain of function)
IFIH1 (MDA5)	dsRNA sensor	AGS, SP, SMS	MAVS	Autosomal dominant (gain of function)
ADAR1 (ADAR1)	RNA editing	AGS, DSH, BSN, SP	MAVS	Autosomal recessive/ dominant negative
DNA-RNA				
SAMHD1 (SAMHD1)	dNTP triphosphohydrolase	AGS, FCL, CVD	cGAS-STING-TBK1-IRF3	Autosomal recessive
TMEM173 (STING)	Pattern-recognition receptor	SAVI, FCL	cGAS-STING-TBK1-IRF3	Autosomal dominant (gain of function)
POLA1 (POLA1)	DNA polymerase	XLPDR	Reduced synthesis of inhibitory DNA/ RNA cytosolic hybrids	X-linked recessive
RNASE H2-A/B/C (ribonuclease H2, subunit A, B,C)	Ribonuclease	AGS	cGAS-STING-TBK1-IRF3	Autosomal recessive
Deregulation of type I IFN pathway				
ACP5 (TRAP)	Dephosphorylation of osteopontin	SPENCD	Increased TLR9-/ Myd88-mediated IRF7 signaling	Autosomal recessive
PSMB8, *PSMA3*, *PSMB4*, *PSMB9*, *POMP* (20S core proteasome)	ATP-dependent protease	CANDLE syndrome	MAVS	Autosomal recessive
USP18 (USP18)	ISG15-specific protease	USP18 deficiency (pseudo-TORCH)	High type I IFN production	Autosomal recessive
ISG15 (ubiquitin-like modifier)	Conjugation to intracellular target proteins/negative type I IFNs regulator	ISG15 deficiency	USP-18-mediated type I IFN overexpression	Autosomal recessive

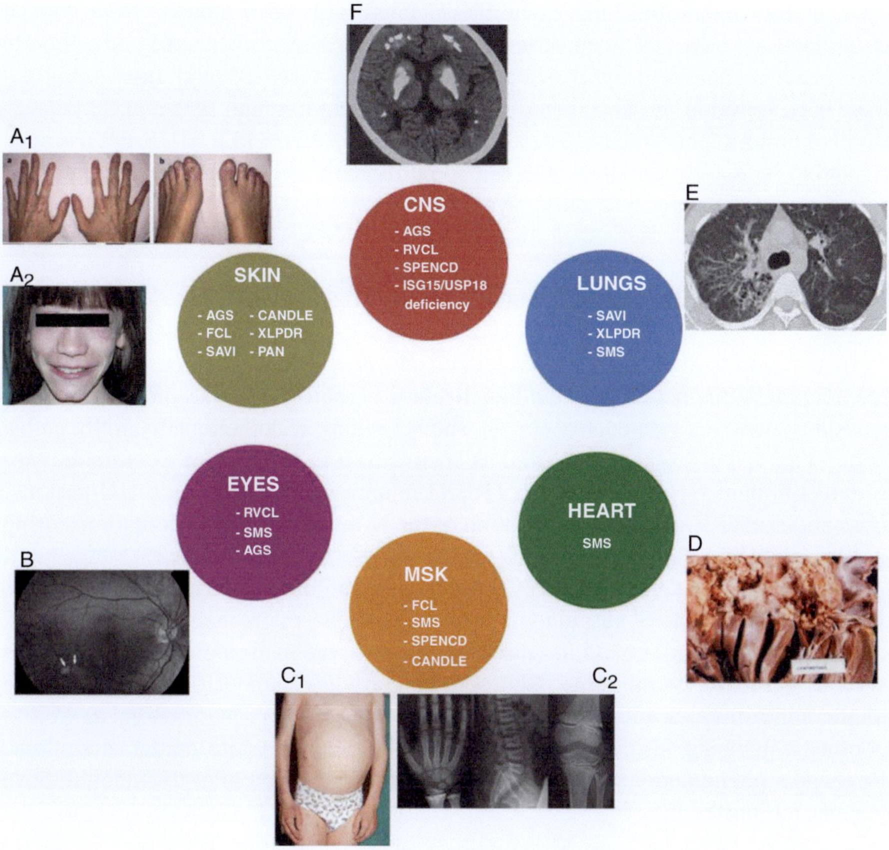

Fig. 10.2 Main organ systems affected in type I interferonopathies. Indicative manifestations are displayed. (**a**$_1$) Vasculitic-like cutaneous lesions in a patient with SAVI syndrome (Source: Manoussakis et al. [101]). (**a**$_2$) Face lipodystrophy in a patient with CANDLE syndrome (Source: Torrelo A et al., *J Am Acad Dermatol*. 2010;62:489–95). (**b**) Cotton woollike spots in a patient with RVCL syndrome (Source: Stam AH et al., *BRAIN*. 2016;139: 2909–22). (**c**$_1$) Growth retardation in a patient suffering from CANDLE syndrome (Source: Torrelo A et al., *J Am Acad Dermatol*. 2010; 62: 489–95). (**c**$_2$) Skeletal dysplasias in a patient with SPENCD syndrome (Source: Lausch et al. [81]). (**d**) Calcifications in the left ventricle, aortic valve and ascending aorta, postmortem specimen in a patient with SMS syndrome (Source: Rutsch et al. [60]). (**e**) Interstitial lung disease-honeycombing-ground gland opacities in a patient with SAVI syndrome (Source: Manoussakis et al. [101]). (**f**) Cerebral calcifications within basal ganglia and the cerebral white matter (Source: Lausch et al. [81]). *AGS* Aicardi-Goutieres syndrome, *CANDLE* chronic atypical neutrophilic dermatosis with lipodystrophy and elevated temperature, *CNS* central nervous system, *FCL* familial chilblain lupus, *ISG15 deficiency* interferon-stimulated gene 15 deficiency, *MSK* musculoskeletal system, *PAN* polyarteritis nodosa, *RVCL* retinal vasculopathy with cerebral leukodystrophy, *SAVI* STING-associated vasculopathy, infantile onset, *SMS* Singleton-Merten syndrome, *SPENCD* spondyloenchondrodysplasia, *USP18 deficiency* ubiquitin-specific peptidase 18 deficiency, *XLPDR* X-linked reticulate pigmentary disorder

well, mainly interstitial lung disease associated with fever attacks. Neurological complications have not been observed so far. Transiently increased autoantibody titers such as anti-neutrophil cytoplasmic antibody (ANCA) and anti-cardiolipin have been reported. Extensive perivascular inflammation with IgM and C3 deposition is a common finding in skin tissues from these patients [52, 53]. SAVI has been related to increased mortality rates due to pulmonary involvement in the context of infections in the lower respiratory system [54].

Retinal Vasculopathy with Cerebral Leukodystrophy (RVCL)

Retinal vasculopathy with cerebral leukodystrophy (*RVCL*) previously considered to encompass distinct clinical entities, namely, cerebroretinal vasculopathy (*CVR*), hereditary vascular retinopathy (*HVR*), and hereditary endotheliopathy, retinopathy, nephropathy, and stroke (*HERNS*), has been shown to result from a common autosomal dominant-type heterozygous TREX1 mutation. The latter leads to C-terminal truncation of TREX1, with preservation of the N-terminal DNAse domain resulting in impaired DNA clearance.

The main characteristics of RVCL include the middle-age onset, the progressive visual loss due to retinal vasculopathy (telangiectasias, microaneurysms, and retinal capillary obliteration around the macula), and variable neurological manifestations such as dementia or migraine. Neuroimaging studies demonstrate cerebral white matter abnormalities, including small infarcts resembling pseudotumors, as well as contrast-enhancing lesions similar to multiple sclerosis white matter alterations. Raynaud's phenomenon, micronodular cirrhosis, and glomerular dysfunction have been also reported [55, 56].

RNA Sensors

Singleton-Merten Syndrome (SMS)

Singleton-Merten syndrome (SMS) – inherited in an autosomal dominant manner – is caused by heterozygous gain-of-function mutations in interferon-induced helicase C domain-containing protein 1 (*IFIH1*) encoding the cytosolic pattern recognition receptors for dsRNA MDA5 or RIG-I, resulting in constitutive type I IFN activation [57–60].

Though there is extensive phenotypic variability, the core characteristics of the syndrome include aortic and valvular calcifications, dental anomalies (early-onset periodontitis and root resorption), abnormal ossification (mainly distal limbs), alveolar bone loss, skeletal abnormalities as well as osteoporosis, osteopenia, and acro-osteolysis. Psoriasis, glaucoma, muscle weakness, abnormal ligaments of joints and muscle, photosensitivity, recurrent respiratory infections and typical face features can also frequently occur [57, 59, 60]. *MDA-5* mutations have been particularly linked to Jaccoud's arthropathy, also observed in patients with systemic lupus erythematosus (SLE) [61].

DNA and RNA Sensors

Aicardi-Goutieres Syndrome (AGS)

Aicardi-Goutieres syndrome (AGS) is a hereditary neurodegenerative disorder of inflammatory etiology, characterized by early-onset progressive encephalopathy with increased levels of IFNα in the CSF. It is regarded as the prototypic disease in the context of interferonopathies [59]. Clinical manifestations occur between 3 and 7 months of age and sometimes during the first week after birth. Especially, in cases of intrauterine onset, newborns are presented with microcephaly.

The main symptoms observed are vomiting, irritability with feeding difficulties, dystonia, epileptic seizures, fever episodes, and a rather subacute onset leading gradually in motor and social skills retardation. With regard to extra-neurological symptoms, patients may present with skin manifestations, like acral chilblain lesions upon cold exposure, raised intraocular pressure and sometimes overlapping lupus-like symptoms, such as hepatosplenomegaly, thrombocytopenia, lymphopenia, and positive antinuclear antibodies (ANA) [62].

Given that mild fever attacks are frequently combined with neurological features, AGS might be misdiagnosed as congenital encephalitis or meningitis caused by TORCH (toxoplasma, other agents, rubella, cytomegalovirus, herpes simplex) or HIV infection. It is estimated that about 25% of patients will die between 1 and 17 years [63].

MRI imaging findings mainly include basal ganglia calcification, white matter abnormalities and brain atrophy, while CSF lymphocytosis and increased IFNα levels are characteristic laboratory manifestations. Similarly to lupus and other autoimmune diseases [8, 64, 65], overexpression of IFN-related genes in peripheral blood samples, known as interferon (IFN)-signature, has been detected in almost every patient at any age [62].

Aberrations of a number of genes have been found to account for AGS. These include TREX1, the three subunits of the ribonuclease H2 (RNAse H2), endonuclease complex (RNase H2A, RNase H2B and RNase H2C), the deoxynucleoside triphosphate triphosphohydrolase and ribonuclease SAM domain and HD domain 1 (SAMHD1), adenosine deaminase acting on RNA (ADAR; also known as DRADA), and the double-stranded RNA (dsRNA) cytosolic sensor IFIH1, also known as MDA5.

Biallelic loss-of-function mutations both for TREX1 and for each subunit of RNAse H2 complex result in intracellular accumulation of endogenous nucleic acid products, whose source is considered to be either chronic DNA damage, especially during DNA replication, or human genome-derived retroelements [66]. Eventually, single-stranded DNA (ssDNA) products trigger the activation of type I IFN axis through cGAS/TBK1/IRF3 pathway [67]. The latter has been also recently shown to be the downstream pathway activated by RNase H2 sensors [68].

Furthermore, biallelic loss-of-function mutations of SAMHD1 lead to chronic DNA damage, activation of type I IFN pathway as well as cerebrovascular aneurysms or stenosis, early-onset strokes and increased malignancy risk [69, 70], through a so far unexplored mechanism. It is of note that SAMHD1 and TREX1 enzymes are implicated in long interspersed nuclear element-1 (LINE-1) retroelements metabolism. Recent findings report activation of the cGAS/STING pathway as the downstream effectors for type I IFN production [71].

With regard to ADAR enzyme, both biallelic and heterozygous mutations lead to excessive recognition of endogenous double-stranded RNA (dsRNA) and to IFN release, via defective editing of short interspersed element (SINES) retroelements, which account for 10% of human genome [72, 73]. In particular, mutations of ADAR1 are implicated in expression of neurological defects, such as bilateral striatal necrosis (*BSN*) and spastic paraparesis (*SP*) as well. Additionally, they are related to dyschromatosis symmetrica hereditaria (*DSH*), a rare autosomal dominant disorder, detected in East Asian population, characterized by mixed hyper- and hypopigmented macules on the dorsal aspect of the hands and feet and freckle-like macules on the face [74].

Lastly, gain-of-function mutations of IFIH1, which encodes the MDA5 sensor, have also an increased affinity to dsRNA molecules and through MAVS activation result eventually in IFN overexpression [75, 76]. Similar to ADAR1 and SAMHD1 mutations, patients demonstrate especially neurological complications, such as SP [66].

Familial Chilblain Lupus (FCL)

Familial chilblain lupus (*FCL*) is a rare monogenic form of cutaneous lupus erythematosus, which is inherited in an autosomal dominant way. It affects patients in early childhood in a more rapidly progressive way compared to spontaneous lupus erythematosus, which is presented in middle-aged women. Patients suffer from partly ulcerating acral lesions or painful bluish-red papules located in the fingers, toes, nose and ears. These lesions are exacerbated by cold exposure and usually improve during summer. They can also be accompanied by arthralgias, affecting mainly large joints, without evidence of true arthritis, photosensitivity, or mouth ulcers.

Laboratory testing revealed slightly elevated antinuclear antibody (ANA) titers and/or lymphopenia, without any other specific serological marker. Given that nailbed alterations seem to be specific in a subset of FCL patients, capillaroscopy may be a promising modality to be implemented. Histopathological findings in affected skin tissues include perivascular inflammatory infiltrates with granular deposits of immunoglobulins and complement along the basement membrane.

Several genetic defects have been so far related to FCL. Heterozygous TREX1 mutations (implicated in AGS and impairment of susceptibility to granzyme-A-mediated cell death) as well as of SAMHD1 and STING molecules lead to FCL, through activation of the known cGAS-cGAMP-STING-TBK1-IRF3 pathway [77–79].

Type I IFN Deregulation

Spondyloenchondrodysplasia (SPENCD)

Spondyloenchondrodysplasia (SPENCD) is inherited in an autosomal recessive manner and it is caused by biallelic mutations in acid phosphatase 5 (ACP5), encoding tartrate-resistant acid phosphatase (TRAP) [80]. TRAP dephosphorylates and inactivates the protein osteopontin (OPN) – a bone matrix protein which upon dephosphorylation by TRAP leads a. to reduced osteoclast binding to different substrates [81], and b. dampened IFNα production by plasmacytoid dendritic cells (pDCs) through disruption of TLR-9/myeloid differentiation factor 88 (MyD88) mediated IFN regulatory factor 7 (IRF-7) activation [82]. Patients with SPENCD present constitutively activated osteopontin, which is probably responsible for increased bone resorption and immune dysregulation that leads to overproduction of type I IFN [59, 83].

Spondyloenchondrodysplasia (SPENCD) – first identified by Schorr et al. in 1976 – is a skeletal dysplasia characterized by enchondromatous radiolucent, irregular spondylar and metaphyseal lesions which represent islands of cartilage tissue within bone leading to platyspondyly. The severity of the lesions varies, but slow progression during childhood is most frequently observed, resulting in significantly short stature. It appears that SPENCD is clinically heterogeneous, as some SPENCD patients are neurologically intact, while others present with neurological dysfunction including spasticity, mental retardation and cerebral calcifications in different combinations. In addition, signs of immune dysregulation and systemic autoimmunity, such as arthritis, antinuclear antibodies and recurrent infections, are often observed in patients with SPENCD [59, 80, 84–87].

Interferon-Stimulated Gene 15 Deficiency (ISG15 Deficiency)

Deficiency of the IFNγ-inducing molecule named interferon-stimulated gene 15 (ISG15) leads to a clinical phenotype characterized by a prominent type I IFN signature in peripheral blood and increased susceptibility to mycobacterial disease possibly as a result of dampened IFNγ production. Absence of intracellular ISG15 prevents the accumulation of ubiquitin-specific peptidase 18 (USP18), a potent negative regulator of type I IFN signaling, resulting in the enhancement and amplification of type I IFN responses [88]. ISG15 deficiency is inherited in an autosomal recessive manner. Similarly to AGS and SPENCD, ISG15-deficient individuals also display marked intracranial calcification [59, 88, 89].

Ubiquitin-Specific Peptidase 18 Deficiency (USP18 Deficiency)

This disorder also known as pseudo-TORCH syndrome is caused by autosomal recessive homozygous mutations of the gene *USP18*, encoding the protein ubiquitin-specific protease 18, which cleaves the ubiquitin-like ISG15 protein from its conjugated proteins [59, 90]. Given the negative regulatory role of this molecule in type I IFN activation, type I IFN overexpression occurs. The clinical spectrum resembling a congenital infection but in the absence of an infectious agent includes microcephaly, enlarged ventricles, and cerebral calcification.

Chronic Atypical Neutrophilic Dermatosis with Lipodystrophy and Elevated Temperature (CANDLE)

CANDLE – a proteasome-associated autoinflammatory syndrome (PRAAS) – has been shown to occur in the context of several defects in catalytic activity of proteasome-immunoproteasome system related to mutations of genes encoding distinct protein subunits (β5i, β7, β1i, α3) [59, 91, 92]. It is inherited in an autosomal recessive pattern and characterized by enhanced peripheral blood ISG expression and constitutive STAT1 phosphorylation [59]. The latter seems to be related to previous observations supporting that proteasome inhibition led to activation of type I IFN pathway through enhancement of MAVS activity [93]. Recurrent fevers in the first months of life, along with characteristic skin lesions, lipodystrophy, violaceous swollen eyelids, arthralgias, extremity contractures, and delayed physical development as well as systemic inflammation markers have been identified as CANDLE-related clinical manifestations [92, 94]. CANDLE has been linked to early mortality rates due to cardiomyopathy, infections, and cardiac arrhythmias [54].

X-Linked Reticulate Pigmentary Disorder (XLPDR)

XLPDR is caused by an intronic mutation of the POLA1 gene, which encodes the catalytic subunit of DNA polymerase-α, an enzyme necessary for the synthesis of RNA-DNA primers during DNA replication. Unexpectedly, it was found that POLA1 is required for the synthesis of cytosolic RNA-DNA hybrids as well, which display an inhibitory action on type I IFN activation. In the setting of XLPDR, missplicing and disruption of POLA1 expression occur, leading to heightened type I IFN production through constitutive activation of IRF- and NF-κB-dependent genes [95] and a constellation of clinical features distinct between male and female carriers. Thus affected male individuals present with generalized hyperpigmentation intermingled with small hypomelanotic macules during early childhood, a distinctive face characterized by an upswept frontal hairline and arched eyebrows, as well as severe photophobia, recurrent respiratory infections and severe gastrointestinal disorders. In female carriers, the type and distribution of the pigmentation mimic that of incontinentia pigmenti (patchy pigmentary skin lesions along the lines of Blaschko), without any systemic manifestations [59, 96, 97].

Childhood-Onset Polyarteritis Nodosa: ADA2 Deficiency

Childhood-onset polyarteritis nodosa (PAN) is an autosomal recessive systemic vascular inflammatory disorder affecting mainly the brain and skin caused by biallelic mutations of the cat eye syndrome chromosome region, candidate 1 (*CECR1*). *CECR1* encodes the enzyme adenosine deaminase 2 (ADA2) which deaminates adenosine to inosine. Patients with ADA2 deficiency exhibit constitutive type I IFN activation in blood, although the underlying mechanism is unclear [59, 98].

Fever, necrotizing vasculitis of the gastrointestinal tract, and renal aneurysms as well as varying degrees of immunodeficiency and autoimmunity have been described and related to this disorder. The ensuing tissue ischemia can affect any organ, including the skin, musculoskeletal system, kidneys, gastrointestinal tract, and the cardiovascular and nervous systems [59, 98].

Therapeutic Implications

The delineation of pathogenetic mechanisms, implicated in type I IFN-related diseases, has provided promising prospects for the development of new therapeutic strategies, given the relative ineffectiveness of conventional immunosuppressive treatment. Since gene expression products of TREX1, SAMHD1, RNAse H2, and ADAR are involved in metabolism of endogenous retrovirus-derived nucleic acids, it has been postulated that the use of reverse transcriptase inhibitors might be effective in controlling inflammatory activity of the disease. In fact, the successful effect of reverse transcriptase inhibitors in an experimental TREX1-deficient mouse model has been reported [99], while a pilot phase II study is in progress, in pediatric population, using as treatment modalities zidovudine, lamivudine, and abacavir [*NCT02363452*].

In the context of interferonopathies, the common pathogenetic mechanism, leading to ISGs upregulation, is the JAK/STAT activation through triggering of the IFNAR receptor. Given the possibility of a potential therapeutic target, in 2016, Fremond and his colleagues described three cases of children, carrying TMEM173 mutations, who were successfully treated with Janus kinase 1/2 inhibitor ruxolitinib [100]. Furthermore, another case of patient with TMEM173-related FCL was treated with JAK (1/3) inhibitor tofacitinib for a very short period of time with doubtful results [101] [102]. Moreover, JAK-inhibitor baricitinib, previously shown to be successful in a case of CANDLE syndrome with alopecia areata [103], is currently tested in an ongoing clinical trial including patients with SAVI, juvenile dermatomyositis, and proteasome-related autoinflammatory syndrome [*NCT01724580*].

In the same context, targeted therapies against IFNAR receptor (anifrolumab) and IFNα itself (sifalimumab) – with promising so far results in lupus populations though [104–106], as well as hydroxychloroquine recently shown to inhibit cGAS stimulation by dsDNA molecules [107] – seem to be additional future options for patients with interferonopathies.

Conclusions

Type I interferonopathies is a recently discovered group of genetic disorders hallmarked by activation of type I IFN pathway and a wide variety of clinical phenotypes possibly related to tissue-specific gene or protein, together with the effects of environmental triggers. Major issues to be resolved also include the underlying mechanistic relationship between type I IFN pathway, tissue damage, and clinical phenotype as well the specific molecules along the extended type I IFN pathway that need to be targeted. To conclude, further investigations to better clarify the underlying mechanisms on excessive activation of type I IFN system are required leading to novel discoveries enabling more effective treatment strategies in the future.

ADAR1 adenosine deaminase acting on RNA 1; *AGS* Aicardi-Goutieres syndrome; *BSN* bilateral striatal necrosis; *CANDLE* chronic atypical neutrophilic dermatosis with lipodystrophy and elevated temperature; *cGAS* cyclic GMP-AMP synthase; *CVD* cerebrovascular disease; *DSH* dyschromatosis symmetrica hereditaria; *FCL* familial chilblain lupus; *IFIH1* interferon-induced helicase C domain-containing protein 1; *IFN* type I interferon; *IRF3* IFN-regulatory factor 3; *IRF7* IFN-regulatory factor 7; *ISG15 deficiency* interferon-stimulated gene 15 deficiency; *ISG15* interferon-stimulated gene 15; *MAVS* mitochondrial antiviral signaling; *MDA5* melanoma differentiation-associated gene 5; *POLA1* polymerase-α1; *RIG-I* retinoic acid-inducible gene I; *RNase H2A, RNase H2B, and RNase H2C* RNAse H2 ribonuclease H2 subunits A, B, and C; *RVCL* retinal vasculopathy with cerebral leukodystrophy; *SAMHD1* deoxynucleoside triphosphate triphosphohydrolase and ribonuclease SAM domain and HD domain 1; *SAVI* STING-associated vasculopathy, infantile onset; *SLE* systemic lupus erythematosus; *SMS* Singleton-Merten syndrome; *SP* spastic paraparesis; *SPENCD* spondyloenchondrodysplasia; *STING* stimulator of IFN genes; *TBK1* TANK-binding kinase 1; *TLR* Toll-like receptor; *TMEM173* transmembrane protein 173; *TORCH* toxoplasma, other agents, rubella, cytomegalovirus, herpes simplex; *TREX1* three prime (3′) repair exonuclease 1; *USP18 deficiency* ubiquitin-specific peptidase 18 deficiency; *USP18* ubiquitin-specific peptidase 18; *XLPDR* X-linked reticulate pigmentary disorder

References

1. Rodero MP, Crow YJ. Type I interferon-mediated monogenic autoinflammation: the type I interferonopathies, a conceptual overview. J Exp Med. 2016;213(12):2527–38.
2. Isaacs A, Lindenmann J. Virus interference. I. The interferon. Proc R Soc Lond B Biol Sci. 1957;147(927):258–67.
3. Isaacs A, Lindenmann J, Valentine RC. Virus interference. II. Some properties of interferon. Proc R Soc Lond B Biol Sci. 1957;147(927):268–73.

4. Mavragani CP, Crow MK. Activation of the type I interferon pathway in primary Sjogren's syndrome. J Autoimmun. 2010;35(3):225–31.
5. Hooks JJ, et al. Immune interferon in the circulation of patients with autoimmune disease. N Engl J Med. 1979;301(1):5–8.
6. Crow MK. Type I interferon in the pathogenesis of lupus. J Immunol. 2014;192(12):5459–68.
7. Kim D, et al. Induction of interferon-alpha by scleroderma sera containing autoantibodies to topoisomerase I: association of higher interferon-alpha activity with lung fibrosis. Arthritis Rheum. 2008;58(7):2163–73.
8. Nezos A, et al. Type I and II interferon signatures in Sjogren's syndrome pathogenesis: contributions in distinct clinical phenotypes and Sjogren's related lymphomagenesis. J Autoimmun. 2015;63:47–58.
9. Vakaloglou KM, Mavragani CP. Activation of the type I interferon pathway in primary Sjogren's syndrome: an update. Curr Opin Rheumatol. 2011;23(5):459–64.
10. Gresser I, et al. Interferon-induced disease in mice and rats. Ann N Y Acad Sci. 1980;350:12–20.
11. Aicardi J, Goutieres F. A progressive familial encephalopathy in infancy with calcifications of the basal ganglia and chronic cerebrospinal fluid lymphocytosis. Ann Neurol. 1984;15(1):49–54.
12. Lebon P, et al. Intrathecal synthesis of interferon-alpha in infants with progressive familial encephalopathy. J Neurol Sci. 1988;84(2–3):201–8.
13. Crow YJ, et al. Cree encephalitis is allelic with Aicardi-Goutieres syndrome: implications for the pathogenesis of disorders of interferon alpha metabolism. J Med Genet. 2003;40(3): 183–7.
14. Akwa Y, et al. Transgenic expression of IFN-alpha in the central nervous system of mice protects against lethal neurotropic viral infection but induces inflammation and neurodegeneration. J Immunol. 1998;161(9):5016–26.
15. Campbell IL, et al. Structural and functional neuropathology in transgenic mice with CNS expression of IFN-alpha. Brain Res. 1999;835(1):46–61.
16. Kavanagh D, et al. Type I interferon causes thrombotic microangiopathy by a dose-dependent toxic effect on the microvasculature. Blood. 2016;128(24):2824–33.
17. Ivashkiv LB, Donlin LT. Regulation of type I interferon responses. Nat Rev Immunol. 2014;14(1):36–49.
18. de Weerd NA, et al. Structural basis of a unique interferon-beta signaling axis mediated via the receptor IFNAR1. Nat Immunol. 2013;14(9):901–7.
19. Mostafavi S, et al. Parsing the interferon transcriptional network and its disease associations. Cell. 2016;164(3):564–78.
20. Muller M, et al. The protein tyrosine kinase JAK1 complements defects in interferon-alpha/beta and -gamma signal transduction. Nature. 1993;366(6451):129–35.
21. Stark GR, Darnell JE Jr. The JAK-STAT pathway at twenty. Immunity. 2012;36(4):503–14.
22. Velazquez L, et al. A protein tyrosine kinase in the interferon alpha/beta signaling pathway. Cell. 1992;70(2):313–22.
23. Blaszczyk K, et al. STAT2/IRF9 directs a prolonged ISGF3-like transcriptional response and antiviral activity in the absence of STAT1. Biochem J. 2015;466(3):511–24.
24. Bluyssen HA, Levy DE. Stat2 is a transcriptional activator that requires sequence-specific contacts provided by stat1 and p48 for stable interaction with DNA. J Biol Chem. 1997;272(7):4600–5.
25. Uddin S, Platanias LC. Mechanisms of type-I interferon signal transduction. J Biochem Mol Biol. 2004;37(6):635–41.
26. Medzhitov R, Preston-Hurlburt P, Janeway CA Jr. A human homologue of the Drosophila Toll protein signals activation of adaptive immunity. Nature. 1997;388(6640):394–7.
27. Lamkanfi M, Dixit VM. Inflammasomes and their roles in health and disease. Annu Rev Cell Dev Biol. 2012;28:137–61.
28. Paludan SR, Bowie AG. Immune sensing of DNA. Immunity. 2013;38(5):870–80.

29. Vidya MK, et al. Toll-like receptors: significance, ligands, signaling pathways, and functions in mammals. Int Rev Immunol. 2018;37(1):20–36.
30. Wu J, Chen ZJ. Innate immune sensing and signaling of cytosolic nucleic acids. Annu Rev Immunol. 2014;32:461–88.
31. Kawai T, Akira S. The role of pattern-recognition receptors in innate immunity: update on Toll-like receptors. Nat Immunol. 2010;11(5):373–84.
32. Yoneyama M, et al. Shared and unique functions of the DExD/H-box helicases RIG-I, MDA5, and LGP2 in antiviral innate immunity. J Immunol. 2005;175(5):2851–8.
33. Seth RB, et al. Identification and characterization of MAVS, a mitochondrial antiviral signaling protein that activates NF-kappaB and IRF 3. Cell. 2005;122(5):669–82.
34. Silverman RH. Viral encounters with 2′,5′-oligoadenylate synthetase and RNase L during the interferon antiviral response. J Virol. 2007;81(23):12720–9.
35. Diebold SS, et al. Viral infection switches non-plasmacytoid dendritic cells into high interferon producers. Nature. 2003;424(6946):324–8.
36. Chiu YH, Macmillan JB, Chen ZJ. RNA polymerase III detects cytosolic DNA and induces type I interferons through the RIG-I pathway. Cell. 2009;138(3):576–91.
37. Ishikawa H, Barber GN. STING is an endoplasmic reticulum adaptor that facilitates innate immune signalling. Nature. 2008;455(7213):674–8.
38. Tanaka Y, Chen ZJ. STING specifies IRF3 phosphorylation by TBK1 in the cytosolic DNA signaling pathway. Sci Signal. 2012;5(214):ra20.
39. Du XX, Su XD. Detection of cyclic dinucleotides by STING. Methods Mol Biol. 2017;1657:59–69.
40. Burdette DL, et al. STING is a direct innate immune sensor of cyclic di-GMP. Nature. 2011;478(7370):515–8.
41. Xiao TS, Fitzgerald KA. The cGAS-STING pathway for DNA sensing. Mol Cell. 2013;51(2):135–9.
42. Sun L, et al. Cyclic GMP-AMP synthase is a cytosolic DNA sensor that activates the type I interferon pathway. Science. 2013;339(6121):786–91.
43. Wu J, et al. Cyclic GMP-AMP is an endogenous second messenger in innate immune signaling by cytosolic DNA. Science. 2013;339(6121):826–30.
44. Stetson DB, et al. Trex1 prevents cell-intrinsic initiation of autoimmunity. Cell. 2008;134(4):587–98.
45. Crow YJ. The story of DNase II: a stifled death-wish leads to self-harm. Eur J Immunol. 2010;40(9):2376–8.
46. Burckstummer T, et al. An orthogonal proteomic-genomic screen identifies AIM2 as a cytoplasmic DNA sensor for the inflammasome. Nat Immunol. 2009;10(3):266–72.
47. Picard C, Belot A. Does type-I interferon drive systemic autoimmunity? Autoimmun Rev. 2017;16(9):897–902.
48. Mavragani CP, et al. Defective regulation of L1 endogenous retroelements in primary Sjogren's syndrome and systemic lupus erythematosus: role of methylating enzymes. J Autoimmun. 2018;88:75–82.
49. Mavragani CP, et al. Expression of long interspersed nuclear element 1 retroelements and induction of type I interferon in patients with systemic autoimmune disease. Arthritis Rheumatol. 2016;68(11):2686–96.
50. Melki I, et al. Disease-associated mutations identify a novel region in human STING necessary for the control of type I interferon signaling. J Allergy Clin Immunol. 2017;140(2): 543–52. e5
51. Warner JD, et al. STING-associated vasculopathy develops independently of IRF3 in mice. J Exp Med. 2017;214:3279–92.
52. Jeremiah N, et al. Inherited STING-activating mutation underlies a familial inflammatory syndrome with lupus-like manifestations. J Clin Invest. 2014;124(12):5516–20.
53. Liu Y, et al. Activated STING in a vascular and pulmonary syndrome. N Engl J Med. 2014;371(6):507–18.

54. Kim H, Sanchez GA, Goldbach-Mansky R. Insights from Mendelian interferonopathies: comparison of CANDLE, SAVI with AGS, monogenic lupus. J Mol Med (Berl). 2016;94(10):1111–27.
55. Richards A, et al. C-terminal truncations in human 3′-5′ DNA exonuclease TREX1 cause autosomal dominant retinal vasculopathy with cerebral leukodystrophy. Nat Genet. 2007;39(9):1068–70.
56. Schuh E, et al. Multiple sclerosis-like lesions and type I interferon signature in a patient with RVCL. Neurol Neuroimmunol Neuroinflamm. 2015;2(1):e55.
57. Feigenbaum A, et al. Singleton-Merten syndrome: an autosomal dominant disorder with variable expression. Am J Med Genet A. 2013;161A(2):360–70.
58. Jang MA, et al. Mutations in DDX58, which encodes RIG-I, cause atypical Singleton-Merten syndrome. Am J Hum Genet. 2015;96(2):266–74.
59. Lee-Kirsch MA. The type I interferonopathies. Annu Rev Med. 2017;68:297–315.
60. Rutsch F, et al. A specific IFIH1 gain-of-function mutation causes Singleton-Merten syndrome. Am J Hum Genet. 2015;96(2):275–82.
61. de Carvalho LM, et al. Musculoskeletal disease in MDA5-related type I interferonopathy: a Mendelian mimic of Jaccoud's arthropathy. Arthritis Rheumatol. 2017;69(10):2081–91.
62. Chahwan C, Chahwan R. Aicardi-Goutieres syndrome: from patients to genes and beyond. Clin Genet. 2012;81(5):413–20.
63. Barth PG. The neuropathology of Aicardi-Goutieres syndrome. Eur J Paediatr Neurol. 2002;6(Suppl A):A27–31; discussion A37–9, A77–86.
64. Ekholm L, et al. Autoantibody specificities and type I interferon pathway activation in idiopathic inflammatory myopathies. Scand J Immunol. 2016;84(2):100–9.
65. Eloranta ML, Ronnblom L. Cause and consequences of the activated type I interferon system in SLE. J Mol Med (Berl). 2016;94(10):1103–10.
66. Crow YJ, Manel N. Aicardi-Goutieres syndrome and the type I interferonopathies. Nat Rev Immunol. 2015;15(7):429–40.
67. Ablasser A, et al. TREX1 deficiency triggers cell-autonomous immunity in a cGAS-dependent manner. J Immunol. 2014;192(12):5993–7.
68. Mackenzie KJ, et al. Ribonuclease H2 mutations induce a cGAS/STING-dependent innate immune response. EMBO J. 2016;35(8):831–44.
69. Clifford R, et al. SAMHD1 is mutated recurrently in chronic lymphocytic leukemia and is involved in response to DNA damage. Blood. 2014;123(7):1021–31.
70. Kretschmer S, et al. SAMHD1 prevents autoimmunity by maintaining genome stability. Ann Rheum Dis. 2015;74(3):e17.
71. Maelfait J, et al. Restriction by SAMHD1 limits cGAS/STING-dependent innate and adaptive immune responses to HIV-1. Cell Rep. 2016;16(6):1492–501.
72. Mannion NM, et al. The RNA-editing enzyme ADAR1 controls innate immune responses to RNA. Cell Rep. 2014;9(4):1482–94.
73. Vitali P, Scadden AD. Double-stranded RNAs containing multiple IU pairs are sufficient to suppress interferon induction and apoptosis. Nat Struct Mol Biol. 2010;17(9):1043–50.
74. Hayashi M, Suzuki T. Dyschromatosis symmetrica hereditaria. J Dermatol. 2013;40(5):336–43.
75. Funabiki M, et al. Autoimmune disorders associated with gain of function of the intracellular sensor MDA5. Immunity. 2014;40(2):199–212.
76. Oda H, et al. Aicardi-Goutieres syndrome is caused by IFIH1 mutations. Am J Hum Genet. 2014;95(1):121–5.
77. Fiehn C. Familial chilblain lupus - what can we learn from type I interferonopathies? Curr Rheumatol Rep. 2017;19(10):61.
78. Lee-Kirsch MA, et al. A mutation in TREX1 that impairs susceptibility to granzyme A-mediated cell death underlies familial chilblain lupus. J Mol Med (Berl). 2007;85(5):531–7.
79. Lee-Kirsch MA, et al. Familial chilblain lupus, a monogenic form of cutaneous lupus erythematosus, maps to chromosome 3p. Am J Hum Genet. 2006;79(4):731–7.

80. Briggs TA, et al. Spondyloenchondrodysplasia due to mutations in ACP5: a comprehensive survey. J Clin Immunol. 2016;36(3):220–34.
81. Lausch E, et al. Genetic deficiency of tartrate-resistant acid phosphatase associated with skeletal dysplasia, cerebral calcifications and autoimmunity. Nat Genet. 2011;43(2):132–7.
82. An J, et al. Tartrate-resistant acid phosphatase deficiency in the predisposition to systemic lupus erythematosus. Arthritis Rheumatol. 2017;69(1):131–42.
83. Briggs TA, et al. Tartrate-resistant acid phosphatase deficiency causes a bone dysplasia with autoimmunity and a type I interferon expression signature. Nat Genet. 2011;43(2):127–31.
84. Navarro V, et al. Two further cases of spondyloenchondrodysplasia (SPENCD) with immune dysregulation. Am J Med Genet A. 2008;146A(21):2810–5.
85. Renella R, et al. Spondyloenchondrodysplasia with spasticity, cerebral calcifications, and immune dysregulation: clinical and radiographic delineation of a pleiotropic disorder. Am J Med Genet A. 2006;140(6):541–50.
86. Roifman CM, Melamed I. A novel syndrome of combined immunodeficiency, autoimmunity and spondylometaphyseal dysplasia. Clin Genet. 2003;63(6):522–9.
87. Schorr S, Legum C, Ochshorn M. Spondyloenchondrodysplasia. Enchondromatomosis with severe platyspondyly in two brothers. Radiology. 1976;118(1):133–9.
88. Zhang X, et al. Human intracellular ISG15 prevents interferon-alpha/beta over-amplification and auto-inflammation. Nature. 2015;517(7532):89–93.
89. Bogunovic D, et al. Mycobacterial disease and impaired IFN-gamma immunity in humans with inherited ISG15 deficiency. Science. 2012;337(6102):1684–8.
90. Meuwissen ME, et al. Human USP18 deficiency underlies type 1 interferonopathy leading to severe pseudo-TORCH syndrome. J Exp Med. 2016;213(7):1163–74.
91. Brehm A, et al. Additive loss-of-function proteasome subunit mutations in CANDLE/PRAAS patients promote type I IFN production. J Clin Invest. 2015;125(11):4196–211.
92. Torrelo A. CANDLE syndrome as a paradigm of proteasome-related autoinflammation. Front Immunol. 2017;8:927.
93. Castanier C, et al. MAVS ubiquitination by the E3 ligase TRIM25 and degradation by the proteasome is involved in type I interferon production after activation of the antiviral RIG-I-like receptors. BMC Biol. 2012;10:44.
94. Tufekci O, et al. CANDLE syndrome: a recently described autoinflammatory syndrome. J Pediatr Hematol Oncol. 2015;37(4):296–9.
95. Starokadomskyy P, et al. DNA polymerase-alpha regulates the activation of type I interferons through cytosolic RNA:DNA synthesis. Nat Immunol. 2016;17(5):495–504.
96. Pezzani L, et al. X-linked reticulate pigmentary disorder with systemic manifestations: a new family and review of the literature. Am J Med Genet A. 2013;161A(6):1414–20.
97. Zhang J, Li M, Yao Z. Updated review of genetic reticulate pigmentary disorders. Br J Dermatol. 2017;177(4):945–59.
98. Navon Elkan P, et al. Mutant adenosine deaminase 2 in a polyarteritis nodosa vasculopathy. N Engl J Med. 2014;370(10):921–31.
99. Beck-Engeser GB, Eilat D, Wabl M. An autoimmune disease prevented by anti-retroviral drugs. Retrovirology. 2011;8:91.
100. Fremond ML, et al. Efficacy of the Janus kinase 1/2 inhibitor ruxolitinib in the treatment of vasculopathy associated with TMEM173-activating mutations in 3 children. J Allergy Clin Immunol. 2016;138(6):1752–5.
101. Manoussakis MN, et al. Type I interferonopathy in a young adult. Rheumatology (Oxford). 2017;56:2241–3.
102. Konig N, et al. Familial chilblain lupus due to a gain-of-function mutation in STING. Ann Rheum Dis. 2017;76(2):468–72.
103. Jabbari A, et al. Reversal of alopecia areata following treatment with the JAK1/2 inhibitor baricitinib. EBioMedicine. 2015;2(4):351–5.
104. Oon S, Wilson NJ, Wicks I. Targeted therapeutics in SLE: emerging strategies to modulate the interferon pathway. Clin Transl Immunol. 2016;5(5):e79.

105. Petri M, et al. Sifalimumab, a human anti-interferon-alpha monoclonal antibody, in systemic lupus erythematosus: a phase I randomized, controlled, dose-escalation study. Arthritis Rheum. 2013;65(4):1011–21.
106. Relle M, et al. Genetics and novel aspects of therapies in systemic lupus erythematosus. Autoimmun Rev. 2015;14(11):1005–18.
107. An J, et al. Cutting edge: antimalarial drugs inhibit IFN-beta production through blockade of cyclic GMP-AMP synthase-DNA interaction. J Immunol. 2015;194(9):4089–93.

Chapter 11
Deficiency of Adenosine Deaminase 2 (DADA2)

Andreas Reiff

Introduction

The past two decades have witnessed an unprecedented expansion of clinically distinct autoinflammatory syndromes through the identification of single-gene defects in different pathways of the innate immune system. In contrast to the traditional mostly monogenic periodic fever syndromes, recently discovered genes and cellular pathways have identified new, often polygenic autoinflammatory syndromes that are L-1 independent and among others can lead to a chronic interferon type I (IFN) overproduction, an aberrant IL-18 production, or impaired endothelial keratinocyte development. Others affect protein misfolding, homeostasis or impaired differentiation, and development of myeloid cells. As a result, the clinical presentation of many patients with autoinflammatory diseases has become much more complex, and a substantial number of patients who are treatment refractory to IL-1 blocking agents remain undiagnosed.

One of these new complex monogenic autoinflammatory syndromes defined by features of autoinflammation, vasculitis, varying degrees of immunodeficiency, bone marrow failure, and autoimmunity is based on a deficiency of adenosine deaminase type 2 (DADA2) and typically presents as childhood-onset vasculopathy resembling polyarteritis nodosa. First described in 2014 in patients with mild immune deficiency, systemic inflammation, and central nervous system vasculopathy, initially suspected to have polyarteritis nodosa (PAN), DADA2 has now been established as a separate disease entity in over 125 patients including children. DADA2 appears not to be limited to any specific ethnic group, although important founder effects for specific mutations in select populations are described [1–3]. Patients with DADA2 characteristically present with an early-onset vasculopathy with livedo racemosa, purpura, leg ulcers, Raynaud's phenomenon, and digital necrosis and in more severe

A. Reiff (✉)
Division Head Rheumatology, Children's Hospital Los Angeles, USC Keck School of Medicine, Los Angeles, CA, USA

P. Efthimiou (ed.), *Auto-Inflammatory Syndromes*,
https://doi.org/10.1007/978-3-319-96929-9_11

cases with peripheral neuropathy or early-onset hemorrhagic and ischemic strokes. Other symptoms include subcutaneous nodules, recurrent fevers, hepatosplenomegaly, ophthalmologic manifestations, hypertension, arthritis, arthralgia, myalgia, and laboratory abnormalities [4–6].

Pathogenesis

The enzyme adenosine deaminase exists in two major isoforms: ADA1, which can be the cause of a severe combined immunodeficiency (SCID) phenotype when deficient or absent [7], and ADA2, which has partial structural homology with ADA1. The two isoforms are mainly differentiated by the fact that ADA2 is a dimer and exocytosed into the extracellular environment, while ADA1 is largely an intracellular monomer [8, 9]. While both isoforms convert adenosine to inosine and 2′-deoxyadenosine to 2′-deoxyinosine, a key step in purine metabolism, the affinity of ADA2 for adenosine is substantially lower than that of ADA1 [10, 11]. Adenosine is an important signaling modulator in inflammation that rises in conditions such as ischemia and cellular stress. The accumulation of adenosine can influence the inflammatory response by binding several receptors leading to inflammation, tissue damage, and fibrosis [10]. Adenosine has been postulated as one of the targets of the anti-inflammatory effects of methotrexate [12, 13].

Whereas ADA1 is expressed in all cell types, ADA2 is mainly produced by myeloid cells [14]. ADA2 belongs to a family of cell growth and differentiation factors that are critical for the maintenance of vascular development and integrity of endothelial cells and leukocytes. ADA2 regulates neutrophil activation and differentiation through its interaction with neutrophil surface receptors and acts as a growth factor for endothelial and leukocyte development and differentiation [15]. Deficiency of ADA2 leads to an upregulation of neutrophil-expressed gene transcripts with a subsequent negative impact on the endogenous anti-inflammatory adenosine feedback loop [15, 16]. Even though the exact pathophysiologic mechanism remains unclear, it is assumed that this chronic uncontrolled activation of neutrophils ultimately leads to endothelial cell dysfunction and secondary release and accumulation of proinflammatory cytokines resulting in tissue injury [9, 16].

Another important aspect in the pathogenesis and clinical presentation of DADA2 is dysregulated macrophage differentiation resulting in reduced numbers of anti-inflammatory M2-like macrophages and divergence toward more proinflammatory M1-like macrophages and monocytes [7, 17, 18] (Fig. 11.1).

DADA2 is caused by autosomal recessive loss-of-function mutations in the *CECR1* gene (cat eye syndrome chromosome region 1), on chromosome 22q11.1, encoding for the enzymatic protein adenosine deaminase 2 (ADA2) [1, 2]. The gene contains a receptor-binding domain, a catalytic domain, a signal sequence domain, and a dimerization domain. So far a total of 39 pathogenic mutations with variable prevalence across various ethnicities have been described [Infevers.com].

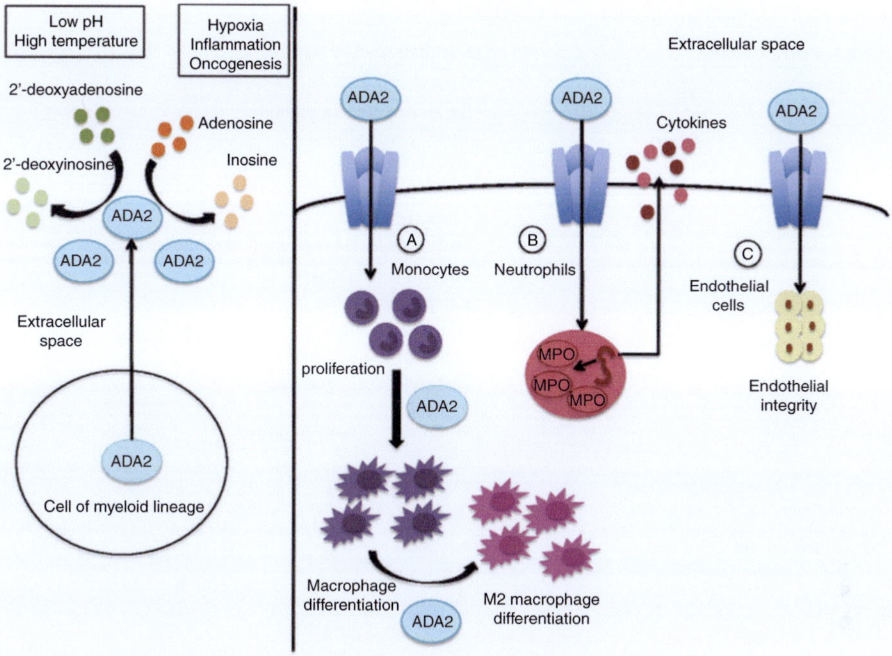

Fig. 11.1 The physiological role of adenosine deaminase type 2 in inflammation, endothelial integrity, and macrophage differentiation. (Adapted from Caorsi et al. [18])

Even though endothelial cells do not express the *CECR1* gene, it has been found to be important for vascular integrity and neutrophil development [15]. Interestingly the knockdown zebrafish model for the *CECR1* gene exhibits cerebral hemorrhages without morphologic alteration in the vascular structure [1, 18]. Ultimately it remains to be determined what exact role ADA2 plays in endothelial homeostasis of the innate and adaptive immune response and next-generation sequencing technologies will be helpful further clarifying its role.

Clinical Presentation

The clinical course of patients with DADA2 appears to evolve over time and is highly variable in regard to age at onset (ranging from 2 months to 59 years), disease severity, and organ involvement suggesting a strong regulatory influence by modifying alleles and epigenetic factors [18]. In a recent case series summarized by Caorsi et al. including 65 DADA2 patients of mainly Russian, Caucasian, or Turkish descent, the median age at onset was 2 years [18]. Disease manifestations can range from mild limited skin disease to severe, often fatal multiorgan involvement that can occur at a very early age (<5 years) [19–21] (Table 11.1). Some patients might only

Table 11.1 Clinical Manifestations of DADA2

Organ involvement	Clinical manifestation
Central nervous system	Transitory ischemic attacks (TIA) Transient mononeuritis Polyneuropathies Cranial nerve involvement Sensorineural hearing loss Optic neuritis Ischemic or hemorrhagic lacunar strokes
Skin	Livedo reticularis Livedo racemosa Maculopapular rash Erythema nodosum Subcutaneous nodules Purpura Raynaud's phenomenon Ulcers Digital necrosis Alopecia
Musculoskeletal	Myalgia Arthralgia Arthritis
Gastrointestinal	Abdominal pain, Chronic gastritis, Weight loss Hepatosplenomegaly Portal hypertension Bowel perforation Bowel obstruction
Renal	Nephrogenic hypertension Focal glomerulosclerosis Amyloidosis
Systemic	Recurrent fevers
Laboratory findings	Anemia, Leukopenia Pancytopenia Neutrophilic leukocytosis Elevated markers of inflammation (ESR, CRP) Hypogammaglobulinemia

be identified in the context of family screening following identification of an index case as they are either asymptomatic or present with very subtle disease manifestations despite confirmed low ADA2 activity.

Interestingly, the clinical presentation of the disease can vary widely even among patients with the same mutations in the *CECR1* gene.

Symptoms at presentation are often clinically undistinguishable from systemic polyarteritis nodosa (PAN), and many children with DADA2 present with symptoms or histological findings fulfilling the criteria of childhood-onset PAN [22]. Similar to other patients with IL-1 independent autoinflammatory diseases, the prior medical history is often noncontributory, but patients may have some evidence of recurrent bacterial and viral infections or a positive family history of consanguinity/endogamy [23].

In early childhood, clinical symptoms typically include recurrent fevers with *skin manifestations* (mainly livedo racemosa) and laboratory evidence of systemic inflammation with elevated acute phase reactants. Other skin manifestations can include maculopapular rashes, erythema nodosum, subcutaneous nodules, purpura, Raynaud's phenomenon, skin ulcers, and digital necrosis [1, 2].

One of the most serious disease manifestations of DADA2 is the involvement of the *peripheral and central nervous system*. Peripheral neurologic involvement can consist of transient mononeuritis or more permanent polyneuropathies. CNS manifestations can vary and range from transitory ischemic attacks (TIA), cranial nerve involvement with transient paralysis or sensorineural hearing loss, and optic neuritis to ischemic or hemorrhagic lacunar strokes. In the case series summarized by Caorsi et al. mentioned above, 60% of the patients had CNS involvement [1, 2, 18]. It has been suggested that patients with strokes appear to have lower ADA2 activity when compared to those without [24].

Gastrointestinal involvement also can vary widely with mild symptoms such as weight loss, abdominal pain, chronic gastritis, and hepatosplenomegaly but can also lead to more serious complications such as portal hypertension, bowel perforation, or stenosis. In the case series summarized by Caorsi et al., 54% of the patients had GI involvement ranging from mild hepatosplenomegaly to bowel perforation [18, 21].

As can be expected based on the nature of an autoinflammatory syndrome, *renal involvement* with focal glomerulosclerosis and renal amyloidosis has been described in few patients. On the other hand, nephrogenic hypertension appears rather common in DADA2 [18, 25].

Pulmonary involvement seems to be rather rare, and to my knowledge only one patient with fatal necrotizing pneumonia has been reported in the literature [25].

Some patients may present with features resembling Castleman's disease with fevers, night sweats, fatigue, nausea, vomiting, weight loss, hepatosplenomegaly, peripheral neuropathy, ascites, renal failure, as well as bruising, bleeding, and risk of infection due to bone marrow failure.

Lastly, the clinical findings in those patients with more predominant features of immunodeficiency who may ultimately require hematopoietic stem cell transplantation, would include delayed growth and development, increased susceptibility to longer lasting more difficult to treat infections, as well as opportunistic infections or development of malignancies [30, 32].

Due to the close clinical similarity, ADA2 deficiency may also account for some patients diagnosed with *Sneddon's syndrome (SS)*, a rare noninflammatory thrombotic vasculopathy [26, 27]. SS is characterized by the combination of livedo racemosa (LR) and TIAs or cerebral infarcts with or without cerebral hemorrhage typically affecting women between the ages of 20 and 42 years. Distinct histopathological findings on skin biopsy and focal neurological deficits are required for the diagnosis. Similar to DADA2, patients may present with multiorgan involvement including renal, cardiac, and ophthalmologic as well as neurological symptoms such as headaches, seizures, and neurocognitive and psychiatric symptoms. However there are also subtle differences when compared to DADA2. The skin pattern of LR in patients with DADA2, which can precede the onset of stroke by years, is broken up in larger irregular branch-like patterns indicative of more localized impairment of blood flow and appears less sensitive to temperature changes [9, 25]. In addition, the presence of antiphospholipid antibodies appears to be more common in SS patients, supporting a hypercoagulable state and intrinsic small-vessel vasculopathy of small- to medium-sized arteries as the underlying cause [26, 27].

Diagnosis

The diagnosis of DAD2 is mainly based on clinical criteria after careful exclusion of other conditions and other vasculitides that can mimic these symptoms as described below.

Genetic testing for autosomal recessive loss-of-function mutations in the *CECR1* gene is essential to confirm the diagnosis. Measurements of serum or plasma adenosine deaminase type 2 activity and/or levels, which according to preliminary data seem to be higher in children than in adults, are not yet commonly available through commercial laboratories [28, 29]. In addition to anemia or pure red cell aplasia mimicking Blackfan-Diamond anemia, neutrophilic leukocytosis, and elevated markers of inflammation (ESR, CRP), laboratory workup can demonstrate hypogammaglobulinemia that may affect all immune globulin subclasses, while other autoantibodies are usually negative. On the other hand, pancytopenia and/or leukopenia was a rather common finding in a recent case series of nine DADA2 patients with a homozygous R169Q mutation [24]. Additional laboratory tests to exclude other conditions should include a basic immunodeficiency and hypercoagulability workup, ANCA titers (negative in DADA2 and PAN), antiphospholipid, anticardiolipin, and beta 2 glycoprotein antibodies.

There are conflicting results regarding the serum profiles of patients with DADA2. While in one study elevated serum levels of IL-1β, IL-6, and TNFα were detected especially in patients with a homozygous deletion of 22q11.1, another study performed at the NIH with cultured whole blood cell supernatants failed to replicate these results when compared to healthy donors [1, 30]. Similar conflicting results have been reported concerning the T cell function in these patients. While the same NIH study mentioned above was not able to ascertain any differences in T lymphocyte numbers and activation, a recent case report in one patient with DADA2 described an increase of regulatory T cells, a decrease of CD8+ and CD4 + memory T cells, and a reduced number of Th1, Th2, and follicular T helper (Tfh) cells [1, 30]. On the other hand, an increased mortality of B cells, decreased numbers of memory B cells, terminally differentiated B cells, and plasma cells has been described in patients with DADA2 [1, 7]. This may explain why patients with DADA2 only present with a mild immune deficiency phenotype when compared to patients with ADA1 deficiency and suggests a role of this protein in the adaptive immune response [1, 37].

While a skin biopsy might be helpful to differentiate DADA2 from other forms of necrotizing vasculitis, histologic findings commonly demonstrate a non-granulomatous small- and midsized vasculitis with the same histopathologic features as polyarteritis nodosa or more unspecific findings such as a small-vessel leukocytoclastic vasculitis or panniculitis [1, 2, 19].

Neuroimaging in the form of conventional angiography, CT and/or MRI, is essential even though findings may initially be negative. MRI appears to be most useful to detect the full extent of smaller lacunar strokes and can demonstrate ventricular hemorrhage, aneurisms, and/or stenoses in the midsized arteries that may otherwise have been missed by CT scan or conventional angiography [21, 24].

As mentioned above, a clinical separation between PAN and especially cutaneous polyarteritis nodosa (cPAN) to DADA2 might be challenging. Polyarteritis nodosa (PAN) is defined as an ANCA-negative necrotizing arteritis of medium or small arteries that does not involve arterioles, capillaries, or venules [22, 23, 32]. While PAN can involve the skin, musculature, gastrointestinal system, kidneys, and the peripheral nervous system, cPAN is typically devoid of systemic organ involvement. Similar to DADA2, cPAN can present as a relapsing-remitting necrotizing, non-granulomatous, medium-sized vessel arteritis with an isolated skin phenotype encompassing subcutaneous nodules, ulcers, and livedo racemosa and/or livedo reticularis.

Angiographic evidence of stenosis and/or aneurysms of the renal, hepatic, celiac, and/or mesenteric artery and its branches might be more common in patients with PAN than in those with DADA2. It has been proposed that based on its genetic nature, DADA2 should be incorporated in the Chapel Hill classification of vasculitides [22, 31]. Other diseases that should be considered in the differential diagnosis include other forms of vasculitis such as Kawasaki's disease, Takayasu's arteritis, or Aicardi-Goutières syndrome, common variable immunodeficiency (CVID), antiphospholipid antibody syndrome, and Castleman's disease.

Treatment

Due to its novelty and the limited experience from small patient series, treatment recommendations for DADA2 remain based on anecdotal evidence. As a result, decisions about therapy should be based on the individual presentation and severity of the disease and made on a case-by-case basis. Similar to other autoinflammatory disorders and patients with PAN, high-dose steroids have been used and are effective to at least control the acute symptoms. With the exception of sirolimus, which reduces M1 macrophage differentiation and IL-6 production, traditional disease-modifying antirheumatic drugs (DMARDs) such as cyclophosphamide, azathioprine, or methotrexate appear to be ineffective [1, 2, 5, 6, 15, 23–25, 33].

Infusion of fresh frozen plasma (which contains ADA2) or direct enzymatic replacement therapy with ADA**1** (ADA2 enzyme replacement is not yet available) has been attempted with mixed results [20, 28]. Treatment results with various biologic agents are controversial, and treatment responses are often partial. Interestingly, treatment with anti-TNF drugs appears to be most beneficial and is probably explained by the skewing toward an M1 pro-inflammatory macrophage immunophenotype, although this requires further study [18, 20, 34, 35]. In one of the published case series examining the role of anti-TNF therapy in DADA2 including nine DADA2 patients treated with either etanercept, adalimumab, or infliximab, a complete response was noted in eight patients, despite prior DMARD failure [24]. Other therapeutic options include anti-interleukin 1 or interleukin 6-blocking agents, which may not work for all but have been reported to be at least partially successful in a few patients with DADA2 [1, 3, 6, 25, 28].

Due to the nature of DADA2 being at least a partial immunodeficiency, hematopoietic stem cell transplantation (HSCT) has been proposed as a potentially curative approach by introducing new cell lines with a subsequent normalization of ADA2 plasma levels. This treatment approach has been performed with a complete and sustained response for up to 13 years in several patients with severe disease. However some patients experienced complications from GVHD and/or cytopenias [36–39].

Similar to DADA2, optimal treatment for patients with SS has also not been established.

For patients with thromboembolic cerebral ischemic complications, long-term anticoagulation has been recommended, while the use of immunomodulatory agents remains controversial [26, 27].

Outcome

Due to the lack of long-term data and the significant variability in the clinical symptomatology ranging from neonatal onset with severe multisystem organ involvement to adult patients with minimal skin involvement, the overall outcome of patients with DADA2 remains unknown. The reported mortality rate in the literature is about 10% citing complications of intracranial hemorrhage with subsequent respiratory failure, necrotizing pneumonia, gastrointestinal perforation, and sepsis as the main causes of death [30, 33].

Conclusion

The discovery of new clinically distinct autoinflammatory syndromes is rapidly expanding. The newer syndromes are far more complex than the traditional mostly monogenic periodic fever syndromes encompassing elements of immunodeficiency, autoinflammation, and autoimmunity.

DADA2 is a relatively young member of this family of genetic conditions that is mainly characterized by an inflammatory vasculopathy resembling PAN. The phenotype of this disease is still emerging, and what we know so far about DADA2 is based on small case series in adult and pediatric patients. DADA2 appears to be highly variable in regard to age at onset, disease severity, and organ involvement. It seems almost apparent that some patients with PAN but especially those with cPAN and younger patients with CNS involvement have probably not been properly recognized as having DADA2. Consequently, testing for ADA2 levels, genetic analysis of *CECR1* gene mutations, and an underlying immunodeficiency should be part of the basic workup facilitating an expedited diagnosis and early treatment. The reason for the phenotypic variability of this condition even among patients with same gene mutations remains to be investigated.

Therapeutic decisions should be based on the individual presentation and severity of the disease since general treatment guidelines do not yet exist.

References

1. Zhou Q, Yang D, Ombrello AK, et al. Early-onset stroke and vasculopathy associated with mutations in ADA2. N Engl J Med. 2014;370:911–20.
2. Navon Elkan P, Pierce SB, Segel R, et al. Mutant adenosine deaminase 2 in a polyarteritis nodosa vasculopathy. N Engl J Med. 2014;370:921–31.
3. van Montfrans J, Zavialov A, Zhou Q. Mutant ADA2 in vasculopathies. N Engl J Med. 2014;371(5):478.
4. Bras J, Guerreiro R, Santo GC. Mutant ADA2 in vasculopathies. N Engl J Med. 2014;371(5):478–80.
5. Van Eyck L, Liston A, Wouters C. Mutant ADA2 in vasculopathies. N Engl J Med. 2014;371(5):480.
6. Garg N, Kasapcopur O, Foster J 2nd, et al. Novel adenosine deaminase 2 mutations in a child with a fatal vasculopathy. Eur J Pediatr. 2014;173(6):827–30.
7. Adenosine HM, Deficiency D. In: Adam MP, Ardinger HH, Pagon RA, et al., editors. Gene reviews. Seattle: University of Washington; 2006. p. 1993–2018.
8. Zavialov AV, Yu X, Spillmann D, et al. Structural basis for the growth factor activity of human adenosine deaminase ADA2. J Biol Chem. 2010;285:12367–77.
9. Giannelou A, Zhou Q, Kastner DL. When less is more: primary immunodeficiency with an autoinflammatory kick. Curr Opin Allergy Clin Immunol. 2014;14(6):491–500.
10. Eltzschig HK, Sitkovsky MV, Robson SC. Purinergic signaling during inflammation. N Engl J Med. 2012;367:2322–33.
11. Savic S, McDermott MF. Clinical genetics in 2014: new monogenic diseases span the immunological disease continuum. Nat Rev Rheumatol. 2015;11(2):67–8.
12. Cronstein BN, Eberle MA, Gruber HE, Levin RI. Methotrexate inhibits neutrophil function by stimulating adenosine release from connective tissue cells. Proc Natl Acad Sci U S A. 1991;88(6):2441–5.
13. Cronstein B. How does methotrexate suppress inflammation? Clin Exp Rheumatol. 2010;28(5 Suppl 61):S21–3. Epub 2010 Oct 28. Review.
14. Zavialov AV, Engstrom A. Human ADA2 belongs to a new family of growth factors with adenosine deaminase activity. Biochem J. 2005;391:51–7.
15. Belot A, Wassmer E, Twilt M, et al. Mutations in CECR1 associated with a neutrophil signature in peripheral blood. Pediatr Rheumatol Online J. 2014;12:44.
16. McColl SR, St-Onge M, Dussault AA, et al. Immunomodulatory impact of the A2A adenosine receptor on the profile of chemokines produced by neutrophils. FASEB J. 2006;20(1):187–9.

17. Zavialov AV, Garcia E, Glaichenhaus N, et al. Human adenosine deaminase 2 induces differentiation of monocytes into macrophages and stimulates proliferation of T helper cells and macrophages. J Leukoc Biol. 2010;88:279–90.
18. Caorsi R, Penco F, Grossi A, Insalaco A, Omenetti A, Alessio M, Conti G, Marchetti F, Picco P, Tommasini A, Martino S, Malattia C, Gallizi R, Podda RA, Salis A, Falcini F, Schena F, Garbarino F, Morreale A, Pardeo M, Ventrici C, Passarelli C, Zhou Q, Severino M, Gandolfo C, Damonte G, Martini A, Ravelli A, Aksentijevich I, Ceccherini I, Gattorno M. Monogenic polyarteritis: the lesson of ADA2 deficiency. Pediatric Rheumatol. 2016;14:51.
19. Gonzalez Santiago TM, Zavialov A, Saarela J, et al. Dermatologic features of ADA2 deficiency in cutaneous polyarteritis nodosa. JAMA Dermatol. 2015;1.
20. Hashem H, Kelly SJ, Ganson NJ, Hershfield MS. Deficiency of adenosine deaminase 2 (DADA2), an inherited cause of polyarteritis nodosa and a mimic of other systemic rheumatologic disorders. Curr Rheumatol Rep. 2017;19(11):70.
21. Sahin S, Adrovic A, Barut K, Ugurlu S, Turanli ET, Ozdogan H, Kasapcopur O. Clinical, imaging and genotypical features of three deceased and five surviving cases with ADA2 deficiency. Rheumatol Int. 2018;38(1):129–36.
22. Ozen S, Pistorio A, Lusan SM, et al. EULAR/PRINTO/PRES criteria for Henoch-Schonlein purpura, childhood polyarteritis nodosa, childhood Wegener granulomatosis and childhood Takayasu arteritis: Ankara 2008. Part II: final classification criteria. Ann Rheum Dis. 2010;69:798–806.
23. Gonzalez Santiago TM, Zavialov A, Saarela J, Seppanen M, Reed AM, Abraham RS, Gibson LE. Dermatologic features of ADA2 deficiency in cutaneous polyarteritis nodosa. JAMA Dermatol. 2015;151(11):1230–4.
24. Van Montfrans JM, Hartman EA, Braun KP, et al. Phenotypic variability in patients with ADA2 deficiency due to identical homozygous R169Q mutations. Rheumatology (Oxford). 2016;55(5):902–10.
25. Batu ED, Karadag O, Taskiran EZ, et al. A case series of adenosine deaminase 2-deficient patients emphasizing treatment and genotype-phenotype correlations. J Rheumatol. 2015;42(8):1532–4.
26. Wu S, Xu Z, Liang H. Sneddon's syndrome: a comprehensive review of the literature. Orphanet J Rare Dis. 2014;9:215.
27. Bolayir E, Yilmaz A, Kugu N, Erdogan H, Akyol M, Akyuz A. Sneddon's syndrome: clinical and laboratory analysis of 10 cases. Acta Med Okayama. 2004;58(2):59–65. Review
28. Nanthapisal S, Murphy C, Omoyinmi E, Hong Y, Standing A, Berg S, Ekelund M, Jolles S, Harper L, Youngstein T, Gilmour K, Klein NJ, Eleftheriou D, Brogan PA. Deficiency of adenosine deaminase type 2: a description of phenotype and genotype in fifteen cases. Arthritis Rheumatol. 2016;68:2314–22.
29. Brogan P, Eleftheriou D. Vasculitis update: pathogenesis and biomarkers. Pediatr Nephrol. 2018;33(2):187–98. https://doi.org/10.1007/s00467-017-3597-4. Epub 2017 Aug 7. Review.
30. Fellmann F, Angelini F, Wassenberg J, et al. IL-17 receptor A and adenosine deaminase 2 deficiency in siblings with recurrent infections and chronic inflammation. J Allergy Clin Immunol. 2016;137(4):1189–96.e2. https://doi.org/10.1016/j.jaci.2015.07.053. Epub 2015 Nov 20.
31. Jennette JC, Falk RJ, Bacon PA, et al. 2012 revised international Chapel Hill consensus conference nomenclature of vasculitides. Arthritis Rheum. 2013;65:1–11.
32. Schepp J, Bulashevska A, Mannhardt-Laakmann W, et al. Deficiency of adenosine deaminase 2 causes antibody deficiency. J Clin Immunol. 2016;36(3):179–86.
33. Caorsi R, Penco F, Grossi A, Insalaco A, Omenetti A, Alessio M, Conti G, Marchetti F, Picco P, Tommasini A, Martino S, Malattia C, Gallizi R, Podda RA, Salis A, Falcini F, Schena F, Garbarino F, Morreale A, Pardeo M, Ventrici C, Passarelli C, Zhou Q, Severino M, Gandolfo C, Damonte G, Martini A, Ravelli A, Aksentijevich I, Ceccherini I, Gattorno M. ADA2 deficiency (DADA2) as an unrecognised cause of early onset polyarteritis nodosa and stroke: a multicentre national study. Ann Rheum Dis. 2017;76(10):1648–56. Epub 2017 May 18.

34. Caorsi R, Omenetti A, Picco P, et al. Long-term efficacy of etanercept in ADA2 deficiency. Pediatr Rheumatol Online J. 2014;12(suppl 1):72.
35. Nihira H, Nakagawa K, Izawa K, Kawai T, Yasumi T, Nishikomori R, Nambu M, Miyagawa-Hayashino A, Nomura T, Kabashima K, Ito M, Iwaki-Egawa S, Sasahara Y, Nakayama M, Heike T. Fever of unknown origin with rashes in early infancy is indicative of adenosine deaminase type deficiency. Scand J Rheumatol. 2017;30:1–3.
36. Van Eyck JL, Hershfield MS, Pombal D, et al. Hematopoietic stem cell transplantation rescues the immunologic phenotype and prevents vasculopathy in patients with adenosine deaminase 2 deficiency. J Allergy Clin Immunol. 2015;135(1):283–7.
37. Schepp J, Proietti M, Frede N, Buchta M, Hübscher K, Rojas Restrepo J, Goldacker S, Warnatz K, Pachlopnik Schmid J, Duppenthaler A, Lougaris V, Uriarte I, Kelly S, Hershfield M, Grimbacher B. Screening of 181 patients with antibody deficiency for deficiency of adenosine deaminase 2 sheds new light on the disease in adulthood. Arthritis Rheumatol. 2017;69(8):1689–700. Epub 2017 Jul 5.
38. Collison J. Autoinflammation: stem cell transplantation for DADA2. Nat Rev Rheumatol. 2017.
39. Hashem H, Kumar AR, Müller I, Babor F, Bredius R, Dalal J, Hsu AP, Holland SM, Hickstein DD, Jolles S, Krance R, Sasa G, Taskinen M, Koskenvuo M, Saarela J, van Montfrans J, Wilson K, Bosch B, Moens L, Hershfield M, Meyts I. Hematopoietic stem cell transplantation rescues the hematological, immunological and vascular phenotype in DADA2. Blood. 2017;130(24):2682–88. https://doi.org/10.1182/blood-2017-07-798660. Epub 2017 Oct 3.

Chapter 12
Yao Syndrome

Qingping Yao

Abbreviations

NOD2	Nucleotide-binding, oligomerization domain 2
SAID	Systemic autoinflammatory disease
YAOS	Yao syndrome

Clinical Phenotype

YAOS was initially reported by us from the Cleveland Clinic, United States, in 2011 [1], and its clinical phenotype has been well characterized since [2–6]. This disease possesses clinical features of systemic autoinflammatory diseases (SAIDs) with absence/lower titer of antinuclear antibodies or antigen specific T cells. YAOS is a polygenic systemic disease, and its phenotype and genotype are described below.

Demographics and Population Genetics

Patients with YAOS are predominantly white adults with a female to male ratio of 2:1 at an estimated disease prevalence of 1–10/100,000 [3]. The disease is relatively common when compared with monogenic SAIDs like cryopyrin-associated

Q. Yao
Department of Medicine, Stony Brook University School of Medicine,
Stony Brook, NY, USA
e-mail: QingPing.Yao@stonybrookmedicine.edu

P. Efthimiou (ed.), *Auto-Inflammatory Syndromes*,
https://doi.org/10.1007/978-3-319-96929-9_12

periodic syndrome in the American adult patient population [7]. Pediatric cases of YAOS have been reported also [8]. Disease occurrence is primarily sporadic, though a minority of patients may have a positive family history.

Fever

Patients usually present with flu-like symptoms, fatigue, and weight loss. Besides these constitutional symptoms, recurrent or intermittent fever of varying degrees is common, and febrile episodes occur every a few weeks to months with a duration of several days to a few weeks with spontaneous resolution.

Dermatitis

Patients present with episodic rash in 90% of cases, and it is described as erythematous patches or plaques on the face, trunk, and limbs (Fig. 12.1). The rash is mostly non-itchy or minimally itchy and occurs every a few weeks to months with a

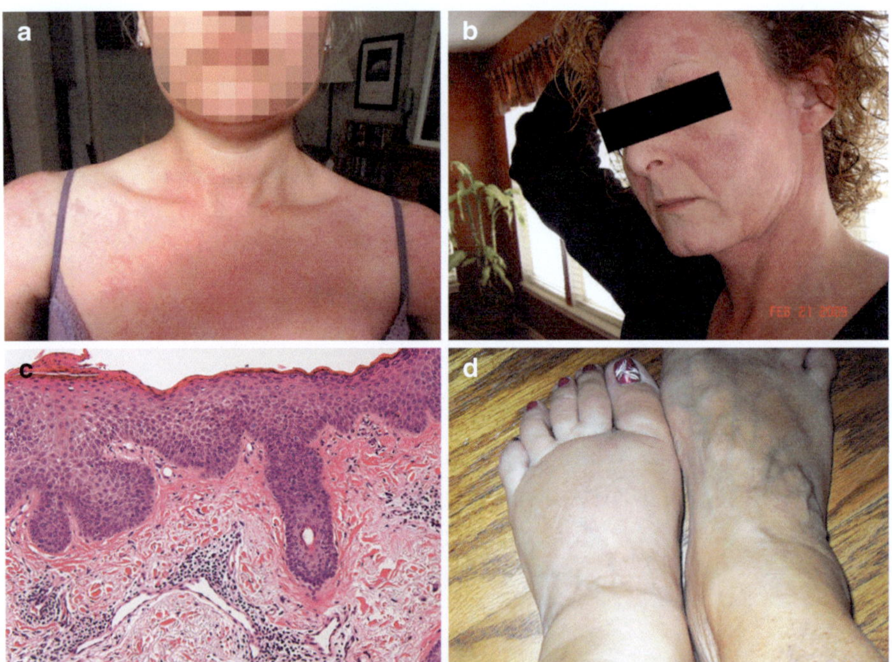

Fig. 12.1 Clinical features of YAOS patients. (**a**) Patchy erythema on upper chest. (**b**) Erythematous plaques on face. (**c**) Subacute spongiotic dermatitis. (**d**) Distal lower extremity swelling

duration of several days to weeks. The cutaneous histopathology is consistent with spongiotic dermatitis in a majority of cases, and granulomatous dermatitis is extremely rare.

Inflammatory Arthritis

Patients (90%) present with intermittent inflammatory arthritis, manifesting as olio- or polyarthralgia with variable morning stiffness in the peripheral joints, particularly in the lower extremities. A quarter of patients have unilateral or bilateral distal lower extremity swelling intermittently. Radiographs of affected joints show soft tissue swelling without erosions or joint narrowing. A magnetic resonance image of the ankle can show periarticular soft tissue swelling.

Gastrointestinal Symptoms

Patients present with gastrointestinal symptoms in 60% of cases, often manifesting as episodic mild to moderate abdominal cramping pain with bloating and non-bloody diarrhea. Upper and lower gastrointestinal endoscopy with pathology reveals no findings of inflammatory bowel disease like Crohn disease, but nonspecific colitis may be seen occasionally.

Sicca-Like Symptoms

Approximately 60% of patients complain of sicca-like symptoms with a positive Schirmer test sometimes, but there is no serological (anti-SSA/SSB antibodies) or pathological evidence of primary Sjögren syndrome on a minor salivary gland biopsy. Patients can present with eyelid rash and swelling but without uveitis. Ocular myositis can rarely happen.

Others

Patients can complain of chest pain, and pleuritis/pericarditis can happen. Recurrent oral ulcers occur in 20% of cases, and these patients generally have no genital ulcers. Lymphadenopathy can occur without evidence of malignancy.

Laboratory and Genetic/Molecular Testing

Generally, white blood cell count is normal; mild leukocytosis and anemia can be seen. Liver and renal functions are generally normal. Urinalysis is pristine. Acute phase reactants, such as erythrocyte sedimentation rate and C-reactive protein, can be elevated in approximately 50% of cases.

All patients carry *NOD2* variants as tested by targeted DNA or next-generation sequencing; nearly all patients carry *NOD2* $IVS8^{+158}$ variant, and up to 25% of patients have concurrent *NOD2* R702W. Haplotype of *NOD2* $IVS8^{+158}$ with L1007 fs or G908R can be seen in some cases. Other rarer *NOD2* variants have been reported as well.

Diagnosis and Differential Diagnosis

YAOS is different than inflammatory bowel disease, Blau syndrome, primary Sjögren syndrome, and monogenic hereditary SAIDs [2] (Table 12.1).

The diagnosis of YAOS is dependent on the characteristic phenotype and genotype, as well as exclusion criteria (Table 12.2) [4].

Pathophysiology

Nucleotide-binding, oligomerization domain 2 (*NOD2*) is an intracellular bacterial sensor protein of the NOD-like receptor (NLR) family [9]. The *NOD2* gene is mapped to chromosome 16q12-21, and several genetic variants are known to predispose individuals to the development of inflammatory diseases, such as Crohn disease, Blau syndrome, and YAOS [10] (Fig. 12.2). *NOD2* as an innate immune receptor in the cytosol detects a component of the bacterial cell wall and muramyl dipeptide (MDP) and stimulates signal transduction cascades. These in turn activate NF-κB and mitogen-activated kinases (MAPKs) and result in the secretion of pro-inflammatory cytokines (Fig. 12.3). Normally, *NOD2* proteins serve as defense against microbial infections, regulation of the inflammatory process, and apoptosis [10], as well as enhance autophagy to dispose damaged organelles and protect cells.

In disease state like YAOS, as a result of the genetic defects, *NOD2* expression and its signal transduction are aberrant, and this in turn leads to imbalanced inflammatory process, such as overproduction of certain pro-inflammatory cytokines like IL-6 [11]. These data underscore the significance of the abnormal innate immune response as a hallmark of the disease. It is postulated that YAOS as a genetically complex disease may occur due to the interplay between the defective *NOD2* and environmental factors or triggers. Future study of a broader immune function in the disease is warranted.

Table 12.1 Differentiating features between the major autoinflammatory diseases

	YAOS	BS	FMF	TRAPS	HIDS	CAPS
Age at onset	Adult	<5 years	<20 years	<20 years	Child	Infancy
Fever	Several days	Rare	<3 days	>7 days	3–7 days	1–2 days
Serositis	Yes	No	Yes	Yes	Yes	Rare
Joints	Oligo- or polyarthritis	Polyarthritis, granulomatous, camptodactyly	Monoarthritis	Mono- or oligoarthritis	Polyarthralgia	Deforming arthritis
Skin	Spongiotic dermatitis, primarily erythematous patches/plaques	Granulomatous dermatitis, mostly papulonodular rash and subcutaneous plaques	Erysipeloid rash on the lower extremities	Various, mostly erythematous patches/plaques, underlying myalgia	Maculopapular rash	Urticaria-like
GI symptoms	Yes	No	Peritonitis-related	Yes	Yes	No
Sicca	Yes	Yes	No	No	No	No
Uveitis	No	Yes	No	No	No	Rare
Inheritance	Unknown, mostly sporadic	Dominant	Recessive	Dominant	Recessive	Dominant
Gene mutations	NOD2: LRR	NOD2: NBD	MEFV	TNFRSF1A	MVK	NLRP3/CIAS1
Therapy	GC, sulfasalazine, IL-1/IL-6 inhibitors	NSAID, GC, infliximab	Colchicine, TNFα inhibitors, IL-1 inhibitors	NSAID, GC, TNFα inhibitors, IL-1 inhibitors	NSAID, TNFα inhibitors, IL-1 inhibitors	IL-1 inhibitors

Reprinted with permission from Yao et al. [2]

YAOS Yao syndrome, *BS* Blau syndrome, *FMF* familial Mediterranean fever, *TRAPS* TNF receptor-associated periodic syndrome, *HIDS* hyper-IgD periodic fever syndrome, *CAPS* cryopyrin-associated periodic syndrome, *GI* gastrointestinal, *LRR* leucine-rich repeat, *NBD* nucleotide-binding domain, *MEFV* Mediterranean fever, *TNFRSF1A* tumor necrosis factor receptor superfamily 1A, *MVK* mevalonate kinase, *NLRP3* NLR family pyrin domain containing 3, *CIAS1* cold-induced autoinflammatory syndrome, *GC* glucocorticoids, *NSAID* nonsteroidal anti-inflammatory drugs, *IL-1/IL-6* interleukin-1/interleukin-6

Table 12.2 The diagnostic criteria for Yao syndrome

Clinical criteria	Comments
Major	
1	Periodic occurrence ≥ twice
2	Recurrent fever and/or dermatitis
Minor	
1	Oligo- or polyarthralgia/inflammatory arthritis or distal extremity swelling
2	Abdominal pain and/or diarrhea
3	Sicca-like symptoms
4	Pericarditis and/or pleuritis
Molecular criterion	*NOD2* IVS8^{+158} and/or R702W or other rare variants
Exclusion criteria	High titer ANAs, inflammatory bowel disease, Blau syndrome, adult sarcoidosis, primary Sjögren syndrome, and monogenic autoinflammatory diseases

Reprinted with permission from Yao and Shen [4]
Yao syndrome is diagnosed if 2 major criteria, ≥1 minor criteria, the molecular criterion, and exclusion criteria are fulfilled

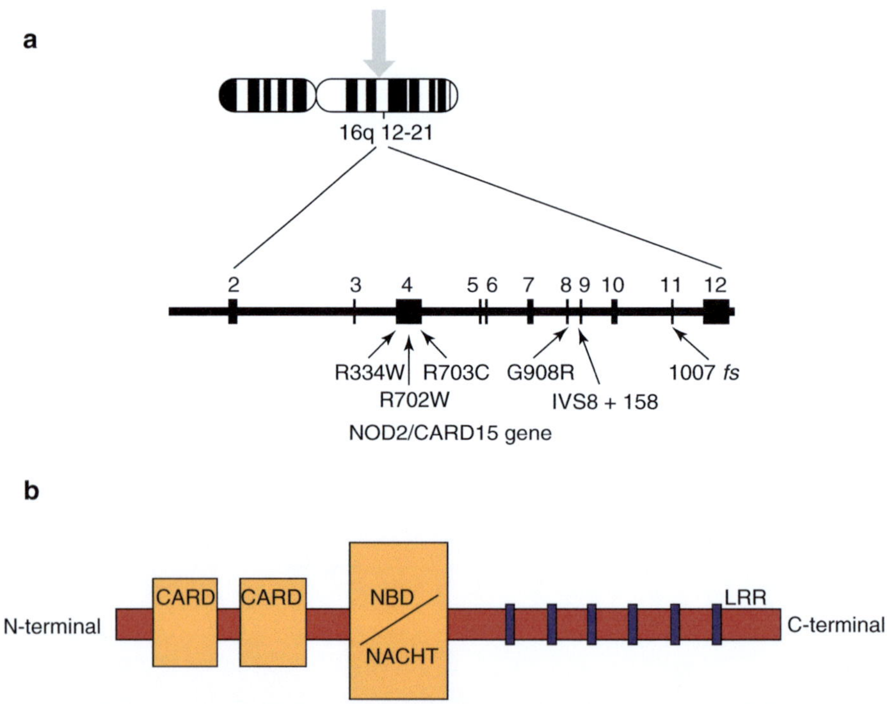

Fig. 12.2 NOD2 protein structure

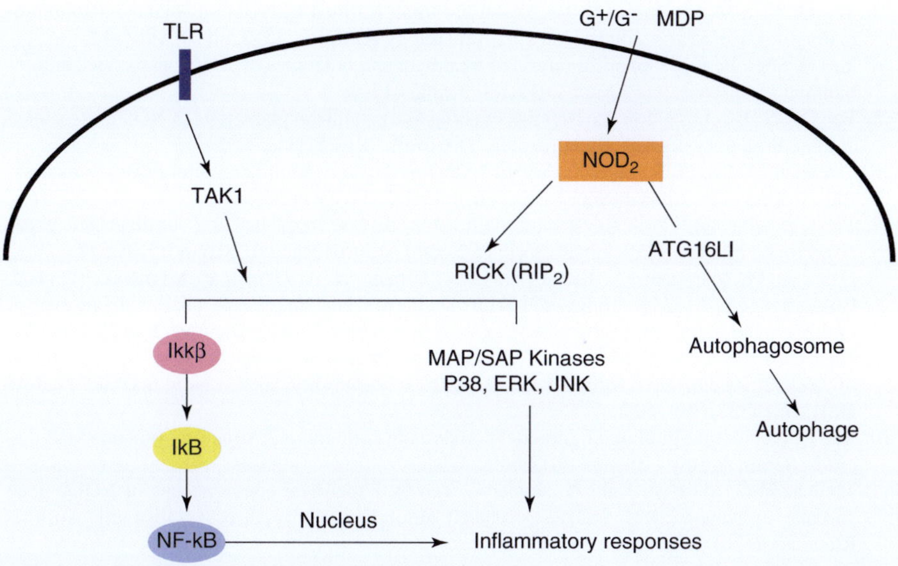

Fig. 12.3 Inflammatory response via NOD2 molecule

Therapy and Prognosis [4]

Therapeutic regimen for YAOS consists of glucocorticoids and/or sulfasalazine in general. For refractory symptoms, both IL-1 and IL-6 antagonists, such as canakinumab and tocilizumab, may be tried with effectiveness. As a systemic inflammatory disease, YAOS involves multiorgans but with rare influence on the internal solid organs. It can cause chronic pain syndrome, fibromyalgia, and even disability in some cases. Relatively common comorbidities are fibromyalgia, asthma, and urinary stones. Early and prompt recognition of the disease can minimize duplication of extensive and expensive testing, and with a correct diagnosis, physicians are able to manage the patients with assurance.

Acknowledgment I am grateful to my collaborators in both clinical and translational studies of the disease over the last several years. I am also thankful to the Cleveland Clinic and Stony Brook University, where the disease was discovered and has been studied.

References

1. Yao Q, Zhou L, Cusumano P, Bose N, Piliang M, Jayakar B, et al. A new category of autoinflammatory disease associated with NOD2 gene mutations. Arthritis Res Ther. 2011;13(5):R148.
2. Yao Q, Su LC, Tomecki KJ, Zhou L, Jayakar B, Shen B. Dermatitis as a characteristic phenotype of a new autoinflammatory disease associated with NOD2 mutations. J Am Acad Dermatol. 2013;68(4):624–31.

3. Yao Q, Shen M, McDonald C, Lacbawan F, Moran R, Shen B. NOD2-associated autoinflammatory disease: a large cohort study. Rheumatology (Oxford). 2015;54(10):1904–12.
4. Yao Q, Shen B. A systematic analysis of treatment and outcomes of NOD2-associated autoinflammatory disease. Am J Med. 2017;130(3):365 e13–8.
5. Yao Q, Schils J. Distal lower extremity swelling as a prominent phenotype of NOD2-associated autoinflammatory disease. Rheumatology (Oxford). 2013;52(11):2095–7.
6. Estephan M, Yao Q, Springer J. Case of NOD2-associated autoinflammatory disease successfully treated with sulfasalazine. J Clin Rheumatol. 2017;23(1):58–9.
7. Yao Q, Lacbawan F, Li J. Adult autoinflammatory disease frequency and our diagnostic experience in an adult autoinflammatory clinic. Semin Arthritis Rheum. 2016;45(5):633–7.
8. Dziedzic M, Marjanska A, Babol-Pokora K, Urbanczyk A, Grzesk E, Mlynarski W, et al. Co-existence of Blau syndrome and NAID? Diagnostic challenges associated with presence of multiple pathogenic variants in NOD2 gene: a case report. Pediatr Rheumatol. 2017;15(1):57.
9. Hugot JP, Chamaillard M, Zouali H, Lesage S, Cezard JP, Belaiche J, et al. Association of NOD2 leucine-rich repeat variants with susceptibility to Crohn's disease. Nature. 2001;411(6837):599–603.
10. Yao Q. Nucleotide-binding oligomerization domain containing 2: structure, function, and diseases. Semin Arthritis Rheum. 2013;68:624–31.
11. McDonald C, Shen M, Kabi A, Homer C, Yao Q. Functional consequences of NOD2 gene variants in patients with NOD2-associated autoinflammatory disease [abstract]. Arthritis Rheumatol. 2015;67(suppl 10):1719–20.

Part II
Polygenic Autoinflammatory Diseases

Chapter 13
Systemic Juvenile Idiopathic Arthritis

Ricardo A. G. Russo and María Martha Katsicas

Introduction

Systemic juvenile idiopathic arthritis (SJIA) is a disease of unknown etiology characterized by arthritis and systemic symptoms such as highly spiking daily fever, evanescent skin rash, organomegaly, and serositis. There is evidence that SJIA represents a diverse group of clinically and genetically distinct illnesses [1]. Due to the prominent abnormalities observed in the innate immunity components, dramatic response to IL-1 inhibitors, occurrence at very young age, equal frequency among males and females, and absence of pathogenic autoantibodies, the disease is considered to be a complex, polygenic autoinflammatory disorder by many researchers [2–5].

In this chapter, pathogenetic mechanisms, clinical features, clues to diagnosis, and classification as well as treatment approaches will be discussed.

Epidemiology

The prevalence of SJIA is 3.5 per 100,000 children, and its incidence ranges between 0.4 and 0.9 per 100,000 children per year [6, 7]. There is no specific ethnic predilection; a large number of studies have demonstrated equal distribution between girls and boys. While the disease can start at any age before the 16th birthday, its onset more common in children below 6 years; the peak age of onset occurs at age 3 years [8, 9]. SJIA represents nearly 5–25% of patients with juvenile idiopathic arthritis (JIA) in

R. A. G. Russo (✉) · M. M. Katsicas
Service of Immunology & Rheumatology, Hospital de Pediatría Prof. Dr. Juan P. Garrahan, Buenos Aires, Argentina
e-mail: rrusso@garrahan.gov.ar

P. Efthimiou (ed.), *Auto-Inflammatory Syndromes*,
https://doi.org/10.1007/978-3-319-96929-9_13

cohort studies, but this proportion differs in different parts of the world. However, SJIA accounts for nearly two-thirds of the total mortality rate in JIA [10, 11].

Classification

SJIA is classified among the complex autoinflammatory diseases of unknown etiology and also as a category of the JIA as defined by the International League of Associations for Rheumatology (ILAR) classification criteria [2, 12]. According to this set of criteria, classification of SJIA requires the presence of arthritis and a documented quotidian fever of at least 2 weeks´ duration, plus one of the following: typical rash, generalized lymphadenopathy, enlargement of liver or spleen, or serositis. The disease spectrum includes both those patients with mild, monocyclic forms and those with a severe, destructive course. SJIA is clinically heterogeneous and involves patients who exhibit the purely systemic features but never develop arthritis (or the joint component appears months or years after the disease onset). These patients cannot be classified according to the ILAR criteria but may fit the Yamaguchi criteria for adult-onset Still's disease [13–15].

Pathogenesis

The pathogenic mechanisms of SJIA are poorly understood. Growing evidence suggests a major disbalance in innate immunity pathways: disturbed proinflammatory cytokine expression patterns and inappropriate downregulation of immune activation are major determinants of the immunological abnormalities of the disease [3].

There is ample evidence supporting the autoinflammatory nature of SJIA, at least in its early phases. Expansion and dysfunction of circulating innate immune effector cells – neutrophils, monocytes, and natural killer (NK) cells – and increased expression of proinflammatory molecules and innate immune receptors, as well as lower expression of regulatory mediators, are frequently reported and proposed as key pathogenic mechanisms of the disease [16–18]. Some authors propose that SJIA could evolve in a biphasic fashion, from a disease of predominantly autoinflammatory features in its early stages to one in which interleukin (IL)-17-mediated autoimmunity may have a role in joint-related outcomes [19–21].

Cytokines Several studies support the predominant pathogenic roles of IL-1β, IL-6, and IL-18 in SJIA. Disbalance of IL-10, IL-17, interferon (IFN)-γ, and tumor necrosis factor (TNF)-α is also involved [22–24]. Shimizu et al. supported the heterogeneity of the disease by describing different plasma cytokine profiles in patients with SJIA: an IL-6-dominant group (with predominant arthritic symptoms and good response to IL-6 inhibitors) and an IL-1β-/IL-18-dominant group (with mainly systemic symptoms, predisposition to develop macrophage activation syndrome [MAS], and good response to IL-1 blockers) [25, 26].

There is substantial evidence that IL-1β plays a major role in SJIA. Pascual et al. not only showed high levels of IL-1β in supernatants of stimulated peripheral blood mononuclear cells (PBMCs) of SJIA patients but also demonstrated that serum of SJIA patients induced transcription and secretion of IL-1β by healthy PBMCs [22]. However, other researchers could not observe the same phenomena [27, 28]. Gene expression profiling in PBMCs demonstrates upregulation of components of the IL-1, IL-18, and toll-like receptor (TLR) signaling pathways and of components of the NLRP3 inflammasome [22, 29, 30]. Moreover, therapeutic benefit of IL-1 blocking agents also supports the pathogenic role of IL-1 [22, 31].

IL-18 – another IL-1 family member – also has a disease-promoting role in SJIA. Excessive IL-18 plasma levels reflect disease activity, and they may persist even during inactive disease phases [23, 24, 28, 32, 33].

IL-6 is also believed to be a central pathogenic cytokine. Elevated IL-6 levels have been demonstrated in synovial fluid as well as in plasma of SJIA patients in several studies. Their levels correlated with disease activity and with systemic symptoms and laboratory abnormalities (anemia and thrombocytosis) [34–36]. Also, IL-6 inhibition through the use of anti-IL-6 receptor-monoclonal antibodies has proven highly efficacious in controlling systemic and arthritic symptoms in SJIA [37]. Additionally, there is in vitro evidence demonstrating a reduced inhibition of IL-6 by IL-10 in patients with SJIA as compared to healthy controls [38, 39].

Animal models of SJIA endorse the pathogenic role of IL-1β, IL-6, and IL-18 as well [40–43]. Finally, while IFNγ levels are not particularly elevated during active phases of SJIA, this cytokine seems to be central in the development of MAS [44].

NK Cells NK cell number and function are abnormal at least in a proportion of patients with SJIA. Some investigators have found decreased numbers of NK cells in whole-blood samples of SJIA patients as compared to patients with other categories of JIA or healthy controls [45–48]. Grom et al. demonstrated reduced perforin expression and suppressed cytolytic activity of NK cells in a number of SJIA patients [47]; the same group also showed that a proportion of patients with SJIA who have not yet had an episode of MAS exhibit decreased NK cytolytic function and absence of circulating $CD56^{bright}$ population [48]. Wulffraat et al. found similar defects in a group of SJIA patients, and these abnormalities were reversible upon autologous stem cell transplantation [49]. Put et al. [50] did not find these defects but demonstrated decreased granzyme K expression in $CD56^{bright}$ NK cells. These authors also analyzed the gene expression in NK cells and found increased expression of components of innate pathways, such as TLR-4 and S100 proteins, and decreased expression of granzyme K and IL-10 receptor, which have immune regulatory properties [50]. It has been proposed that the characteristic inflammatory environment of SJIA (with abundant IL-6 and IL-18) alters NK cell function leading to decreased NK cell numbers, decreased production of IFNγ, perforin and granzyme K, and the simultaneous increased production of proinflammatory cytokines [51, 52]. Interestingly, de Jager et al. found that the decreased NK cell responses to IL-18 are associated with decreased phosphorylation of the IL-18 receptor [53].

Monocytes/Macrophages Monocytes seem to be a key effector cell in the pathogenesis of the disease. Expansion and activation of monocytes in active SJIA, likely related to increased monocyte resistance to apoptosis, have been clearly demonstrated by Macaubas et al. [54]. Monocytes from SJIA patients appear to have a mixed polarization phenotype, with features of both classically (M1) and alternatively (M2) activated populations [55]. Activated macrophages with M1 phenotype are potential sources of proinflammatory cytokines, while those with M2 phenotype would be responsible for an anti-inflammatory, compensatory, regulatory mechanism during inactive state. According to one study, the microRNA miR-125a-5p contributes to regulatory macrophage polarization with expression of both inflammatory cytokines and M2-associated markers [56].

The predominant role of the innate immune system in SJIA is also demonstrated by the uniquely high serum concentrations of products of activated granulocytes and monocytes, the proteins S100A8 (or myeloid-related protein [MRP]8) and S100A9 (or MRP14) and the neutrophil-derived S100A12, which may act as endogenous TLR ligands [57–59].

Genetics

There are few demonstrated HLA associations with SJIA. A large genome-wide association study of SJIA has showed an association with the HLA class II locus, consistent with T cell autoimmunity. This study of 988 SJIA patients from different regions of the world identified several SJIA-associated risk loci: the MHC locus on chromosome 6 (HLA-DRB1*11 was strongly associated with SJIA) and another susceptibility locus on the short arm of chromosome 1 (1p36.32) [60]. Another study on a smaller sample supported the HLA-DRB1*11 association [61]. On the other hand, polymorphisms in non-HLA genes such as *TNF*, *IL-1*, *IL-6*, macrophage inhibitory factor (*MIF*), interferon regulatory factor (*IRF*) 1, and IL-10 have been reported to be associated with the disease [62–69]. Similarly, polymorphisms in *IRF5* have been associated with susceptibility to MAS [70]. Additional genetic abnormalities affecting other components of the innate immune system, such as *P2X7* (encoding an ATP receptor involved in IL-1 regulation), have also been reported [28].

Polymorphisms in the *MEFV* gene and duplications in the *NLRP* gene cluster have been reported in patients with SJIA [71–73]. The implications of such associations on the phenotypical expression of SJIA are still unknown.

Several polymorphisms and protein-altering variants in gene coding for proteins involved in the cytolytic pathway have been described in patients with SJIA. Variants in *perforin, LYST, MUNC13–4,* and *STXBP2* genes may be related to susceptibility to develop MAS [16, 74–77].

Finally, a monogenic, autosomal-recessive form of SJIA has been described in six consanguineous families from southern Saudi Arabia and Lebanon. A missense mutation in the gene *FAMIN* (Fatty Acid Metabolism-Immunity Nexus, formerly also referred to as *LACC1*) was found by whole-exome sequencing and confirmed by Sanger sequencing in patients with a SJIA-like disease that satisfied ILAR classification criteria [78, 79].

Clinical Features

Typical clinical features are fever, arthritis, rash, lymphadenopathy, serositis, and hepatosplenomegaly.

Fever Fever is present in 95–98% of patients [8]. In many cases, it may precede the onset of arthritis by weeks or months. The fever pattern is typically quotidian, and it occurs once or twice daily, more often during the evening. Commonly reaching 39 °C axillary, temperature exceeding 40,5 °C is rare. Fever is coincident with the rash in 80% of patients. The classic fever pattern is only present in 37% of patients; morning (12%), bi-daily (15%), intermittent (27%), and unremitting (5%) fever patterns are also observed [8].

Arthritis Arthritis is present at onset in 88% of patients, and it may appear months or years after disease onset [8, 80]. The most frequently involved joints at presentation are wrists, knees, ankles, cervical spine, and hips. The joint pattern is usually symmetrical, polyarticular (45%), or oligoarticular (40%), while involvement of a single joint is extremely infrequent [7.8]. Synovial cysts are frequent [81]. At least 40% of patients will show a chronically active arthritic course, and bilateral, destructive changes in hips and wrists may occur [82].

Rash Nearly 80% of patients exhibit skin rash at onset (Fig. 13.1). Macular papules are usually salmon pink-colored or erythematous and morbilliform, surrounded by a pallor zone; purpuric lesions are not seen and pruritus may accompany in 5% of cases. The diameter of the individual lesions usually ranges between 2 and 5 mm, also larger, coalescent lesions may occur [7]. Its most distinctive feature is evanescence; it may be coincident with fever and migratory. Sites where rash is most common are trunk and proximal extremities. Pathology usually demonstrates subdermal, perivascular infiltrates of neutrophils and monocytes, accompanied by a marked expression of endothelial adhesion molecules. Keratinocytes are activated and express MRP 8 and MRP 14 [83].

Lymphadenopathy Generalized lymphadenopathy is observed in 25% of patients [6, 8, 82]. It usually consists in mobile nodes on the cervical, axillary, inguinal, epithroclear, mesenteric, and mediastinal groups. They may mimic malignances like lymphomas; biopsy often reveals reactive changes [84].

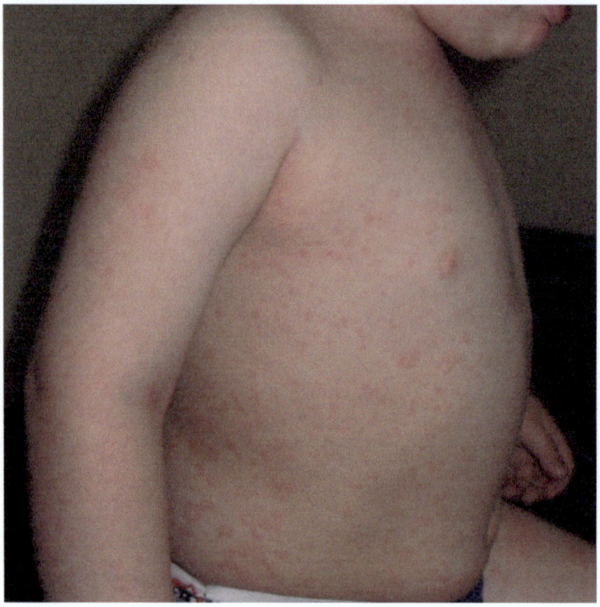

Fig. 13.1 Erythematous, salmon-pink colored, morbilliform rash in a 3-year-old patient with active systemic juvenile idiopathic arthritis

Hepatomegaly/Splenomegaly Splenomegaly has been described in 50% of patients, and it is usually evident during active phases. Hepatomegaly does not occur as often as splenomegaly, though abnormal liver enzymes may be observed irrespective of the presence of hepatomegaly. Liver biopsy usually exhibits periportal infiltrates. Hepatosplenomegaly may be the initial sign of MAS or amyloidosis [82].

Serositis Pericarditis is the most common form of serositis, and it can be detected in nearly 10–15% patients; pleuritis and peritonitis are rare [11].

Less frequent manifestations are aseptic meningitis, pseudotumor cerebri, encephalopathy and CNS hemorrhage (as part of MAS), myocarditis, endocarditis, congestive heart failure, coronary artery dilatation, pulmonary artery hypertension, interstitial lung disease, lipoid pneumonia, orbital tenosynovitis (Brown's Syndrome), uveitis, glomerulonephritis, and nasal septal perforation [85–90].

Radiological Features Radiographic changes are not specific. Early changes include soft tissue involvement and juxta-articular osteoporosis. Abnormalities in the development and maturation of ossification centers, joint space narrowing due to cartilage damage, bony erosions, and growth abnormalities usually appear later during the disease course. Joint damage is more frequent in the hips, wrists, temporomandibular joints, and cervical spine [91, 92]. A meaningful proportion of patients with SJIA develop joint damage within 2 years, while 75% of patients show radiographic damage at 5 years after diagnosis [93, 94]. Rapid progression can be observed despite aggressive treatment, particularly in the hips [95].

Complications

Macrophage Activation Syndrome MAS, a form of secondary or reactive hemophagocytic lymphohistiocytosis, is a serious complication of SJIA, and it is associated with a mortality rate approaching 10–20% [96, 97]. Even though MAS may develop during active SJIA in the absence of a recognizable trigger, different factors such as infections (remarkably EBV-related) or changes in therapy have been associated to its onset [97–99]. The syndrome occurs in 5–20% of SJIA patients, but this proportion may reach 50% if cases of subclinical MAS are included [96]. MAS represents the most severe end of a continuous clinical spectrum of disease activity in SJIA. Its hallmark is an uncontrolled dysfunctional immune response with massive expansion of T lymphocytes and macrophage populations leading to marked hypercytokinemia and multiorgan failure [100]. The syndrome may develop either abruptly or progressively over the course of several days; clinical suspicion and timely diagnosis should occur before the full-blown picture is overt and chances of organ failure increase (Table 13.1). Typical features are continuous fever (as opposed to the intermittent fever occurring during active SJIA), fixed rash that may include petechiae or purpura, encephalopathy, hepatosplenomegaly, and a paradoxical improvement in the joint symptoms. Laboratory abnormalities include pancytopenia

Table 13.1 Clinical features and laboratory abnormalities during active systemic juvenile idiopathic arthritis (SJIA), transition to macrophage activation syndrome, and macrophage activation syndrome (MAS)

Feature	SJIA	Transition	MAS
Skin rash	Evanescent	Mixed	Fixed
Arthritis	++	+	+/–
Lymphadenopathy	++	+++	++++
Hepatosplenomegaly	++	+++	++++
Edema	–	+	++
Fever	Intermittent	Continuous	Continuous
Neurologic symptoms	–	+/–	+
Hemorrhage	–	Petechiae	++
Anemia	++	++	+++
WBC	↑↑	Normal	Normal or ↓
Platelet count	↑↑↑	Normal	Normal or ↓
ESR	↑↑↑	Normal	Normal
Ferritin	↑	↑↑	↑↑↑
LDH	Normal or ↑	↑	↑↑
Fibrinogen	↑↑	Normal or ↓	↓↓
AST	Normal or ↑	↑	↑↑

Table 13.2 Classification criteria for SJIA-associated macrophage activation syndrome

A febrile patient with known or suspected SJIA is classified as having MAS if the following criteria are met	
Criteria	Required value
Ferritin	>684 ng/ml
And any two of the following	
Platelet count	$<181 \times 10^9$/liter
Aspartate aminotransferase	>45 units/liter
Triglycerides	>156 mg/dl
Fibrinogen	≤360 mg/dl

From Ravelli et al. [102]
Laboratory abnormalities should not be otherwise explained by the patient's condition, such as concomitant immune-mediated thrombocytopenia, infectious hepatitis, visceral leishmaniasis, or familial hyperlipidemia

(or decreasing white blood cell and platelet counts), elevated liver enzymes, coagulopathy, hyperferritinemia, hypertriglyceridemia, normal or falling erythrocyte sedimentation rate (ESR), hypofibrinogenemia, elevated D-dimers, reduced NK-cell numbers and cytotoxic activity, and increased serum sCD25 (or interleukin-2 receptor α-chain) [97, 101]. Recently, classification criteria for SJIA-associated MAS were developed by an international panel of experts [102] (Table 13.2). Evidence of hemophagocytosis is commonly found in bone marrow aspirates, but it is not a mandatory criterion for diagnosis [103].

Growth Delay Growth delay is associated to active disease, corticosteroids treatment, and poor nutrition. Catch up growth is incomplete in 30% and mean final height is −2 SD [92, 104].

Amyloidosis Amyloidosis is a rare complication. It typically occurs late in patients with persistent active disease and elevated levels of serum amyloid-A (SAA) and other inflammatory proteins [72, 105]. Lately, the use of efficacious biologic agents has led to better control of inflammation and a dramatic decrease in the frequency of this complication [106].

Osteoporosis Longer disease duration, persistent inflammatory activity, use of corticosteroids, biologic action of proinflammatory cytokines, muscle atrophy, and sedentarism predispose SJIA patients to osteoporosis. Vertebral fractures are frequent, while bone mineral density catch up is usually incomplete [107–110].

Laboratory Examination and Biomarkers

Laboratory findings reflect systemic inflammation during active phases. There are no specific tests, but typically high C-reactive protein and ESR, leukocytosis with neutrophilia, marked thrombocytosis, and microcytic anemia are present during active phases. Autoantibodies are absent, and complement levels may be normal or elevated.

Serum biomarkers that reflect disease activity include ferritin, S100A8, S100A9 (or the S100A8/S100A9 complex, calprotectin), and S100A12. The serum levels of these proteins are significantly higher in patients with SJIA than in patients with confounding conditions (such as Kawasaki disease [KD] or infections) and correlate well -and early- with disease activity and response to treatment, which has led some investigators to propose them as predictors of relapses [58, 111–115]. Increased transaminase levels, abnormal coagulation screen, a fall in fibrinogen and platelet count, and increasing serum ferritin levels may precede the onset of MAS [101]. Serum levels of soluble CD163 and sCD25 (markers of activation and expansion of macrophages and T cells, respectively) may aid with the diagnosis of MAS and assessment of treatment response [116].

Other proposed biomarkers of disease activity are serum follistatin-like protein 1 (FSTL-1), IL-18, and SAA [117–120]. Interestingly, SAA levels may persist elevated during inactive phases, probably revealing subclinical ongoing inflammation. Additionally, plasma and urine proteomic profiling may exhibit a "signature" associated to the active phases of the disease [121–123]. One study demonstrated that programmed death ligand-1 (PD-L1) expression on monocytes was significantly lower in SJIA than in patients with febrile illnesses such as infections or KD [115]. Finally, gene expression analysis may discriminate between active and inactive phases and provide additional predictors of flares or MAS [16].

Diagnosis: Differential Diagnosis

Diagnosis is made on the basis of clinical features and exclusion of infections, malignances, autoimmune diseases, and monogenic autoinflammatory syndromes [8]. Although serum levels of MRP proteins or IL-18 may support the clinical suspicion, there are no specific biomarkers that allow the differentiation of the disease from other conditions or JIA categories [112, 124]. The spectrum of clinical manifestations is wide and may overlap with those that are common in other febrile diseases of childhood (Table 13.3). Children with SJIA may fulfill criteria for KD at presentation. It has been estimated that 0.2% of patients with a diagnosis of KD will later be diagnosed as SJIA. Features suggestive of SJIA are MAS, an incomplete KD phenotype, and persistence of arthritis [90].

Treatment

The optimal management of SJIA requires a multidisciplinary team that includes, but is not limited to, pediatric rheumatologists, nurses, physiotherapists, occupational therapists, social workers, and psychologists.

Table 13.3 Differential diagnosis in SJIA

Confounding disease	Clinical features
Infections	
Bacterial endocarditis	Heart murmurs, low-grade fever
Acute rheumatic fever	Migratory polyarthritis, carditis, chorea
Cat scratch disease	Lymphadenopathy, arthritis
Lyme disease	Arthritis, erythema migrans
Brucellosis	Arthritis, rash, visceromegaly
Mycoplasma	Arthritis, rash
Leishmaniasis	Arthritis, rash, visceromegaly
Parvovirus	Arthritis, fixed rash
Malignancy	
Acute lymphoblastic leukemia	Arthritis, usually periarthritis or pseudoarthritis, and bone pain
Lymphoma	Lymphadenopathy, visceromegaly
Rheumatic Diseases	
Systemic lupus erythematosus	Rash, arthritis, low-grade fever, lymphadenopathy, nephritis
Polyarteritis nodosa	Arthralgia/arthritis, nodules, fever
Kawasaki disease	Conjunctivitis, cracked lips, rash, fever, edema
Autoinflammatory Syndromes	
Familial Mediterranean fever	Abdominal pain, arthralgia, fever
Mevalonate kinase deficiency	Arthritis, visceromegaly, rash
Periodic fever, aphthous stomatitis, pharyngitis, and adenitis (PFAPA)	Aphthous stomatitis, pharyngitis, fever
TNF receptor-associated periodic syndrome (TRAPS)	Conjunctivitis, rash, arthritis, fever, fasciitis
Cryopyrin-associated periodic syndrome (CAPS)	Rash, arthralgia, fever, hearing loss
Blau's syndrome	Arthritis, ichthyosiform rash, uveitis
Familial HLH	Rash, fever, visceromegaly, recurrent MAS

Corticosteroids The initial pharmacological therapy consists in nonsteroidal anti-inflammatory drugs supplemented with corticosteroids in variable amounts according to the severity of the disease [125], but the more ample availability of anti-IL-1 agents has led some groups to use the IL-1R antagonist, anakinra (ANK) very early during the disease course, even before or instead of the prescription of corticosteroids [126–129]. Indications for the use of steroids are presence of anemia, myocarditis, pericarditis, pleuritis, peritonitis, and MAS. Recommendations for steroid dosing and tapering have been developed [130]. Pulse methylprednisolone may be useful in certain circumstances, such as MAS.

DMARDs Traditional disease-modifying agents have not demonstrated consistent efficacy in SJIA. Methotrexate may be effective in patients with no systemic features, although it is not as effective as in other forms of JIA [131].

Thalidomide and atorvastatin have been modestly effective in small series or single, refractory cases [132, 133].

Biologics The use of biologic agents has dramatically changed the outcome of SJIA patients (Table 13.4). The first biologic agents that were approved for the treatment of JIA have been used for the treatment of SJIA with conflicting results. SJIA patients with systemic features were excluded from the pivotal clinical trials of anti-TNF agents and abatacept in JIA [134–136], and they have usually failed to show sustained efficacy in children with SJIA in routine clinical practice, especially in patients with active systemic features [137–142]. However, these agents might be

Table 13.4 Effective biologic agents in systemic juvenile idiopathic arthritis

Agent	Molecule	Mechanism of action	Half-life	Dosing	Route	References
Etanercept[a]	IgG1Fc/TNF receptor p75 fusion protein	Inhibition of TNFα and TNFβ	4 days	0.4 mg/kg (up to 1 mg /kg) twice weekly or up to 50 mg once weekly	SQ	[134]
Adalimumab[a]	Human anti-TNFα monoclonal antibody	Inhibition of TNFα	15–19 days	BW ≤ 30 kg: 20 mg every 14 days. BW > 30 kg: 40 mg every 14 days	SQ	[136]
Abatacept[a]	IgG1Fc/CTLA-4 fusion protein	Inhibition of T cell activation	14 days	10 mg/kg every 28 days	IV (SQ)[b]	[135]
Anakinra	IL-1 receptor antagonist	Inhibition of IL-1α and IL-1β	4–6 hours	2–4 mg/kg (up to 100 mg) daily	SQ	[28, 126, 127, 129, 144–150, 152, 153, 168]
Canakinumab	Human anti-IL-1β monoclonal antibody	Inhibition of IL-1β	26 days	4 mg/kg every 28 days	SQ	[31, 154, 155]
Rilonacept	IgG1Fc/IL-1 receptor fusion protein	Inhibition of IL-1α and IL-1β	7 days	Loading: 4.4 mg/kg; maintenance 2.2 mg/kg once weekly	SQ	[156, 157]
Tocilizumab	Humanized anti-IL-6 receptor monoclonal antibody	Inhibition of IL-6 through blockade of IL-6R and sIL-6R	8 days	BW ≤ 30 kg: 12 mg/kg every 14 days. BW > 30 kg: 8 mg/kg every 14 days	IV (SQ)[b]	[37, 158–160]

[a]In patients without systemic features
[b]In clinical trials

useful in patients without systemic features or during the late, predominantly arthritic phases of the disease [143].

Several observational studies and clinical trials have shown efficacy and safety of ANK in the treatment of SJIA, at least in the first year of therapy [144–150]. Most studies have demonstrated that ANK is effective in suppressing systemic signs more than joint inflammation. Gattorno et al. showed that SJIA patients can be divided into two different groups according to their response to ANK: good responders (about 40% of treated patients) and incomplete or nonresponders [28]. In a French multicenter, randomized, double-blind, placebo-controlled trial, ANK demonstrated rapid efficacy in 8 of 12 SJIA patients during the double-blind phase of the trial, while 7 out of 16 patients reached 30% improvement in a composite score (ACR 30) during the12-month-long, open-label, extension phase [151]. Interestingly, one patient was diagnosed with Crohn's disease after receiving ANK during the trial [149]. Observational, non-controlled, retrospective, and prospective studies have shown that ANK (both in combination with steroids and DMARDs and alone) is effective as a first-line therapy, is associated with rapid resolution of systemic symptoms, and could probably alter the course of SJIA [126, 127, 129]. Interestingly, treatment with ANK has been demonstrated to induce normalization of soluble inflammatory markers as well as gene expression abnormalities [29, 126, 149]. Besides, ANK has showed efficacy in the treatment of SJIA-associated MAS [152]. Toxicity has been reported in several cases: infections, severe skin reaction at the injection site, and hepatitis (or subtle MAS) have occurred in several patients [147, 153].

Canakinumab (CNK), an anti-IL-1 monoclonal antibody, was rapidly effective in a preliminary, phase II, multicenter, open-label, dosage-escalation study involving 24 children [154]. CNK was more effective in children with fewer swollen joints. A larger phase III trial including 177 SJIA patients with active systemic symptoms demonstrated its rapid efficacy in the vast majority of treated children, allowing dose reduction or discontinuation of corticosteroids [31]. After 15 days of treatment, ACR30 was achieved by 84% of patients on CNK, and inactive disease state was observed in 33%. At the end of the withdrawal phase, 62% of CNK-treated patients and 34% of patients in the placebo group had inactive disease. The agent was well tolerated, but MAS occurred in seven patients. Additionally, CNK therapy proved to induce downregulation of innate immune response genes in SJIA patients [155].

Rilonacept (RLN), an anti-IL-1 soluble decoy receptor protein, was tested in a controlled clinical trial where no significant differences in efficacy between the RLN- and the placebo-treated patients were observed in the double-blind phase, but fever and rash subsided during the open-label phase [156]. Another trial involving 71 SJIA patients with a long-standing disease and paucity of systemic features demonstrated that shorter time to response occurred in the RLN arm as compared to the placebo arm. Liver enzyme elevation and MAS were among the reported severe adverse events [157].

Tocilizumab (TCZ), a humanized anti-IL-6 receptor monoclonal antibody, showed marked efficacy and safety in a double-blind, placebo-controlled, withdrawal, phase III trial enrolling 56 patients [37]. ACR 30, 50, and 70 responses were achieved by 91%, 86%, and 68% patients, respectively, at the end of the open-label phase of the study. These results were confirmed in a larger trial involving 112 patients [158]. Of interest, TCZ allowed improved growth and normalization of insulin-like growth factor 1 (IGF-1) in the majority of these patients [159]. One surveillance study on TCZ performed in Japan demonstrated a more frequent occurrence of MAS and serious infusion-related adverse in routine clinical practice than in clinical trials [160].

ANK, CNK, and TCZ have been included in recently developed clinical practice recommendations and treatment plans [128, 161, 162]. Patients whose disease is refractory to IL-1 therapies may respond to IL-6 inhibitors and vice versa [163]. Some anecdotal reports show that combination biological therapy may be successful in the treatment of refractory cases [164, 165].

Although its use has decreased since the advent of effective biologic agents, autologous stem cell transplantation represented an option for severe, refractory cases of SJIA during the 1990s, when anti-IL-1 and anti-IL-6 therapies were not available. However, high morbidity and mortality (due to MAS or infections) progressively led to the abandoning of this therapeutic procedure, which is now reserved for patients whose disease is refractory to conventional and biologic therapies [166].

Finally, MAS requires a rapid and intense treatment. The combination of high-dose intravenous corticosteroid pulses and cyclosporine has showed efficacy [167]. Noteworthy, early addition of ANK at higher doses has been effective in several published cases [168].

Disease Course and Outcome

Classically, the disease course pattern of SJIA is classified into monocyclic (a single phase lasting up to 24 months), polycyclic (disease flares separated by months or years of inactive disease), or persistent (chronic persistent arthritis requiring treatment often into adulthood) [169, 170]. According to published series, these courses have variable frequencies: monocyclic 11–45%, polycyclic 7–35%, and persistent 51–55% [169, 171]. Similarly, the disease may show persistent active systemic features ("systemic" course) or it may progress into an exclusively arthritic disease ("polyarticular" course) after the initial months or years. However, flares that include active systemic symptoms may occur, even after years of remission or purely arthritic involvement. Patients with very early onset (before age 18 months) are characterized by a serious and aggressive disease course [9].

Disability is proportional to the disease duration and affects a greater proportion of patients with longer follow-up [94, 105, 172]. Predictive factors for poor functional capacity and/or joint damage are persistently active systemic features, use of corticosteroids and thrombocytosis at 6 months after onset, male sex, polyarticular involvement, cervical and hip involvement, and younger age at onset [92, 173–179]. The general outcome is variable, ranging from very good in the monocyclic course to a more serious, progressive disease carrying considerable morbidity and mortality in the persistently active disease. However, nowadays clinically inactive disease and sustained remission are attainable in a significant proportion of cases [180–182].

Conclusion

Systemic-onset juvenile idiopathic arthritis is a polygenic autoinflammatory disease or diverse group of clinically and genetically distinct illnesses, in which innate immunity components drive the inflammatory response and create a multiorganic inflammatory scenario frequently leading to chronic synovitis and extra-articular manifestations. Spiking daily fever, evanescent skin rash, organomegaly, and serositis are the clinical hallmarks of the active phases of the disease, often evolving into the severe MAS. Dramatic response to IL-1 and IL-6 inhibitors occurs in a high proportion of patients, who may reach inactive disease or even clinical remission status.

References

1. Woo P. Anakinra treatment for systemic juvenile idiopathic arthritis and adult onset Still disease. Ann Rheum Dis. 2008;67:281–2.
2. Masters SL, Simon A, Aksentijevich I, et al. Horror autoinflammaticus: the molecular pathophysiology of autoinflammatory disease. Annu Rev Immunol. 2009;27:621–68.
3. Mellins ED, Macaubas C, Grom AA. Pathogenesis of systemic juvenile idiopathic arthritis: some answers, more questions. Nat Rev Rheumatol. 2011;7:416–26.
4. Hedrich CM, Tsokos GC. Bridging the gap between autoinflammation and autoimmunity. Clin Immunol. 2013;147:151–4.
5. Nigrovic PA. Autoinflammation and autoimmunity in systemic juvenile idiopathic arthritis. PNAS. 2015;112:15785–6.
6. Modesto C, Antón J, Rodriguez B, Bou R, Arnal C, Ros J, et al. Incidence and prevalence of juvenile idiopathic arthritis in Catalonia (Spain). Scand J Rheumatol. 2010;39:472–9.
7. Gurion R, Lehman TJ, Moorthy LN. Systemic arthritis in children: a review of clinical presentation and treatment. Int J Inflam. 2012;2012:271569.
8. Behrens EM, Beukelman T, Gallo L, Spangler J, Rosenkranz M, Arkachaisri T, et al. Evaluation of the presentation of systemic onset juvenile rheumatoid arthritis: data from the Pennsylvania Systemic Onset Juvenile Arthritis Registry. (PASOJAR). J Rheumatol. 2008;35:343–8.
9. Russo R, Katsicas MM. Patients with very early-onset systemic juvenile idiopathic arthritis exhibit more inflammatory features and a worse outcome. J Rheumatol. 2013;40:329–34.
10. Wallace CA, Levinson JE. Juvenile rheumatoid arthritis: outcome and treatment for the 1990s. Rheum Dis Clin North Am. 1991;17:891–905.
11. Woo P. Systemic juvenile idiopathic arthritis: diagnosis, management, and outcome. Nat Clin Pract Rheumatol. 2006;2:28–34.
12. Petty RE, Southwood TR, Manners P, Baum J, Glass DN, Goldenberg J, et al. International League of Associations for Rheumatology classification of juvenile idiopathic arthritis: second revision, Edmonton, 2001. J Rheumatol. 2004;31:390–2.

13. Kumar S, Kunhiraman DS, Rajam L. Application of the Yamaguchi criteria for classification of "suspected" systemic juvenile idiopathic arthritis (sJIA). Pediatr Rheumatol. 2012;10:40.
14. Martini A. It is time to rethink juvenile idiopathic arthritis classification and nomenclature? Ann Rheum Dis. 2012;71:1437–9.
15. Deslandre C. Juvenile idiopathic arthritis: definition and classification. Arch Pediatr. 2016;23:437–41.
16. Fall N, Barnes M, Thornton S, et al. Gene expression profiling of peripheral blood from patients with untreated new-onset systemic juvenile idiopathic arthritis reveals molecular heterogeneity that may predict macrophage activation syndrome. Arthritis Rheum. 2007;56:3793–804.
17. Cepika AM, Banchereau R, Segura E, et al. A multidimensional blood stimulation assay reveals immune alterations underlying systemic juvenile idiopathic arthritis. J Exp Med. 2017;214:3449–66.
18. Hinze CH, Fall N, Thornton S, et al. Immature cell populations and an erythropoiesis gene-expression signature in systemic juvenile idiopathic arthritis: implications for pathogenesis. Arthritis Res Ther. 2010;12:R123.
19. Omoyinmi E, Hamaoui R, Pesenacker A, et al. Th1 and Th17 cell subpopulations are enriched in the peripheral blood of patients with systemic juvenile idiopathic arthritis. Rheumatology. 2012;51:1881–6.
20. Nigrovic PA. Is there a window of opportunity for treatment of systemic juvenile idiopathic arthritis? Arthritis Rheum. 2014;66:1405–13.
21. Kessel C, Lippitz A, Weinhage T, et al. Proinflammatory cytokine environments can drive Interleukin-17 overexpression by γ/δ T cells in systemic juvenile idiopathic arthritis. Arthritis Rheum. 2017;69:1480–94.
22. Pascual V, Allantaz F, Arce E, Punaro M, Banchereau J. Role of interleukin-1 (IL-1) in the pathogenesis of systemic onset juvenile idiopathic arthritis and clinical response to IL-1 blockade. J Exp Med. 2005;201:1479–86.
23. de Jager W, Hoppenreijs EP, Wulffraat NM, Wedderburn LR, Kuis W, Prakken BJ. Blood and synovial fluid cytokine signatures in patients with juvenile idiopathic arthritis: a cross-sectional study. Ann Rheum Dis. 2007;66:589–98.
24. Frosch M, Roth J. New insights in systemic juvenile idiopathic arthritis-from pathophysiology to treatment. Rheumatology. 2008;47:121–5.
25. Shimizu M, Nakagishi Y, Kasai K, Yamasaki Y, Miyoshi M, Takei S, et al. Tocilizumab masks the clinical symptoms of systemic juvenile idiopathic arthritis-associated macrophage activation syndrome: the diagnostic significance of interleukin-18 and interleukin-6. Cytokine. 2012;58:287–94.
26. Shimizu M, Nakagishi Y, Yachie A. Distinct subsets of patients with systemic juvenile idiopathic arthritis based on their cytokine profiles. Cytokine. 2013;61:345–8.
27. Muller K, Herner EB, Stagg A, Bendtzen K, Woo P. Inflammatory cytokines and cytokine antagonists in whole blood cultures of patients with systemic juvenile chronic arthritis. Br J Rheumatol. 1998;37:562–9.
28. Gattorno M, Piccini A, Lasiglie D, et al. The pattern of response to anti-interleukin-1 treatment distinguishes two subsets of patients with systemic-onset juvenile idiopathic arthritis. Arthritis Rheum. 2008;58:1505–15.
29. Allantaz F, Chaussabel D, Stichweh D, et al. Blood leukocyte microarrays to diagnose systemic onset juvenile idiopathic arthritis and follow the response to IL-1 blockade. J Exp Med. 2007;204:2131–44.
30. Quartier P, Allantaz F, Cimaz R, et al. A multicentre, randomised, double-blind, placebo-controlled trial with the interleukin-1 receptor antagonist anakinra in patients with systemic-onset juvenile idiopathic arthritis (ANAJIS trial). Ann Rheum Dis. 2011;70:747–54.
31. Ruperto N, Brunner HI, Quartier P, et al. Two randomized trials of Canakinumab in systemic juvenile idiopathic arthritis. N Engl J Med. 2012;367:2396–406.
32. Lotito AP, Campa A, Silva CA, Kiss MH, Mello SB. Interleukin 18 as a marker of disease activity and severity in patients with juvenile idiopathic arthritis. J Rheumatol. 2007;34:823–30.

33. Shimizu M, Yokoyama T, Yamada K, Kaneda H, Wada H, Wada T, et al. Distinct cytokine profiles of systemic-onset juvenile idiopathic arthritis-associated macrophage activation syndrome with particular emphasis on the role of interleukin-18 in its pathogenesis. Rheumatology (Oxford). 2010;49:1645–53.
34. de Benedetti F, Massa M, Robbioni P, Ravelli A, Burgio GR, Martini A. Correlation of serum interleukin-6 levels with joint involvement and thrombocytosis in systemic juvenile rheumatoid arthritis. Arthritis Rheum. 1991;34:1158–63.
35. Cazzola M, Ponchio L, de Benedetti F, Ravelli A, Rosti V, Beguin Y, et al. Defective iron supply for erythropoiesis and adequate endogenous erythropoietin production in the anemia associated with systemic-onset juvenile chronic arthritis. Blood. 1996;87:4824–30.
36. de Benedetti F, Meazza C, Oliveri M, Pignatti P, Vivarelli M, Alonzi T, et al. Effect of IL-6 on IGF binding protein-3: a study in IL-6 transgenic mice and in patients with systemic juvenile idiopathic arthritis. Endocrinology. 2001;142:4818–26.
37. Yokota S, Imagawa T, Mori M, et al. Efficacy and safety of tocilizumab in patients with systemic-onset juvenile idiopathic arthritis: a randomised, double-blind, placebo-controlled, withdrawal phase III trial. Lancet. 2008;371:998–1006.
38. Raziuddin S, Bahabri S, al-Dalaan A, Siraj AK, al-Sedairy S. A mixed Th1/Th2 cell cytokine response predominates in systemic onset juvenile rheumatoid arthritis: immunoregulatory IL-10 function. Clin Immunol Immunopathol. 1998;86:192–8.
39. Pignatti P, Vivarelli M, Meazza C, Rizzolo MG, Martini A, De BF. Abnormal regulation of interleukin 6 in systemic juvenile idiopathic arthritis. J Rheumatol. 2001;28:1670–6.
40. de Benedetti F, Alonzi T, Moretta A, Lazzaro D, Costa P, Poli V, et al. Interleukin-6 causes growth impairment in transgenic mice through a decrease in insulin-like growth factor-I. A model for stunted growth in children with chronic inflammation. J Clin Invest. 1997;99:643–50.
41. Strippoli R, Carvello F, Scianaro R, Pasquale LD, Vivarelli M, Petrini S, et al. Amplification of the response to toll-like receptor ligands by prolonged exposure to interleukin-6 in mice: implications for the pathogenesis of macrophage activation syndrome. Arthritis Rheum. 2012;64:1680–8.
42. Canna SW, Wrobel J, Chu N, Kreiger PA, Paessler M, Behrens EM. Interferon-gamma mediates anemia but is dispensable for fulminant toll-like receptor 9- induced macrophage activation syndrome and hemophagocytosis in mice. Arthritis Rheum. 2013;65:1764–75.
43. Avau A, Mitera T, Put S, Put K, Brisse E, Filtjens J, et al. Systemic juvenile idiopathic arthritis-like syndrome in mice following stimulation of the immune system with Freund's complete adjuvant: regulation by interferon- gamma. Arthritis Rheum. 2014;66:1340–51.
44. Bracaglia C, de Graaf K, Marafon DP, et al. Elevated circulating levels of interferon-γ and interferon-γ-induced chemokines characterize patients with macrophage activation syndrome complicating systemic juvenile idiopathic arthritis. Ann Rheum Dis. 2017;76:166–72.
45. Wouters CH, Ceuppens JL, Stevens EA. Different circulating lymphocyte profiles in patients with different subtypes of juvenile idiopathic arthritis. Clin Exp Rheumatol. 2002;20: 239–48.
46. Zhou J, Tang X, Ding Y, An Y, Zhao X. Natural killer cell activity and frequency of killer cell immunoglobulin-like receptors in children with different forms of juvenile idiopathic arthritis. Pediatr Allergy Immunol. 2013;24:691–6.
47. Grom AA, Villanueva J, Lee S, Goldmuntz EA, Passo MH, Filipovich A. Natural killer cell dysfunction in patients with systemic-onset juvenile rheumatoid arthritis and macrophage activation syndrome. J Pediatr. 2003;142:292–6.
48. Villanueva J, Lee S, Giannini EH, et al. Natural killer cell dysfunction is a distinguishing feature of systemic onset juvenile rheumatoid arthritis and macrophage activation syndrome. Arthritis Res Ther. 2005;7:R30–7.
49. Wulffraat NM, Rijkers GT, Elst E, Brooimans R, Kuis W. Reduced perforin expression in systemic juvenile idiopathic arthritis is restored by autologous stem-cell transplantation. Rheumatology (Oxford). 2003;42:375–9.

50. Put K, Vandenhaute J, Avau A, et al. Inflammatory gene expression profile and defective interferon-γ and Granzyme K in natural killer cells from systemic juvenile idiopathic arthritis patients. Arthritis Rheum. 2017;69:213–24.
51. Brady J, Carotta S, Thong RP, Chan CJ, Hayakawa Y, Smyth MJ, et al. The interactions of multiple cytokines control NK cell maturation. J Immunol. 2010;185:6679–88.
52. Cifaldi L, Prencipe G, Caiello I, Bracaglia C, Locatelli F, de Benedetti F, et al. Inhibition of natural killer cell cytotoxicity by interleukin-6: implications for the pathogenesis of macrophage activation syndrome. Arthritis Rheum. 2015;67:3037–46.
53. de Jager W, Vastert SJ, Beekman JM, Wulffraat NM, Kuis W, Coffer PJ, et al. Defective phosphorylation of interleukin-18 receptor b causes impaired natural killer cell function in systemic onset juvenile idiopathic arthritis. Arthritis Rheum. 2009;60:2782–93.
54. Macaubas C, Nguyen K, Deshpande C, et al. Distribution of circulating cells in systemic juvenile idiopathic arthritis across disease activity states. Clin Immunol. 2010;134:206–16.
55. Macaubas C, Nguyen KD, Peck A, Buckingham J, Deshpande C, Wong E, et al. Alternative activation in systemic juvenile idiopathic arthritis monocytes. Clin Immunol. 2012;142:362–72.
56. Schulert GS, Fall N, Harley JB, et al. Monocyte MicroRNA expression in active systemic juvenile idiopathic arthritis implicates MicroRNA-125a-5p in polarized monocyte phenotypes. Arthritis Rheum. 2016;68:2300–13.
57. Frosch M, Vogl T, Seeliger S, et al. Expression of myeloid-related proteins 8 and 14 in systemic-onset juvenile rheumatoid arthritis. Arthritis Rheum. 2003;48:2622–6.
58. Foell D, Wittkowski H, Hammerschmidt I, et al. Monitoring neutrophil activation in juvenile rheumatoid arthritis by S100A12 serum concentrations. Arthritis Rheum. 2004;50:1286–95.
59. Foell D, Roth J. Proinflammatory S100 proteins in arthritis and autoimmune disease. Arthritis Rheum. 2004;50:3762–71.
60. Ombrello MJ, Remmers EF, Tachmazidou I, et al. HLA-DRB1*11 and variants of the MHC class II locus are strong risk factors for systemic juvenile idiopathic arthritis. PNAS. 2015;112:15970–5.
61. Hinks A, Bowes J, Cobb J, et al. Fine-mapping the MHC locus in juvenile idiopathic arthritis (JIA) reveals genetic heterogeneity corresponding to distinct adult inflammatory arthritic diseases. Ann Rheum Dis. 2017;76:765–72.
62. Stock CJ, Ogilvie EM, Samuel JM, Fife M, Lewis CM, Woo P. Comprehensive association study of genetic variants in the IL-1 gene family in systemic juvenile idiopathic arthritis. Genes Immun. 2008;9:349–57.
63. de Benedetti F, Meazza C, Vivarelli M, et al. Functional and prognostic relevance of the −173 polymorphism of the macrophage migration inhibitory factor gene in systemic-onset juvenile idiopathic arthritis. Arthritis Rheum. 2003;48:1398–407.
64. Fishman D, Faulds G, Jeffery R, et al. The effect of novel polymorphisms in the interleukin-6 (IL-6) gene on IL-6 transcription and plasma IL-6 levels, and an association with systemic-onset juvenile chronic arthritis. J Clin Invest. 1998;102:1369–76.
65. Ogilvie EM, Fife MS, Thompson SD, et al. The -174G allele of the Interleukin-6 gene confers susceptibility to systemic arthritis in children. Arthritis Rheum. 2003;48:3202–6.
66. Donn RP, Barrett JH, Farhan A, et al. Cytokine gene polymorphisms and susceptibility to juvenile idiopathic arthritis. British Paediatric rheumatology study group. Arthritis Rheum. 2001;44:802–10.
67. Donn RP, Shelley E, Ollier WE, et al. A novel 5′-flanking region polymorphism of macrophage migration inhibitory factor is associated with systemic-onset juvenile idiopathic arthritis. Arthritis Rheum. 2001;44:1782–5.
68. Fife MS, Gutierrez A, Ogilvie EM, Stock CJ, Samuel JM, Thomson W, et al. Novel IL10 gene family associations with systemic juvenile idiopathic arthritis. Arthritis Res Ther. 2006;8:R148.
69. Moller JC, Paul D, Ganser G, Range U, Gahr M, Kelsch R, et al. IL10 promoter polymorphisms are associated with systemic onset juvenile idiopathic arthritis (SoJIA). Clin Exp Rheumatol. 2010;28:912–8.

70. Yanagimachi M, Goto H, Miyamae T, et al. Association of IRF5 polymorphisms with susceptibility to Hemophagocytic Lymphohistiocytosis in children. J Clin Immunol. 2011;31:946–51.
71. Ayaz NA, Ozen S, Bilginer Y, et al. MEFV mutations in systemic onset juvenile idiopathic arthritis. Rheumatology. 2009;48:23–5.
72. Cantarini L, Lucherini OM, Simonini G, Galeazzi M, Baldari CT, Cimaz R. Systemic-onset juvenile idiopathic arthritis complicated by early onset amyloidosis in a patient carrying a mutation in the MEFV gene. Rheumatol Int. 2012;32:465–7.
73. Tadaki H, Saitsu H, Nishimura-Tadaki A, et al. De novo 19q13.42 duplications involving NLRP gene cluster in a patient with systemic-onset juvenile idiopathic arthritis. J Human Gen. 2011;56:343–7.
74. Hazen MM, Woodward AL, Hofmann I, et al. Mutations of the Hemophagocytic Lymphohistiocytosis-associated gene UNC13D in a patient with systemic juvenile idiopathic arthritis. Arthritis Rheum. 2008;58:567–70.
75. Vastert SJ, van Wijk R, D'Urbano LE, de Vooght KM, de Jager W, Ravelli A, et al. Mutations in the perforin gene can be linked to macrophage activation syndrome in patients with systemic onset juvenile idiopathic arthritis. Rheumatology (Oxford). 2010;49:441–9.
76. Zhang K, Biroschak J, Glass DN, et al. Macrophage activation syndrome in patients with systemic juvenile idiopathic arthritis is associated with MUNC13-4 polymorphisms. Arthritis Rheum. 2008;58:2892–6.
77. Kaufman KM, Linghu B, Szustakowski JD, et al. Whole-exome sequencing reveals overlap between macrophage activation syndrome in systemic juvenile idiopathic arthritis and familial hemophagocytic lymphohistiocytosis. Arthritis Rheum. 2014;66:3486–95.
78. Wakil SM, Monies DM, Abouelhoda M, et al. Association of a mutation in LACC1 with a monogenic form of systemic juvenile idiopathic arthritis. Arthritis Rheum. 2015;67:288–95.
79. Kallinich T, Thorworth A, von Stuckrad SL, et al. Juvenile arthritis caused by a novel FAMIN (LACC1) mutation in two children with systemic and extended oligoarticular course. Pediatr Rheumatol. 2016;14:63.
80. Calabro JJ. Other extraarticular manifestations of juvenile rheumatoid arthritis. Arthritis Rheum. 1977;20:237–40.
81. Shimizu M, Yokoyama T, Wada T, Yachie A. Bicipital synovial cyst in systemic-onset juvenile idiopathic arthritis. J Pediatr. 2010;157:168.
82. Schneider R, Laxer RM. Systemic onset juvenile rheumatoid arthritis. Baillieres Clin Rheumatol. 1998;12:245–71.
83. Frosch M, Metze D, Foell D, Vogl T, Sorg C, Sunderkötter C, et al. Early activation of cutaneous vessels and epithelial cells is characteristic of acute systemic onset juvenile idiopathic arthritis. Exp Dermatol. 2005;14:259–65.
84. Ramanan AV, Wynn RF, Kelsey A, Baildam EM. Systemic juvenile idiopathic arthritis, Kikuchi's disease and haemophagocytic lymphohistiocytosis - is there a link? Case report and literature review. Rheumatology (Oxford). 2003;42:596–8.
85. Tabak F, Tanverdi M, Ozaras R, Mert A, Tartan Z, Ozturk R, et al. Neutrophilic pleocytosis in cerebrospinal fluid: adult-onset Still's disease. Intern Med. 2003;42:1039–41.
86. Heyd J, Glaser J. Early occurrence of aortic valve regurgitation in a youth with systemic-onset juvenile rheumatoid arthritis. Am J Med. 1990;89:123–4.
87. Kimura Y, Weiss JE, Haroldson KL, Lee T, Punaro M, Oliveira S, et al. Pulmonary hypertension and other potentially fatal pulmonary complications in systemic juvenile idiopathic arthritis. Arthritis Care Res. 2013;65(5):745–52.
88. Wang FM, Wertenbaker C, Behrens MM, Jacobs JC. Acquired Brown's syndrome in children with juvenile rheumatoid arthritis. Ophthalmology. 1984;91:23–6.
89. Avcin T, Silverman ED, Forte V, Schneider R. Nasal septal perforation: a novel clinical manifestation of systemic juvenile idiopathic arthritis/adult onset Still's disease. J Rheumatol. 2005;32:2429–31.
90. Dong S, Bout-Tabaku S, Texter K, Jaggi P. Diagnosis of systemic-onset juvenile idiopathic arthritis after treatment for presumed Kawasaki disease. J Pediatr. 2015;166:1283–8.

91. Solari N, Viola S, Pistorio A, Magni-Manzoni S, Vitale R, Ruperto N, et al. Assessing current outcomes of juvenile idiopathic arthritis: a cross-sectional study in a tertiary center sample. Arthritis Rheum. 2008;15(59):1571–9.
92. Russo RAG, Katsicas MM. Global damage in systemic juvenile idiopathic arthritis: preliminary early predictors. J Rheumatol. 2008;35:1151–6.
93. Oen K, Reed M, Malleson PN, Cabral DA, Petty RE, Rosenberg AM, et al. Radiologic outcome and its relationship to functional disability in juvenile rheumatoid arthritis. J Rheumatol. 2003;30:832–40.
94. Bowyer SL, Roettcher PA, Higgins GC, Adams B, Myers LK, Wallace C, et al. Health status of patients with juvenile rheumatoid arthritis at 1 and 5 years after diagnosis. J Rheumatol. 2003;30:394–400.
95. Sudoł-Szopińska I, Matuszewska G, Gietka P, Płaza M, Walentowska-Janowicz M. Imaging of juvenile idiopathic arthritis. Part I: clinical classifications and radiographs. J Ultrason. 2016;16:225–36.
96. Behrens EM, Beukelman T, Paessler M, Cron RQ. Occult macrophage activation syndrome in patients with systemic juvenile idiopathic arthritis. J Rheumatol. 2007;34:1133–8.
97. Minoia F, Davì S, Horne A, Demirkaya E, Bovis F, Li C, Lehmberg K, et al. Clinical features, treatment, and outcome of macrophage activation syndrome complicating systemic juvenile idiopathic arthritis: a multinational, multicenter study of 362 patients. Arthritis Rheum. 2014;66:3160–9.
98. Stéphan JL, Koné-Paut I, Galambrun C, Mouy R, Bader-Meunier B, Prieur AM. Reactive haemophagocytic syndrome in children with inflammatory disorders. A retrospective study of 24 patients. Rheumatology (Oxford). 2001;40:1285–92.
99. Russo RAG, Rosenzweig S, Katsicas MM. Hepatitis A-associated macrophage activation syndrome in children with systemic juvenile idiopathic arthritis: report of 2 cases. J Rheumatol. 2008;35:166–8.
100. Schulert GS, Grom AA. Pathogenesis of macrophage activation syndrome and potential for cytokine-directed therapies. Annu Rev Med. 2015;66:18.1–18.15.
101. Ravelli A, Minoia F, Davi S, et al. Expert consensus on dynamics of laboratory tests for diagnosis of macrophage activation syndrome complicating systemic juvenile idiopathic arthritis. RMD Open. 2016;2:e000161.
102. Ravelli A, Minoia F, Davi S, et al. 2016 classification criteria for macrophage activation syndrome complicating systemic juvenile idiopathic arthritis. Ann Rheum Dis. 2016;75:481–9.
103. Ravelli A, Magni-Manzoni S, Pistorio A, et al. Preliminary diagnostic guidelines for macrophage activation syndrome complicating systemic juvenile idiopathic arthritis. J Pediatr. 2005;146:598–604.
104. Simon D. Management of growth retardation in juvenile idiopathic arthritis. Horm Res. 2007;68(Suppl 5):122–5.
105. Packham JC, Hall MA. Long-term follow-up of 246 adults with juvenile idiopathic arthritis: functional outcome. Rheumatology (Oxford). 2002;41:1428–35.
106. Saha A, Chopra Y, Theis JD, Vrana JA, Sethi S. AA amyloidosis associated with systemic -onset juvenile idiopathic arthritis. Am J Kidney Dis. 2013;62:834–8.
107. Murray KJ, Boyle RJ, Woo P. Pathological fractures and osteoporosis in a cohort of 103 systemic onset juvenile idiopathic arthritis patients. Arthritis Rheum. 2000;43:S119.
108. Stagi S, Masi L, Capannini S, Cimaz R, Tonini G, Matucci-Cerinic M, et al. Cross- sectional and longitudinal evaluation of bone mass in children and young adults with juvenile idiopathic arthritis: the role of bone mass determinants in a large cohort of patients. J Rheumatol. 2010;37:1935–43.
109. Rodd C, Lang B, Ramsay T, Alos N, Huber AM, Cabral DA, et al. Incident vertebral fractures among children with rheumatic disorders 12 months after glucocorticoid initiation: a national observational study. Arthritis Care Res (Hoboken). 2012;64:122–31.
110. Lien G, Flatø B, Haugen M, Vinje O, Sørskaar D, Dale K. Frequency of osteopenia in adolescents with early-onset juvenile idiopathic arthritis: a long-term outcome study of one hundred five patients. Arthritis Rheum. 2003;48:2214–23.

111. Foell D, Wittkowski H, Hammerschmidt I, Wulffraat N, et al. Monitoring neutrophil activation in juvenile rheumatoid arthritis by S100A12 serum concentrations. Arthritis Rheum. 2004;50:1286–95.
112. Wittkowski H, Frosch M, Wulffraat N, Goldbach-Mansky R, et al. S100A12 is a novel molecular marker differentiating systemic-onset juvenile idiopathic arthritis from other causes of fever of unknown origin. Arthritis Rheum. 2008;58:3924–31.
113. Gerss J, Roth J, Holzinger D, et al. Phagocyte-specific S100 proteins and high-sensitivity C reactive protein as biomarkers for a risk-adapted treatment to maintain remission in juvenile idiopathic arthritis: a comparative study. Ann Rheum Dis. 2012;71:1991–7.
114. Holzinger D, Frosch M, Kastrup A, et al. The toll-like receptor 4 agonist MRP8/14 protein complex is a sensitive indicator for disease activity and predicts relapses in systemic-onset juvenile idiopathic arthritis. Ann Rheum Dis. 2012;71:974–80.
115. Shenoi S, Ou JN, Ni C, et al. Comparison of biomarkers for systemic juvenile idiopathic arthritis. Pediatr Res. 2015;78:554–9.
116. Bleesing J, Prada A, Siegel DM, et al. The diagnostic significance of soluble CD163 and soluble Interleukin-2 receptor α-chain in macrophage activation syndrome and untreated new-onset systemic juvenile idiopathic arthritis. Arthritis Rheum. 2007;56:965–71.
117. Wilson DC, Marinov AD, Blair HC, et al. Follistatin-like protein 1 is a mesenchyme-derived inflammatory protein and may represent a biomarker for systemic-onset juvenile rheumatoid arthritis. Arthritis Rheum. 2010;62:2510–6.
118. de Jager W, Hoppenreijs EP, Wulffraat NM, Wedderburn LR, et al. Blood and synovial fluid cytokine signatures in patients with juvenile idiopathic arthritis: a cross-sectional study. Ann Rheum Dis. 2007;66:589–98.
119. Jelusic M, Lukic IK, Tambic-Bukovac L, Dubravcic K, et al. Interleukin-18 as a mediator of systemic juvenile idiopathic arthritis. Clin Rheumatol. 2007;26:1332–4.
120. Nguyen KD, Macaubas C, Nadeau KC, et al. Serum amyloid a overrides Treg anergy via monocyte-dependent and Treg-intrinsic, SOCS3-associated pathways. Blood. 2011;117:3793–8.
121. Ling XB, Park JL, Carroll T, et al. Plasma profiles in active systemic juvenile idiopathic arthritis: biomarkers and biological implications. Proteomics. 2010;10:4415–30.
122. Miyamae T, Malehorn DE, Lemster B, et al. Serum protein profile in systemic-onset juvenile idiopathic arthritis differentiates response versus nonresponse to therapy. Arthritis Res Ther. 2005;7:R746–55.
123. Ling XB, Lau K, Deshpande C, et al. Urine Peptidomic and targeted plasma protein analyses in the diagnosis and monitoring of systemic juvenile idiopathic arthritis. Clin Proteomics. 2010;6:175–93.
124. Gohar F, Kessel C, Lavric M, Holzinger D, Foell D. Review of biomarkers in systemic juvenile idiopathic arthritis: helpful tools or just playing tricks? Arthritis Res Ther. 2016;18:163.
125. Kimura Y, Fieldston E, Devries-Vandervlugt B, et al. High dose, alternate day corticosteroids for systemic onset juvenile rheumatoid arthritis. J Rheumatol. 2000;27:2018–24.
126. Nigrovic P, Mannion M, Prince FHM, et al. Anakinra as first-line disease-modifying therapy in systemic juvenile idiopathic arthritis. Arthritis Rheum. 2011;63:545–55.
127. Hedrich CM, Bruck N, Fiebig B, Gahr M. Anakinra: a safe and effective first-line treatment in systemic onset juvenile idiopathic arthritis (SoJIA). Rheumatol Int. 2012;32:3525–30.
128. DeWitt EM, Kimura Y, Beukelman T, et al. Consensus treatment plans for new-onset systemic juvenile idiopathic arthritis. Arthritis Care Res. 2012;64:1001–10.
129. Vastert SJ, de Jager W, Noordman BJ, et al. Effectiveness of first-line treatment with recombinant Interleukin-1 receptor antagonist in steroid-naive patients with new-onset systemic juvenile idiopathic arthritis. Arthritis Rheum. 2014;66:1034–43.
130. Ilowite NT, Sandborg CI, Feldman BM, et al. Algorithm development for corticosteroid management in systemic juvenile idiopathic arthritis trial using consensus methodology. Pediatr Rheumatol. 2012;10:31.

131. Woo P, Southwood TR, Prieur A-M, et al. Randomized, placebo-controlled crossover trial of low-dose oral methotrexate in children with extended oligoarticular or systemic arthritis. Arthritis Rheum. 2000;43:1849–57.
132. Lehman TJ, Schechter SJ, Sundel RP, et al. Thalidomide for severe systemic onset juvenile rheumatoid arthritis: a multicenter study. J Pediatr. 2004;145:856–7.
133. ten Cate R, Nibbering PH, Bredius RG. Therapy-refractory systemic juvenile idiopathic arthritis successfully treated with statins. Rheumatology (Oxford). 2004;43:934–5.
134. Lovell DJ, Giannini EH, Reiff A, et al. Etanercept in children with polyarticular juvenile rheumatoid arthritis. N Engl J Med. 2000;342:763–9.
135. Ruperto N, Lovell DJ, Quartier P, et al. Abatacept in children with juvenile idiopathic arthritis: a randomised, double-blind, placebo-controlled withdrawal trial. Lancet. 2008;372:383–91.
136. Lovell DJ, Ruperto N, Goodman S, et al. Adalimumab with or without methotrexate in juvenile rheumatoid arthritis. N Engl J Med. 2008;359:810–20.
137. Russo RAG, Katsicas MM, Zelazko M. Etanercept in systemic juvenile idiopathic arthritis. Clin Exp Rheumatol. 2002;20:723–6.
138. Quartier P, Taupin P, Bordeaut F, et al. Efficacy of etanercept for the treatment of juvenile idiopathic arthritis according to the onset type. Arthritis Rheum. 2003;48:1093–101.
139. Horneff G, Schmeling H, Biederman T, et al. The German etanercept registry for treatment of juvenile idiopathic arthritis. Ann Rheum dis 2004;63:1638-44.Katsicas MM and Russo R. Use of infliximab in patients with systemic juvenile idiopathic arthritis refractory to etanercept. Clin Exp Rheumatol. 2005;23:545–8.
140. Kimura Y, Pinho P, Walco G, et al. Etanercept treatment in patients with refractory systemic onset juvenile rheumatoid arthritis. J Rheumatol. 2005;32:935–42.
141. Katsicas MM, Russo RAG. Use of adalimumab in patients with juvenile idiopathic arthritis refractory to etanercept and/or infliximab. Clin Rheumatol. 2009;28:985–8.
142. Russo RA, Katsicas MM. Clinical remission in patients with systemic juvenile idiopathic arthritis treated with anti-tumor necrosis factor agents. J Rheumatol. 2009;38:1078–82.
143. Lovell DJ, Reiff A, Ilowite NT, et al. Safety and efficacy of up to eight years of continuous etanercept therapy in patients with juvenile rheumatoid arthritis. Arthritis Rheum. 2008;58:1496–504.
144. Verbsky JW, White AJ. Effective use of the recombinant interleukin 1 receptor antagonist anakinra in therapy resistant systemic onset juvenile rheumatoid arthritis. J Rheumatol. 2004;31:2071–5.
145. Pascual V, Allantaz F, Arce E, et al. Role of interleukin-1 (IL-1) in the pathogenesis of systemic onset juvenile idiopathic arthritis and clinical response to IL-1 blockade. J Exp Med. 2005;201:1479–86.
146. Ohlsson V, Balldam E, Foster H, et al. Anakinra treatment for systemic onset juvenile idiopathic arthritis (SOJIA). Rheumatology (Oxford). 2008;47:555–6.
147. Lequerre T, Quartier P, Rosellini D, et al. Interleukin-1 receptor antagonist (anakinra) treatment in patients with systemic-onset juvenile idiopathic arthritis or adult onset still disease: preliminary experience in France. Ann Rheum Dis. 2008;67:302–8.
148. Zeft A, Hollister R, LaFleur B, et al. Anakinra for systemic juvenile arthritis: the Rocky Mountain experience. J Clin Rheumatol. 2009;15:161–4.
149. Quartier P, Allantaz F, Cimaz R, et al. A multicentre, randomised, double-blind, placebo-controlled trial with the interleukin-1 receptor antagonist anakinra in patients with systemic-onset juvenile idiopathic arthritis (ANAJIS trial). Ann Rheum Dis. 2011;70:747–54.
150. Pardeo M, Marafon DP, Insalaco A, et al. Anakinra in systemic juvenile idiopathic arthritis: a single-center experience. J Rheumatol. 2015;42:1523–7.
151. Giannini EH, Ruperto N, Ravelli A, et al. Preliminary definition of improvement in juvenile arthritis. Arthritis Rheum. 1997;40:1202–9.
152. Miettunen PM, Narendran A, Javanthan A, et al. Successful treatment of severe paediatric rheumatic disease-associated macrophage activation syndrome with interleukin-1 inhi-

bition following conventional immunosuppressive therapy: case series with 12 patients. Rheumatology (Oxford). 2011;50:417–9.
153. Canna S, Frankovich J, Higgins G, et al. Acute hepatitis in three patients with systemic juvenile idiopathic arthritis taking interleukin-1 receptor antagonist. Pediatr Rheum. 2009;7:21.
154. Ruperto N, Quartier P, Wulffraat N, et al. A phase II, multicenter, open-label study evaluating dosing and preliminary safety and efficacy of Canakinumab in systemic juvenile idiopathic arthritis with active systemic features. Arthritis Rheum. 2012;64:557–67.
155. Brachat AH, Grom AA, Wulffraat N, et al. Early changes in gene expression and inflammatory proteins in systemic juvenile idiopathic arthritis patients on canakinumab therapy. Arthritis Res Ther. 2017;19:13.
156. Lovell DJ, Giannini EH, Reiff AO, et al. Long-term safety and efficacy of rilonacept in patients with systemic juvenile idiopathic arthritis. Arthritis Rheum. 2013;65:2486–96.
157. Ilowite NT, Prather K, Lokhnuyina Y, et al. Randomized, double-blind, placebo-controlled trial of the efficacy and safety of rilonacept in the treatment of systemic juvenile idiopathic arthritis. Arthritis Rheum. 2014;66:2570–9.
158. De Benedetti F, Brunner H, Ruperto N, et al. Randomized trial of tocilizumab in systemic juvenile idiopathic arthritis. N Engl J Med. 2012;67:2385–95.
159. De Benedetti F, Brunner H, Ruperto N, et al. Catch-up growth during tocilizumab therapy for systemic juvenile idiopathic arthritis. Results from a phase III trial. Arthritis Rheum. 2015;67:840–8.
160. Yokota S, Itoh Y, Morio T, et al. Tocilizumab in systemic juvenile idiopathic arthritis in a real-world clinical setting: results from 1 year of postmarketing surveillance follow-up of 417 patients in Japan. Ann Rheum Dis. 2016;75:1654–60.
161. Ringold S, Weiss PF, Beukelman T, et al. 2013 update of the 2011 American College of Rheumatology recommendations for the treatment of juvenile idiopathic arthritis: recommendations for the medical therapy of children with systemic juvenile idiopathic arthritis and tuberculosis screening among children receiving biologic medications. Arthritis Care Res. 2013;65:1551–63.
162. Kimura Y, DeWitt EM, Beukelman T, et al. Adding Canakinumab to the childhood arthritis and rheumatology research alliance consensus treatment plans for systemic juvenile idiopathic arthritis [letter]. Arthritis Care Res. 2014;66:1430–1.
163. Woerner A, Uettwiller F, Melki I, et al. Biological treatment in systemic juvenile idiopathic arthritis: achievement of inactive disease or clinical remission on a first, second or third biological agent. RMD Open. 2015;1:e000036. https://doi.org/10.1136/rmdopen-2014-000036.
164. Record JL, Beukelman T, Cron RQ. Combination therapy of abatacept and anakinra in children with refractory systemic juvenile idiopathic arthritis: a retrospective case series. J Rheumatol. 2011;38:180–1.
165. Lee M, Isaacs J. The novel use of combined IL-1 and IL-6 inhibition in a patient with severe, aggressive, erosive, systemic-onset juvenile idiopathic arthritis. Eur J Rheumatol. 2017;4:68–9.
166. Brinkman BMC, de Kleer M, ten Cate R, et al. Autologous stem cell transplantation in children with severe progressive systemic or polyarticular juvenile idiopathic arthritis. Arthritis Rheum. 2007;56:2410–21.
167. Ravelli A, De Benedetti F, Viola S, et al. Macrophage activation syndrome in systemic juvenile rheumatoid arthritis successfully treated with cyclosporine. J Pediatr. 1996;128:275–8.
168. Ravelli A, Grom AA, Behrens EM, Cron RQ. Macrophage activation syndrome as part of systemic juvenile idiopathic arthritis: diagnosis, genetics, pathophysiology and treatment. Genes Immun. 2012;13:289–98.
169. Lomater C, Gerloni V, Gattinara M, Mazzotti J, Cimaz R, Fantini F. Systemic onset juvenile idiopathic arthritis: a retrospective study of 80 consecutive patients followed for 10 years. J Rheumatol. 2000;27:491–6.
170. Nigrovic PA, White PH. Care of the adult with juvenile rheumatoid arthritis. Arthritis Rheum. 2006;15(55):208–16.

171. Singh-Grewal D, Schneider R, Bayer N, Feldman BM. Predictors of disease course and remission in systemic juvenile idiopathic arthritis: significance of early clinical and laboratory features. Arthritis Rheum. 2006;54:1595–601.
172. Magni-Manzoni S, Pistorio A, Labo E, et al. A longitudinal analysis of physical functional disability over the course of juvenile idiopathic arthritis. Ann Rheum Dis. 2008;67:1159–64.
173. Schneider R, Lang BA, Reilly BJ, et al. Prognostic indicators of joint destruction in systemic onset juvenile rheumatoid arthritis. J Pediatr. 1992;120:200–5.
174. Spiegel LR, Schneider R, Lang BA, et al. Early predictors of poor functional outcome in systemic-onset juvenile rheumatoid arthritis. A multicenter cohort study. Arthritis Rheum. 2000;43:2402–9.
175. Modesto C, Woo P, García-Consuegra J, et al. Systemic onset juvenile chronic arthritis: polyarticular pattern and hip involvement as markers for a bad prognosis. Clin Exp Rheumatol. 2001;19:211–7.
176. Magni-Manzoni S, Rossi F, Pistorio A, et al. Prognostic factors for radiographic progression, radiographic damage, and disability in juvenile idiopathic arthritis. Arthritis Rheum. 2003;48:3509–17.
177. Oen K, Malleson PN, Cabral DA, et al. Early predictors of longterm outcome in patients with juvenile rheumatoid arthritis: subset-specific correlations. J Rheumatol. 2003;30:585–93.
178. Viola S, Felici E, Magni-Manzoni S, et al. Development and validation of a clinical index for assessment of long-term damage in juvenile idiopathic arthritis. Arthritis Rheum. 2005;52:2092–102.
179. Sandborg C, Holmes TH, Lee T, et al. Candidate early predictors for progression to joint damage in systemic juvenile idiopathic arthritis. J Rheumatol. 2006;33:2322–9.
180. Wallace CA, Huang B, Bandeira M, et al. Patterns of clinical remission in select categories of juvenile idiopathic arthritis. Arthritis Rheum. 2005;52:3554–62.
181. Guzman J, Oen K, Tucker LB, et al. The outcomes of juvenile idiopathic arthritis in children managed with contemporary cohort treatments: results from the ReACCh-Out. Ann Rheum Dis. 2015;74:1854–60.
182. Simonini G, Ferrara G, Pontikaki I, et al. Flares after withdrawal of biologic therapies in juvenile idiopathic arthritis: clinical and laboratory correlates of remission duration. Arthritis Care Res (Hoboken). 2018;70:1046–51.

Chapter 14
Macrophage Activation Syndrome (MAS)

Bella Mehta and Petros Efthimiou

Introduction

Macrophage activation syndrome (MAS), sometimes referred to as "cytokine storm," is a life-threatening condition and a catastrophic complication of adult-onset Still's disease (AOSD), systemic juvenile idiopathic arthritis (SJIA), systemic lupus erythematosus, or other autoimmune or autoinflammatory diseases [1–8]. In AOSD it has a mortality rate between 10% and 22% [9–11]. MAS is considered a subtype of hemophagocytic lymphohistiocytosis (HLH) when the clinical syndrome is associated with rheumatologic disorders. The syndrome of HLH is characterized by acute fever, hepatosplenomegaly, lymphadenopathy, pancytopenia, and extremely elevated levels of serum ferritin, triglycerides, and liver enzymes while being associated with a paradoxically low ESR.

Classification

HLH is classified as primary or secondary to triggering factors [12–14]. Primary HLH occurs in the setting of genetic disorders, such as autosomal recessive familial HLH (FHL) and familial erythrophagocytic lymphohistiocytosis, with multiple causal genes identified [15, 16]. Secondary HLH is associated with underlying

B. Mehta (✉)
Weill Cornell Medicine, New York, NY, USA

Hospital for Special Surgery, New York, NY, USA

P. Efthimiou
New York University School of Medicine, New York, NY, USA

NYU/Langone Health, New York, NY, USA
e-mail: petros.efthimiou@nyumc.org

P. Efthimiou (ed.), *Auto-Inflammatory Syndromes*,
https://doi.org/10.1007/978-3-319-96929-9_14

conditions, such as viral infections (29%), non-viral infections (20%), malignancies (27%), rheumatologic disorders (referred to as MAS) (7%), or immunodeficiency syndromes (6%) [1]. Viral infections include EBV, cytomegalovirus, parvovirus B19, human immunodeficiency virus (HIV), and human herpes virus 6. The most common malignancies that are associated with secondary HLH are the lymphomas (lymphoma-associated hemophagocytic syndrome, LAHS) [17, 18].

Cellular Pathology

On a cellular level, HLH/MAS is characterized by defective cytotoxic cell function coupled with unbridled macrophage activation and cytokine secretion, with the end result being cellular and organ damage. Several pro-inflammatory cytokines including interferon γ (INF-γ); interleukin (IL)-6, IL-8, IL-10, IL-12, and IL-18; tumor necrosis factor a (TNF-a); and macrophage inflammatory protein (MIP 1-a) are elevated in HLH/MAS [2, 18–23]. NK cells directly destroy damaged or infected cells, independent of the major histocompatibility complex (MHC) [24]. Therefore, the combination of a cytokine storm together with uncontrolled hemophagocytosis is established in a vicious cycle of self-perpetuating, feed-forward, unopposed inflammation [25, 26]. Severe IL-18/IL-18BP imbalance results in Th-1 lymphocyte and macrophage activation, which escapes control by NK cell cytotoxicity and may allow for the development of MAS [27].

Studies demonstrate that the amount of hemophagocytosis in the bone marrow of suspected HLH /MAS patients does not reliably correlate with disease probability [28–30]. Therefore, some experts consider extreme inflammation, rather than extensive hemophagocytosis, as the key cellular pathology of HLH/MAS [31]. An unconfirmed theory claimed that a state of immunodeficiency, induced by treatment of rheumatologic conditions, could reactivate latent viruses, such as Epstein-Barr virus, which could potentially lead to MAS [32]. However, MAS can be seen in the absence of immunomodulatory treatments. There is also a possibility that certain therapeutic agents, such as sulfasalazine, may be capable of provoking MAS [33].

Clinical Features

Most patients with HLH/MAS are acutely ill when they are diagnosed, typically with multiple organs affected. Since the definitive genetic expression profiles of peripheral blood mononuclear cells may not be readily available and can delay diagnosis, several attempts have been made to solve this diagnostic challenge [6, 34]. The most widely used diagnostic criteria for HLH were described by Henter et al. [35]. The diagnosis is established by either molecular diagnosis of HLH (e.g., pathologic mutations of

Table 14.1 Preliminary diagnostic guidelines for macrophage activation system complicating systemic juvenile idiopathic arthritis

Diagnostic criteria: Any two or more laboratory criteria or of any two or three or more clinical and/or laboratory criteria	
Laboratory criteria	**Clinical criteria**
Decreased platelet count ($\leq 262 \times 10^9$/L)	Central nervous system dysfunction (irritability, disorientation, lethargy, headache, seizures, coma)
Elevated levels of aspartate aminotransferase (>59 U/L)	Hemorrhages (purpura, easy bruising, mucosal bleeding)
Decreased white blood cell count ($\leq 4.0 \times 10^9$/L)	Hepatomegaly ($\geq$3 cm below the costal arch)
Hypofibrinogenemia ($\leq$2.5 g/L)	

Modified from Ravelli et al. [13]

PRF1, UNC13D, or STX11) or fulfillment of five out of eight criteria: (1) fever; (2) splenomegaly; (3) cytopenias (affecting at least two of three lineages in the peripheral blood); (4) hypertriglyceridemia (fasting, ≥265 mg/100 ml) and/or hypofibrinogenemia (≤150 mg/100 ml); (5) hemophagocytosis in BM, spleen, or lymph nodes; (6) low or absent NK cell activity; (7) ferritin ≥500 ng/ml; and (8) soluble CD25 (i.e, soluble IL-2 receptor) >2400 U/ml (or per local reference laboratory) [36]. Although these criteria use ferritin >500 ng/mL, many experts view ferritin >3000 ng/mL (some use a cutoff of 2000 ng/mL) as concerning for HLH/MAS and ferritin >10,000 as highly suspicious [37].

There are no established definitive diagnostic criteria for MAS; however, a preliminary diagnostic guideline for MAS complicating SJIA based on retrospective laboratory and clinical criteria is published [13]. The presence of any two or more of the laboratory or clinical criteria was found to be highly suggestive of MAS in patients with SJIA (Table 14.1) [13]. A bone marrow aspirate for the demonstration of hemophagocytosis may be required only in doubtful cases. These guidelines are limited by the non-specific nature of some of the laboratory criteria in the setting of autoimmune disease and by their omission of biopsy proven hemophagocytosis in the liver, lymph nodes, and spleen sites where hemophagocytosis is more frequently demonstrated at early stages of the syndrome than the bone marrow. Furthermore, given the retrospective nature of the study, these are not established guidelines and require further validation.

Association of Viral Infections with HLH and Malignancy

There is a complex relationship between viral infections, autoimmune diseases, HLH/MAS, and malignancy (Fig. 14.1). Some case reports suggest that activation of viruses like HHV8 and EBV in the setting of HLH lead to lymphoma [38]. EBV,

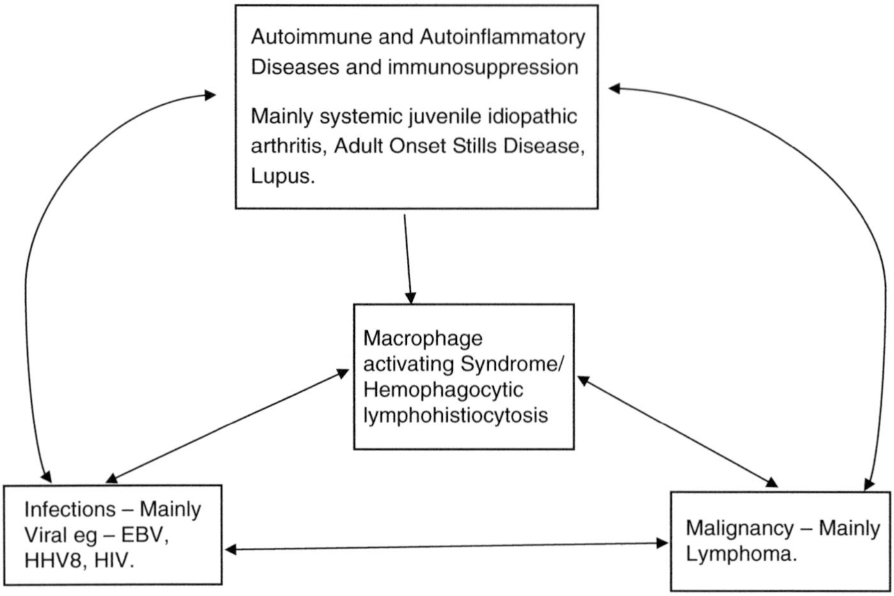

Fig. 14.1 Complex associations – macrophage activation syndrome and hemophagocytic lymphohistiocytosis syndrome

also called human herpes virus 4 (HHV-4) has been the most consistently reported virus associated with HLH [39–43]. It may be the cause or effect of patients with rheumatologic diseases on immunosuppressive therapy [44].

EBV reactivation in immunosuppressed and HIV patients has been shown to trigger HLH [45]. No single sub-strain of EBV has been identified as particularly associated with HLH as of yet [46].

Moreover, EBV is known to reactivate in immunosuppressed states and may have a causal association with malignancy [47]. There are several reports that HIV is associated with HLH [48, 49]. HHV8 has been shown to be associated with lymphomas [50–52]. Immunosuppressive medications like tocilizumab (IL-6 inhibitor) have been associated with MAS in patients with autoimmune diseases [32]. Anakinra (IL-1 inhibitor) was not associated with increased risk of lymphoma, and there have been no reports of EBV activation [53]. In the pediatric literature, there have been reports of anakinra use being associated with HLH [54, 55]. It is known that lymphomas are associated with HLH [56–58]. There is the argument that reports of immunomodulators used for autoinflammatory diseases, such as SJIA/AOSD, being associated with MAS development do not take into consideration the level of the underlying disease activity and the inflammatory response, which is a lot higher in MAS. The same treatments, albeit in much higher doses, have been reported to be effective in MAS cases.

Treatment

The mainstay treatment of MAS/HLH is control of hyperinflammation, and in cases where the trigger is known, elimination is necessary along with supportive therapy. Janka et al. detailed the principles as the Table 14.2 [59]. Pulse steroids could be considered the most important treatment for MAS/HLH. Addition of another agent can be used for steroid sparing. Chemotherapeutic regimens include etoposide, cyclosporin A (CSA), immunoglobulins, and anti-thymocyte globulin. Targeted biologic response modulators (BRMs) are used particularly when suspected underlying rheumatologic disease as the cause of HLH/MAS.

BRMs include IL-1 inhibitors, anti-TNF agents, anti-CD-52, and rituximab.

Anakinra blocks the biologic activity of naturally occurring IL-1, by competitively inhibiting the binding of IL-1 to the interleukin-1 type receptor, which is expressed in many tissues and organs. Anakinra has dramatically benefitted in patients with MAS [60, 61].

Canakinumab is a human monoclonal antibody targeted at IL-1β. Theoretically patients responding to anakinra should respond to canakinumab however that may not be the case as per some reports [62].

Anti-TNF agents in some cases have showed promising response in the initial stages [63, 64]. However a lot of cases of MAS are described in patients on anti-TNFs also a few where MAS worsened when anti-TNFs were given [65–67]. Thus, anti-TNFs are not a recommended treatment option. Alemtuzumab, an antibody against CD52 that is present not only on T cells but also on histiocytes, has been shown to be beneficial in patients with refractory HLH [68].

Table 14.2 Treatment principles

First-line medication	Corticosteroids – usually high doses of
Suppression of hyperinflammation (immunosuppression or immunomodulation)	IV immunoglobulins, cyclosporin A, anticytokine agents
Removal of cytokines	Plasmapheresis
Elimination of infectious trigger	Anti-infection therapy (antibiotics, antifungals, etc.)
Elimination of autoimmune/autoinflammatory trigger	Biologic response modulators (BRMs) mainly IL 1 blockade – anakinra
Supportive therapy (neutropenia, coagulopathy)	Blood products, coagulation factors, granulocyte stimulation factor
Removal of activated immune cells and (infected) antigen-presenting cells	Corticosteroids, etoposide, T cell antibodies (anti-thymocyte globulin, alemtuzumab), rituximab
Replacement of defective immune system	Hematopoietic stem cell transplant

Derived from Janka et al. [59]

Rituximab, an anti-CD20 antibody that depletes B lymphocytes, has been successfully used in EBV-induced lymphoproliferative disease and could be considered in EBV-driven MAS/HLH [69, 70].

Quantitative determination of EBV genome copy numbers in peripheral blood may be useful in predicting prognosis and effectiveness of therapy [71, 72].

Etoposide forms a ternary complex with DNA and the topoisomerase II enzyme (which aids in DNA unwinding), prevents religation of the DNA strands, and by doing so causes DNA strands to break. Etoposide appears to interfere with EBV-induced lymphocyte transformation and suppresses formation of EBV nuclear antigen. In more serious or resistant cases of EBV-associated HLH, etoposide is particularly helpful [73].

Cyclosporin A (CSA) inhibits calcineurin, which, under normal circumstances, is responsible for activating the transcription of interleukin 2. CSA likely inhibits the cytokine storm of MAS/HLH.

A pulse of high-dose corticosteroids with or without CSA is effective in most patients. Early introduction of etoposide improved survival [74].

In patients with severe kidney and liver disease, anti-thymocyte globulin (ATG) might be a safer alternative to etoposide [75, 76]. ATG depletes both CD4þ and CD8þ T cells through complement-dependent cell lysis thus effective however is associated with infusion reactions [77]. Plasma exchange, a historical treatment for removal of cytokines, may still be of use for patients who do not respond to standard treatment or to buy time until other therapies reach therapeutic effect [78, 79]. Definitive treatment with bone marrow transplant has been proposed [80]. Early recognition and prompt treatment initiation is the key to treatment.

References

1. Dhote R, et al. Reactive hemophagocytic syndrome in adult systemic disease: report of twenty-six cases and literature review. Arthritis Rheum. 2003;49(5):633–9.
2. Felix FH, Leal LK, Fontenele JB. Cloak and dagger: the case for adult onset still disease and hemophagocytic lymphohistiocytosis. Rheumatol Int. 2009;29(8):973–4.
3. Kirino Y, et al. Increased serum HO-1 in hemophagocytic syndrome and adult-onset Still's disease: use in the differential diagnosis of hyperferritinemia. Arthritis Res Ther. 2005;7(3):R616–24.
4. Wang Z, et al. Early diagnostic value of low percentage of glycosylated ferritin in secondary hemophagocytic lymphohistiocytosis. Int J Hematol. 2009;90(4):501–5.
5. Pringe A, et al. Macrophage activation syndrome in juvenile systemic lupus erythematosus: an under-recognized complication? Lupus. 2007;16(8):587–92.
6. Davi S, et al. An international consensus survey of diagnostic criteria for macrophage activation syndrome in systemic juvenile idiopathic arthritis. J Rheumatol. 2011;38(4):764–8.
7. Donn R, et al. Genetic loci contributing to hemophagocytic lymphohistiocytosis do not confer susceptibility to systemic-onset juvenile idiopathic arthritis. Arthritis Rheum. 2008;58(3):869–74.
8. Hazen MM, et al. Mutations of the hemophagocytic lymphohistiocytosis-associated gene UNC13D in a patient with systemic juvenile idiopathic arthritis. Arthritis Rheum. 2008;58(2):567–70.

9. Durand M, et al. Macrophage activation syndrome treated with anakinra. J Rheumatol. 2010;37(4):879–80.
10. Tristano AG. Macrophage activation syndrome: a frequent but under-diagnosed complication associated with rheumatic diseases. Med Sci Monit. 2008;14(3):RA27–36.
11. Kumakura S, Murakawa Y. Clinical characteristics and treatment outcomes of autoimmune-associated hemophagocytic syndrome in adults. Arthritis Rheumatol. 2014;66(8):2297–307.
12. Arlet JB, et al. Reactive haemophagocytic syndrome in adult-onset Still's disease: a report of six patients and a review of the literature. Ann Rheum Dis. 2006;65(12):1596–601.
13. Ravelli A, et al. Preliminary diagnostic guidelines for macrophage activation syndrome complicating systemic juvenile idiopathic arthritis. J Pediatr. 2005;146(5):598–604.
14. Sawhney S, Woo P, Murray KJ. Macrophage activation syndrome: a potentially fatal complication of rheumatic disorders. Arch Dis Child. 2001;85(5):421–6.
15. Zhang K, et al. Hypomorphic mutations in PRF1, MUNC13-4, and STXBP2 are associated with adult-onset familial HLH. Blood. 2011;118(22):5794–8.
16. Meeths M, et al. Familial hemophagocytic lymphohistiocytosis type 3 (FHL3) caused by deep intronic mutation and inversion in UNC13D. Blood. 2011;118(22):5783–93.
17. Falini B, et al. Peripheral T-cell lymphoma associated with hemophagocytic syndrome. Blood. 1990;75(2):434–44.
18. Jaffe ES, et al. Malignant lymphoma and erythrophagocytosis simulating malignant histiocytosis. Am J Med. 1983;75(5):741–9.
19. Henter JI, et al. Hypercytokinemia in familial hemophagocytic lymphohistiocytosis. Blood. 1991;78(11):2918–22.
20. Osugi Y, et al. Cytokine production regulating Th1 and Th2 cytokines in hemophagocytic lymphohistiocytosis. Blood. 1997;89(11):4100–3.
21. Takada H, et al. Oversecretion of IL-18 in haemophagocytic lymphohistiocytosis: a novel marker of disease activity. Br J Haematol. 1999;106(1):182–9.
22. Schneider EM, et al. Hemophagocytic lymphohistiocytosis is associated with deficiencies of cellular cytolysis but normal expression of transcripts relevant to killer-cell-induced apoptosis. Blood. 2002;100(8):2891–8.
23. Teruya-Feldstein J, et al. MIP-1alpha expression in tissues from patients with hemophagocytic syndrome. Lab Investig. 1999;79(12):1583–90.
24. George MR. Hemophagocytic lymphohistiocytosis: review of etiologies and management. J Blood Med. 2014;5:69–86.
25. Behrens EM, et al. Repeated TLR9 stimulation results in macrophage activation syndrome-like disease in mice. J Clin Invest. 2011;121(6):2264–77.
26. Terrell CE, Jordan MB. Perforin deficiency impairs a critical immunoregulatory loop involving murine CD8(+) T cells and dendritic cells. Blood. 2013;121(26):5184–91.
27. Mazodier K, et al. Severe imbalance of IL-18/IL-18BP in patients with secondary hemophagocytic syndrome. Blood. 2005;106(10):3483–9.
28. Ho C, et al. Marrow assessment for hemophagocytic lymphohistiocytosis demonstrates poor correlation with disease probability. Am J Clin Pathol. 2014;141(1):62–71.
29. Goel S, Polski JM, Imran H. Sensitivity and specificity of bone marrow hemophagocytosis in hemophagocytic lymphohistiocytosis. Ann Clin Lab Sci. 2012;42(1):21–5.
30. Gupta A, et al. The role of the initial bone marrow aspirate in the diagnosis of hemophagocytic lymphohistiocytosis. Pediatr Blood Cancer. 2008;51(3):402–4.
31. Weaver LK, Behrens EM. Hyperinflammation, rather than hemophagocytosis, is the common link between macrophage activation syndrome and hemophagocytic lymphohistiocytosis. Curr Opin Rheumatol. 2014;26(5):562–9.
32. Yokota S, et al. Macrophage activation syndrome in patients with systemic juvenile idiopathic arthritis under treatment with tocilizumab. J Rheumatol. 2015;42:712.
33. Singh S, Samant R, Joshi VR. Adult onset Still's disease: a study of 14 cases. Clin Rheumatol. 2008;27(1):35–9.
34. Sumegi J, et al. Gene-expression signatures differ between different clinical forms of familial hemophagocytic lymphohistiocytosis. Blood. 2013;121(7):e14–24.

35. Henter JI, et al. HLH-2004: diagnostic and therapeutic guidelines for hemophagocytic lymphohistiocytosis. Pediatr Blood Cancer. 2007;48(2):124–31.
36. Stephan JL, et al. Reactive haemophagocytic syndrome in children with inflammatory disorders. A retrospective study of 24 patients. Rheumatology (Oxford). 2001;40(11):1285–92.
37. Allen CE, et al. Highly elevated ferritin levels and the diagnosis of hemophagocytic lymphohistiocytosis. Pediatr Blood Cancer. 2008;50(6):1227–35.
38. Shah NN, et al. Extracavitary primary effusion lymphoma initially presenting with hemophagocytic lymphohistocytosis. Clin Lymphoma Myeloma Leuk. 2014;14(5):e157–60.
39. Belyea B, et al. Spontaneous resolution of Epstein-Barr virus-associated hemophagocytic lymphohistiocytosis. Pediatr Blood Cancer. 2010;55(4):754–6.
40. Imashuku S. Treatment of Epstein-Barr virus-related hemophagocytic lymphohistiocytosis (EBV-HLH); update 2010. J Pediatr Hematol Oncol. 2011;33(1):35–9.
41. George TI, et al. Epstein-Barr virus-associated peripheral T-cell lymphoma and hemophagocytic syndrome arising after liver transplantation: case report and review of the literature. Pediatr Blood Cancer. 2005;44(3):270–6.
42. Fox CP, et al. Epstein-Barr virus-associated hemophagocytic lymphohistiocytosis in adults characterized by high viral genome load within circulating natural killer cells. Clin Infect Dis. 2010;51(1):66–9.
43. Chellapandian D, et al. Treatment of Epstein Barr virus-induced haemophagocytic lymphohistiocytosis with rituximab-containing chemo-immunotherapeutic regimens. Br J Haematol. 2013;162(3):376–82.
44. Parvaneh N, Filipovich AH, Borkhardt A. Primary immunodeficiencies predisposed to Epstein-Barr virus-driven haematological diseases. Br J Haematol. 2013;162(5):573–86.
45. Thoden J, et al. Fatal hemophagocytic syndrome in a patient with a previously well-controlled asymptomatic HIV infection after EBV reactivation. J Infect. 2012;64(1):110–2.
46. Kelesidis T, et al. Epstein-Barr virus-associated hemophagocytic lymphohistiocytosis in Los Angeles County. J Med Virol. 2012;84(5):777–85.
47. Tse E, Kwong YL. Epstein Barr virus-associated lymphoproliferative diseases: the virus as a therapeutic target. Exp Mol Med. 2015;47:e136.
48. Park KH, et al. Acute human immunodeficiency virus syndrome presenting with hemophagocytic lymphohistiocytosis. Yonsei Med J. 2008;49(2):325–8.
49. Safdar SM, et al. Fatal hemophagocytic syndrome as a manifestation of immune reconstitution syndrome in a patient with acquired immunodeficiency syndrome. Saudi Med J. 2013;34(8):861–4.
50. Yamada M, et al. Unique expression pattern of viral proteins in human herpesvirus 8-positive plasmablastic lymphoma: a case report. Int J Clin Exp Pathol. 2014;7(9):6415–8.
51. Kaplan LD. Human herpesvirus-8: Kaposi sarcoma, multicentric Castleman disease, and primary effusion lymphoma. Hematology Am Soc Hematol Educ Program. 2013;2013:103–8.
52. Fernandes F, et al. Simultaneous presentation of Kaposi sarcoma and HHV8-associated large B-cell lymphoma in the same lymph node: a rare diagnosis in an HIV-negative patient. Am J Case Rep. 2013;14:263–6.
53. Fleischmann RM, et al. Safety of extended treatment with anakinra in patients with rheumatoid arthritis. Ann Rheum Dis. 2006;65(8):1006–12.
54. Nigrovic PA, et al. Anakinra as first-line disease-modifying therapy in systemic juvenile idiopathic arthritis: report of forty-six patients from an international multicenter series. Arthritis Rheum. 2011;63(2):545–55.
55. Zeft A, et al. Anakinra for systemic juvenile arthritis: the Rocky Mountain experience. J Clin Rheumatol. 2009;15(4):161–4.
56. Mehta B, Kasturi S, Teruya-Feldstein J, Horwitz S, Bass AR, Erkan D. Adult-Onset Still's Disease and Macrophage-Activating Syndrome Progressing to Lymphoma: a Clinical Pathology Conference Held by the Division of Rheumatology at Hospital for Special Surgery. HSS J. 2018;14(2):214–21. https://doi.org/10.1007/s11420-018-9606-8. Epub 2018 Mar 26.
57. Balwierz W, Czogala M, Czepko E. Anaplastic large cell lymphoma associated with hemophagocytic lymphohistiocytosis: a case report and review of the literature. Przegl Lek. 2010;67(6):436–8.

58. Hagihara M, et al. Lymphocyte-depleted Hodgkin lymphoma complicating hemophagocytic lymphohistiocytosis as an initial manifestation: a case report and review of the literature. Intern Med. 2012;51(21):3067–72.
59. Janka GE, Lehmberg K. Hemophagocytic lymphohistiocytosis: pathogenesis and treatment. Hematology Am Soc Hematol Educ Program. 2013;2013:605–11.
60. Kelly A, Ramanan AV. A case of macrophage activation syndrome successfully treated with anakinra. Nat Clin Pract Rheumatol. 2008;4(11):615–20.
61. Bruck N, et al. Rapid and sustained remission of systemic juvenile idiopathic arthritis-associated macrophage activation syndrome through treatment with anakinra and corticosteroids. J Clin Rheumatol. 2011;17(1):23–7.
62. De Benedetti F, et al. Randomized trial of tocilizumab in systemic juvenile idiopathic arthritis. N Engl J Med. 2012;367(25):2385–95.
63. Aeberli D, et al. Inhibition of the TNF-pathway: use of infliximab and etanercept as remission-inducing agents in cases of therapy-resistant chronic inflammatory disorders. Swiss Med Wkly. 2002;132(29–30):414–22.
64. Prahalad S, et al. Etanercept in the treatment of macrophage activation syndrome. J Rheumatol. 2001;28(9):2120–4.
65. Ramanan AV, Schneider R. Macrophage activation syndrome following initiation of etanercept in a child with systemic onset juvenile rheumatoid arthritis. J Rheumatol. 2003;30(2):401–3.
66. Atteritano M, et al. Haemophagocytic syndrome in rheumatic patients. A systematic review. Eur Rev Med Pharmacol Sci. 2012;16(10):1414–24.
67. Stern A, Riley R, Buckley L. Worsening of macrophage activation syndrome in a patient with adult onset Still's disease after initiation of etanercept therapy. J Clin Rheumatol. 2001;7(4):252–6.
68. Marsh RA, et al. Salvage therapy of refractory hemophagocytic lymphohistiocytosis with alemtuzumab. Pediatr Blood Cancer. 2013;60(1):101–9.
69. Bosman G, et al. The role of rituximab in a case of EBV-related lymphoproliferative disease presenting with haemophagocytosis. Neth J Med. 2009;67(8):364–5.
70. Balamuth NJ, et al. Use of rituximab in conjunction with immunosuppressive chemotherapy as a novel therapy for Epstein Barr virus-associated hemophagocytic lymphohistiocytosis. J Pediatr Hematol Oncol. 2007;29(8):569–73.
71. Sonke GS, et al. Poor outcomes of chronic active Epstein-Barr virus infection and hemophagocytic lymphohistiocytosis in non-Japanese adult patients. Clin Infect Dis. 2008;47(1):105–8.
72. Rouphael NG, et al. Infections associated with haemophagocytic syndrome. Lancet Infect Dis. 2007;7(12):814–22.
73. Imashuku S, et al. Recent developments in the management of haemophagocytic lymphohistiocytosis. Expert Opin Pharmacother. 2001;2(9):1437–48.
74. Imashuku S, et al. Requirement for etoposide in the treatment of Epstein-Barr virus-associated hemophagocytic lymphohistiocytosis. J Clin Oncol. 2001;19(10):2665–73.
75. Coca A, et al. Macrophage activation syndrome: serological markers and treatment with anti-thymocyte globulin. Clin Immunol. 2009;132(1):10–8.
76. Mahlaoui N, et al. Immunotherapy of familial hemophagocytic lymphohistiocytosis with antithymocyte globulins: a single-center retrospective report of 38 patients. Pediatrics. 2007;120(3):e622–8.
77. Schulert GS, Grom AA. Macrophage activation syndrome and cytokine-directed therapies. Best Pract Res Clin Rheumatol. 2014;28(2):277–92.
78. Matsumoto Y, et al. The efficacy of therapeutic plasmapheresis for the treatment of fatal hemophagocytic syndrome: two case reports. Ther Apher. 1998;2(4):300–4.
79. Raschke RA, Garcia-Orr R. Hemophagocytic lymphohistiocytosis: a potentially underrecognized association with systemic inflammatory response syndrome, severe sepsis, and septic shock in adults. Chest. 2011;140(4):933–8.
80. Jordan MB, Filipovich AH. Hematopoietic cell transplantation for hemophagocytic lymphohistiocytosis: a journey of a thousand miles begins with a single (big) step. Bone Marrow Transplant. 2008;42(7):433–7.

Chapter 15
Schnitzler Syndrome

Paolo Sfriso and Paola Galozzi

The Schnitzler syndrome is a late-onset autoinflammatory disease firstly reported in 1972 by Liliane Schnitzler, a French dermatologist [1]. Its main clinical features are neutrophilic urticarial rash, lymphadenopathy, arthralgia, bone pain, fatigue and systemic inflammatory response [2]. It is associated with a monoclonal gammopathy, typically of immunoglobulin M (IgM) type but sometimes of immunoglobulin G (IgG) type [3]. Schnitzler syndrome patients may also develop an inflammatory anaemia and AA amyloidosis, if untreated, and about 20% can evolve in a lymphoproliferative disorder. Treatment of the Schnitzler syndrome is based on IL-1 blocking agents, even though the disease reappears as soon as treatment is stopped [4].

Epidemiology

Schnitzler syndrome is a rare acquired autoinflammatory disorder. Prevalence is unknown; however, it is likely to be an underdiagnosed condition with about 300 cases reported in literature so far. During the 1970s to early 1990s, Schnitzler syndrome was reported solely in Western European countries, especially in France, presumably due to a better knowledge of this entity. In the last decades, however, cases have been reported in countries all over the world, without ethnic prevalence [5].

The Schnitzler syndrome has a slight male predominance and is basically a disease of middle-aged adults. Few cases have been reported with onset before age of 35 [6].

P. Sfriso (✉) · P. Galozzi
Unit of Rheumatology, Department of Medicine – DIMED, University of Padova, Padova, Italy
e-mail: paolo.sfriso@unipd.it

P. Efthimiou (ed.), *Auto-Inflammatory Syndromes*,
https://doi.org/10.1007/978-3-319-96929-9_15

Pathogenesis

The pathogenesis of the Schnitzler syndrome is not completely understood. Many features indicate that it is an acquired autoinflammatory disorder [7]. The Schnitzler syndrome shares many features with genetically determined autoinflammatory syndromes, as the recurrent fever of unknown cause, the peculiar eruption very similar to the one observed in cryopyrinopathies (CINCA/NOMID syndrome, Muckle-Wells syndrome and FCAS), a significant increase of neutrophils in blood and tissues and an increased interleukin (IL)-1β production in LPS-stimulated peripheral blood monocytes [8]. Recently, Noster et al. demonstrated that systemic overproduction of IL-1β in the Schnitzler syndrome results in a decreased ability of anti-inflammatory T-helper (Th)17 cells to produce IL-10 once stimulated [9]. IL-1β blocking therapy seems to restore the regulatory properties of Th17. Furthermore, the spectacular response to the IL-1 inhibitor agents within hours after the first injection suggests a direct pathogenic effect of IL-1.

A genetic predisposition involving an activating mutation in the *NLRP3* (nucleotide-binding oligomerization domain-leucine-rich repeats containing pyrin domain 3) gene, the same gene involved in CAPS, has been reported in Schnitzler syndrome patients. Using targeted deep resequencing of the *NLRP3* gene, de Koning et al. identified 2 out of 11 patients as NLRP3 mosaics. The authors suggested that Schnitzler syndrome can be caused by mosaic mutations in the *NLRP3* gene in myeloid cells that drive inflammation. Mosaicism explains the later onset of the disease and a slightly different phenotypic spectrum from patients with germline mutations [10].

The role of the monoclonal IgM component in the pathogenesis of the Schnitzler syndrome remains unclear. It is still not known if IgM is the cause or the consequence of the disease: it could be a natural proliferation or the result of a continuous antigenic stimulation or could directly act in a particular biological activity. Interestingly, a few cases of Schnitzler's syndrome without monoclonal gammopathy have been reported [11, 12].

Clinical Manifestations

The first clinical signs of the Schnitzler syndrome are generally urticarial rash, mainly associated with recurrent fever or joint pain (Table 15.1).

The recurrent rash is present mostly on the trunk and limbs. The eruption consists of rose pale or red macules or slightly raised papules and plaques (Fig. 15.1). The frequency of flares is variable from patient to patient, lasts less than 24 h and is usually moderately itchy. Oedematous swelling of the face (angioedema) is very rare, and significant mucosal swelling with dyspnoea and/or dysphonia is exceptional. The rash can be exacerbated by heat/cold exposure, alcohol consumption, stress or physical exercise.

Table 15.1 Clinical and biological findings in patients with Schnitzler syndrome

Clinical findings	Biological findings
Urticarial rash	Monoclonal IgM gammopathy
Fever	Elevated ESR and/or CRP
Arthralgia/arthritis	Leucocytosis (PMN > 10,000/mm^3)
Bone pain	
Abnormal bone morphology	
Palpable lymph nodes	
Liver and/or spleen enlargement	

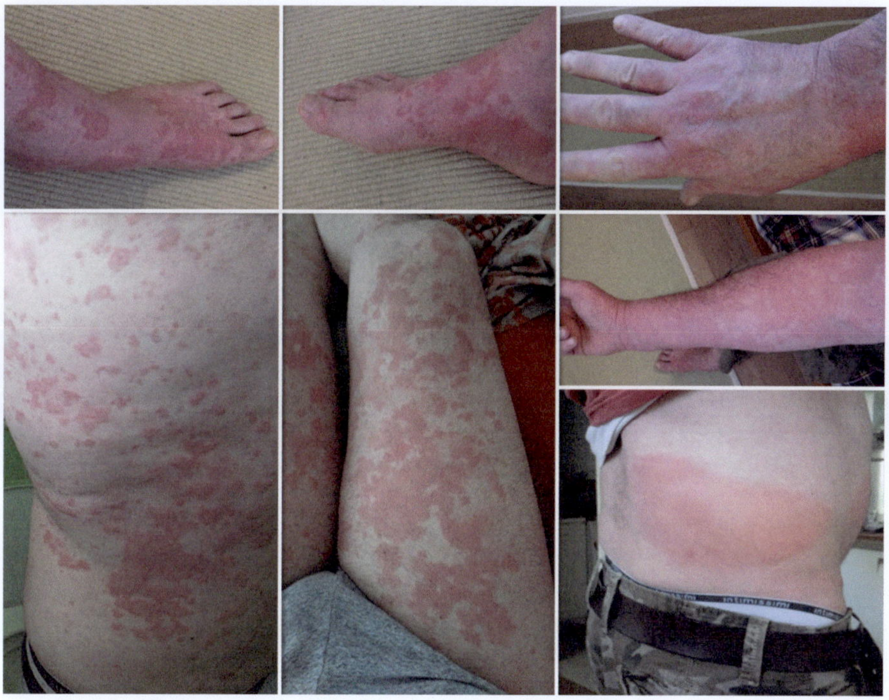

Fig. 15.1 Clinical aspect of the urticarial recurrent rash in patients with the Schnitzler syndrome

A biopsy of a typical plaque at a relatively early stage shows a neutrophilic dermal infiltrate with variable density. The histopathological findings are important for the diagnosis. The epidermis is usually normal. There are no vasculitis and no significant dermal oedema but a perivascular and interstitial infiltrate of neutrophils with leucocytoclasia. Clustering of neutrophils around sweat glands can be found. Vasculitis has been reported in up to 20% of patients, but it might be overestimated as reported by Lipsker that reviewed some published pictures without seen fibrinoid necrosis of vessel wall [7]. Immunofluorescence and immunoelectron microscopic studies show deposition of immunoreactants, mainly IgM, around the superficial dermal vessels, in the epidermis and at the dermal-epidermal junction [13, 14]. The pathogenetic role of these deposits is unclear, but they probably could trigger a local inflammation.

The majority of patients present intermittent fever, rising above 40°C. The fever does not always occur together with the skin rash.

Musculoskeletal involvement is another important feature of the Schnitzler syndrome. About 80% of patients complain of bone pain and arthralgias and sometimes develop nonerosive arthritis. The large joints are mainly affected, including the hips, knees, wrists and ankles.

Bone pain affects mostly the pelvis, the femurs and the tibias. The spine, the clavicles and the forearms are less often involved [15].

Radiographic studies show abnormal bone morphology in about 60% of patients [4]. Bone lesions characteristically are sclerotic, whereas lytic lesions are uncommon [16].

The most frequent radiological pattern is a sclerotic bone marrow involvement with bilateral periostitis of the bones of the knee joint. Bone scintigraphy is the most sensitive test for Schnitzler lesions, showing focal increased tracer uptake. MRI frequently shows the areas of bone marrow oedema, suggesting a primary osteitis.

None of the imaging findings are specific, and several differential diagnoses should be considered. The imaging differential diagnosis primarily includes hypertrophic osteoarthropathy, infectious osteitis, SAPHO (synovitis-acne-pustulosis-hyperostosis-osteitis), POEMS (polyneuropathy, organomegaly, endocrinopathy, monoclonal protein, skin lesions), metastatic disease, CRMO (chronic recurrent multifocal osteomyelitis), Erdheim-Chester disease, mastocytosis, enchondroma and bone infarction [15, 17].

Other common clinical signs are asthenia, loss of weight, myalgia and headache.

Lymphadenopathy is found in 50% of patients. Splenomegaly and/or hepatomegaly could be also present in about 30% of patients. PET/CT imaging is perhaps the most sensitive technique to demonstrate the presence of lymphadenopathy and hepatic or splenic enlargement. Enlarged lymph nodes are usually located at the axillary and inguinal sites. As they can be multiple, permanent and measure up to 3 cm, a biopsy is often required to exclude a lymphoma. Histology shows nonspecific inflammation.

Biological Findings

The monoclonal component is a defining criterion of the Schnitzler syndrome and therefore presents in all patients. A monoclonal IgM gammopathy is recognized in about 90% of cases, while monoclonal IgG gammopathy has been reported in less than 10% of cases. This percentage could be underestimated, as IgG component was

Table 15.2 Lipsker diagnostic criteria of Schnitzler syndrome

Urticarial rash
Monoclonal IgM component
At least 2 of the following criteria:
Fever
Arthralgia or arthritis
Bone pain
Palpable lymph nodes
Liver or spleen enlargement
Elevated ESR
Leucocytosis
Abnormal findings on bone morphologic investigations

not initially included in the definition of the disease. In more than 90% of patients, the monoclonal IgM gammopathy is associated to a kappa light chain.

Patients with monoclonal IgA gammopathy have also been reported but in addition to IgM κ gammopathy [18]. At the moment of diagnosis, the level of the monoclonal component is highly variable. It can be almost undetectable or, conversely, very high (up to 41 g/l) [19]. During the course of the disease, the level of the monoclonal component can remain stable or progressively increase at 0.5 to 1 g/L per year.

Inflammatory markers, such as erythrocyte sedimentation rate (ESR) and C-reactive protein (CRP), are elevated. Leucocytosis is recognized in 90% of cases with a persistent increase of neutrophils (>10,000/mm^3). Complement levels are generally normal. Inflammatory anaemia and sometimes thrombocytosis can also be observed [20].

Diagnosis

There is no specific test for Schnitzler syndrome. Thus, diagnosis is based on a combination of clinical, biological and radiological findings and can be made after the exclusion of other autoimmune, infectious, neoplastic and idiopathic conditions.

The differential diagnosis must include in particular adult-onset Still's disease (AOSD), cryopyrin-associated periodic syndrome (especially Muckle-Wells syndrome) and other monogenic autoinflammatory syndromes, hypocomplementemic urticarial vasculitis, acquired C1 inhibitor deficiency, lymphoma, and Waldenström's disease.

The widely accepted diagnostic criteria were established in 2001 by Lipsker et al. (Table 15.2) [13]. Based on these criteria, the diagnosis of Schnitzler syndrome could be made if the patient presents a combination of an urticarial skin rash, a monoclonal IgM component and at least two of the following criteria: recurrent fever, arthralgia or arthritis, bone pain, lymphadenopathy, hepato- or splenomegaly, leucocytosis, elevated ESR and abnormal findings on bone morphologic investigations.

Clinicians have to be careful in the presence of monoclonal gammopathy of undetermined significance (MGUS) that could exist in association with chronic urticaria of other causes, mimicking the Schnitzler syndrome. However, MGUS and Schnitzler syndrome differ in the possible complications [21].

The Lipsker criteria were revised in 2012 during an expert meeting in Strasbourg (Table 15.3). The Strasbourg criteria introduced the presence of the monoclonal IgG component, which the previous criteria did not, and the dermal neutrophilic infiltrate on skin biopsy. Furthermore, the Strasbourg criteria added the possibility to distinguish between patients with definite Schnitzler syndrome and probable Schnitzler syndrome [4]. In 2016, a multicentric study validated the two sets of criteria, confirming their reliability and validity in clinical practice; however, the efficiency of the diagnostic criteria was not tested in patients with recent-onset disease. The specificity of the Lipsker and the Strasbourg criteria is similar (97%, 100%), but the Lipsker criteria are more sensitive (100% vs 81% and 93% for definite and probable diagnosis, respectively) [19].

Prognosis and Complications

The overall prognosis of Schnitzler syndrome depends on progression to haematological malignancy and the occurrence of AA amyloidosis. Thus, the disease requires long-term follow-up due to the potential development of lymphoproliferative disorders.

Waldenström's disease occurs in about 15% of cases after 10–20 years of evolution [22]. There is neither specific predictive factor nor therapy clearly associated with a reduction of the risk of a lymphoproliferative disorder.

Table 15.3 Strasbourg diagnostic criteria of Schnitzler syndrome

Obligate criteria	Minor criteria
Chronic urticarial rash	Recurrent fever (>38 °C and unexplained) together with skin rash
Monoclonal IgM or IgG	Abnormal bone remodelling with or without bone pain (assessed by bone scintigraphy, MRI or elevation of bone alkaline phosphatase)
	A neutrophilic dermal infiltrate on skin biopsy (absence of fibrinoid necrosis and significant dermal oedema)
	Leucocytosis (neutrophils >10,000/mm^3) and/or elevated CRP (>30 mg/l)
A *definite diagnosis* occurs with two obligate criteria and at least two minor criteria if IgM and three minor criteria if IgG	
A *probable diagnosis* occurs with two obligate criteria and at least one minor criteria if IgM and two minor criteria if IgG	

Also severe anaemia and AA amyloidosis are potential complications in untreated patients [23].

A few cases have reported kidney involvement in the disease, which can be a severe complication [24].

Diffuse aortitis has recently been described in a typical case of Schnitzler syndrome, a condition that can lead to severe aneurysm or arterial thrombosis. Schnitzler syndrome manifestations and aortitis both responded to treatment with anakinra suggesting that aortitis was directly related to Schnitzler syndrome in this patient [25].

Treatments

Before the introduction of IL-1 inhibitors, several drugs have been used to treat the Schnitzler syndrome, but none could induce remission for a long time of all symptoms [7]. Although patients often responded to high doses of steroids, the effects were incomplete, with disease flares on drug discontinuation. Immunosuppressive agents such as cyclophosphamide, azathioprine and methotrexate have proved ineffective. Intravenous immunoglobulin or tumour necrosis factor-α blocking agents are also substantially ineffective. Colchicine and dapsone can provide relief in mild cases, while hydroxychloroquine may be effective on joint symptoms [26]. Pefloxacin, a quinolone antibiotic, was successfully used in some patients, even though the mechanism of its action is not known [27].

To date, IL-1 blockade is the most effective therapy [4]. The efficacy of anakinra, the IL-1 receptor antagonist, was first reported in 2005, and it was subsequently confirmed by many case reports and also a multicentre retrospective cohort study [28, 29]. More than 80% of patients treated with IL-1 inhibitors present a complete remission; the remaining patients have the persistence of joint pain [30]. IL-1 blocking agents are efficient on the inflammation-linked symptoms but not on the monoclonal component. They probably do not reduce the risk of the development of lymphoproliferative disorders that remains the main prognostic issue.

Among the IL-1 blocking agents, the most commonly used is anakinra. Anakinra is the non-glycosylated recombinant soluble antagonist of the IL-1 receptor (IL-1R) that acts preventing activation of this receptor and inhibiting both IL-1α and IL-1β activities. Anakinra has a short half-life (approximately 6 h) and generally is given daily at 100 mg/day subcutaneously [7]. Some patients seem to be able to maintain disease control with alternate-day therapy, while in other cases, to achieve good control of the disease, it is necessary to increase the dose up to 300 mg/day. Anakinra rapidly relieves all clinical symptoms within the hours that follow the first injection. If the patient skips a dose, symptoms quickly reappear. The drug is generally well tolerated apart from local erythematous reaction at the injection site. Neutropenia can also occur especially soon after the introduction of anakinra. Once normalize the neutrophil count, the drug can be reintroduced [31].

The efficacy of other IL-1 inhibitors has also been reported. Canakinumab, a recombinant human monoclonal antibody specifically targeting IL-1β, induces complete remission with disappearance of fever and arthralgias, near abolishment of fatigue and rash and substantial reduction of CRP levels. As for anakinra, interruption of canakinumab can lead to a flare, which can be countered as soon as injections are resumed [32–34]. A phase II randomized placebo-controlled multicentre study was performed to assess the effects of canakinumab in Schnitzler syndrome [35]. Patients received single subcutaneous canakinumab 150 mg or placebo injections for 7 days, followed by a 16-week open-label phase with canakinumab injections on confirmed relapse of symptoms. The results showed good efficacy of canakinumab against placebo in reducing both clinical symptoms and inflammation markers and enhancing quality of life in patients. Even with the limited 4-month duration of the study, canakinumab treatment appears to be safe and well tolerated. Adverse events were controllable and included respiratory tract infections, gastrointestinal symptoms, hypertension, injection-site reactions and neutropenia.

Rilonacept (IL-1 TRAP) is a recombinant chimeric protein consisting of extracellular domains of the human IL-1R complex fused to the Fc-portion of human IgG1. This protein is able to bind IL-1α and IL-1β with high affinity. Patients received a subcutaneous loading dose of rilonacept 320 mg followed by weekly subcutaneous doses of 160 mg for up to 1 year. Rilonacept results effective in reducing clinical symptoms and inflammatory markers. No treatment-related adverse events were reported except mild injection site reactions, upper airway infections, headache and neutropenia [36].

In patients who do not respond to IL-1 inhibitors, if the diagnosis of Schnitzler syndrome is confirmed, an anti-IL-6 treatment should be considered [37]. Tocilizumab treatment (8 mg/kg/month) showed rapid and complete remission of clinical symptoms and inflammatory markers.

References

1. Schnitzler L. Lésions urticariennes chroniques permanentes (érythème pétaloïde?). Journées Dermatologiques d'Angers. 1972; Cas Clinique. N°46b.
2. Schnitzler L, Schubert B, Verret JL, Simon L, Alquier P. Cutaneous manifestations in disseminated intravascular coagulation syndrome. Ann Dermatol Syphiligr. 1976;103:124–34.
3. Lipsker D. Monoclonal gammopathy of cutaneous significance: review of a relevant concept. J Eur Acad Dermatol Venereol. 2017;31:45–52.
4. Simon A, Asli B, Braun-Falco M, De Koning H, Fermand JP, Grattan C, et al. Schnitzler's syndrome: diagnosis, treatment, and follow-up. Allergy. 2013;68:562–8.
5. de Koning HD. Schnitzler's syndrome: lessons from 281 cases. Clin Transl Allergy. 2014;4:41.
6. de Koning HD, Bodar EJ, van der Meer JW, Simon A. Schnitzler Syndrome Study Group: Schnitzler syndrome: beyond the case reports: review and follow-up of 94 patients with an emphasis on prognosis and treatment. Semin Arthritis Rheum. 2007;37(3):137–48.
7. Lipsker D. The Schnitzler syndrome. Orphanet J Rare Dis. 2010;5:38.
8. Pizzirani C, Falzoni S, Govoni M, La Corte R, Donadei S, Di Virgilio F, et al. Dysfunctional inflammasome in Schnitzler's syndrome. Rheumatology (Oxford). 2009;48(10):1304–8.

9. Noster R, de Koning HD, Maier E, Prelog M, Lainka E, Zielinski CE. Dysregulation of proinflammatory versus anti-inflammatory human TH17 cell functionalities in the autoinflammatory Schnitzler syndrome. J Allergy Clin Immunol. 2016;138:1161–9.
10. de Koning HD, van Gijn ME, Stoffels M, Jongekrijg J, Zeeuwen PL, Elferink MG, et al. Myeloid lineage–restricted somatic mosaicism of NLRP3 mutations in patients with variant Schnitzler syndrome. J Allergy Clin Immunol. 2015;135:561–4.
11. Varella TC, Nishimura MY, Machado MC, de Moraes-Vasconcelos D, Rivitti EA. Schnitzler's syndrome without monoclonal gammopathy. Acta Derm Venereol. 2005;85:272–3.
12. Urbanski M, Holfeld K, Milne A, Abbas M. Schnitzler syndrome without a monoclonal gammopathy: a case report. J Cutan Med Surg. 2016;20:575–8.
13. Lipsker D, Veran Y, Grunenberger F, Cribier B, Heid E, Grosshans E. The Schnitzler syndrome. Four new cases and review of the literature. Medicine (Baltimore). 2001;80(1):37–44.
14. Olsen E, Forre O, Lea T, Langeland T. Unique antigenic determinants (idiotypes) used as markers in a patient with macroglobulinemia urticaria: similar idiotypes demonstrated in the skin and on peripheral blood lymphocytes. Acta Med Scan. 1980;207:379–84.
15. Niederhauser BD, Dingli D, Kyle RA, Ringler MD. Imaging findings in 22 cases of Schnitzler syndrome: characteristic para-articular osteosclerosis, and the "hot knees" sign differential diagnosis. Skelet Radiol. 2014;43:905–15.
16. Ferrando FJ, Pujol J, Hortells JR, et al. Schnitzler's syndrome: report of a case with bone osteolysis. J Investig Allergol Clin inmunol. 1994;4:203–5.
17. Willekens I, Walgraeve N, Goethals L, De Geeter F. Correlative bone imaging in a case of Schnitzler's syndrome and brief review of the literature. Hell J Nucl Med. 2015;18:71–3.
18. Carlesimo M, Abruzzese C, Narcisi A, La Verde G, De Marco G, Verga E, et al. Chronic vasculitis urticaria associated to a monoclonal gammopathy of IgM and IgA type, a Schnitzler syndrome? Eur J Dermatol. 2010;20:838–9.
19. Gusdorf L, Asli B, Barbarot S, Neel A, Masseau A, Puechal X, et al. Schnitzler syndrome: validation and applicability of diagnostic criteria in real-life patients. Allergy. 2017;72:177–82.
20. Berdy SS, Bloch KJ. Schnitzler's syndrome: a broader clinical spectrum. J Allergy Clin Immunol. 1991;87:849–54.
21. van de Donk NW, Palumbo A, Johnsen HE, Engelhardt M, Gay F, Gregersen H, et al. The clinical relevance and management of monoclonal gammopathy of undetermined significance and related disorders: recommendations from the European Myeloma Network. Haematologica. 2014;99(6):984–96.
22. Machet L, Vaillant L, Machet MC, Reisenleiter M, Goupille P, Lorette G. Schnitzler ' s syndrome (urticaria and macroglobulinemia): evolution to Waldenström's disease is not uncommon. Acta Derm Venereol (Stockh). 1996;76:413.
23. Claes K, Bammens B, Delforge M, Evenepoel P, Kuypers D, Vanrenterghem Y. Another devastating complication of the Schnitzler syndrome: AA amyloidosis. Br J Dermatol. 2008;158(1):182–4.
24. Basile C, Rossi L, Casucci F, Teutonico A, Libutti P, Lisi P, et al. Kidney involvement in the Schnitzler syndrome, a rare disease. Clin Kidney J. 2017;10(6):723–7.
25. Bursztejn AC, Imperiale A, Lipsker D. Aortitis: a new feature of Schnitzler syndrome. JAAD Case Rep. 2017;3:454–6.
26. Lipsker D, Lenormand C. Management of Schnitzler's syndrome. Expert Opin Orphan Drugs. 2014;2:947–55.
27. Kastritis E, Katoulis A, Terpos E, Panayiotides I, Gavriatopoulopu M, Dimopopoulos MA. Schnitzler's syndrome: increased levels of bone formation and angiogenesis factors are reduced after successful pefloxacin treatment. Clin Lymphoma Myeloma. 2008;8:359–62.
28. Martinez-Taboada VM, Fontalba A, Blanco R, Fernández-Luna JL. Successful treatment of refractory Schnitzler syndrome with anakinra: comment on the article by Hawkins et al. Arthritis Rheum. 2005;52(7):2226–7.
29. Cascavilla N, Bisceglia M, D'Arena G. Successful treatment of Schnitzler's syndrome with anakinra after failure of rituximab trial. Int J Immunopathol Pharmacol. 2010;23(2):633–6.

30. Neel A, Henry B, Barbarot S, Masseau A, Perrin F, Bernier C, et al. Long-term effectiveness and safety of interleukin-1 receptor antagonist (anakinra) in Schnitzler's syndrome: a French multicenter study. Autoimmun Rev. 2014;13:1035–41.
31. Perrin F, Neel A, Graveleau J, Ruellan AL, Masseau A, Hamidou M. Two cases of anakinra-induced neutropenia during auto-inflammatory diseases: drug reintroduction can be successful. Presse Med. 2014;43:319–21.
32. Pesek R, Fox R. Successful treatment of Schnitzler syndrome with canakinumab. Cutis. 2014;94:E11–2.
33. De Koning HD, Schalkwijk J, van der Ven-Jongekrijg J, Stoffels M, van der Meer JWM, Simon A. Sustained efficacy of the monoclonal anti-interleukin-1 beta antibody canakinumab in a 9-month trial in Schnitzler's syndrome. Ann Rheum Dis. 2013;72:1634–8.
34. Vanderschueren S, Knockaert D. Canakinumab in Schnitzler syndrome. Semin Arthritis Rheum. 2013;42:413–6.
35. Krause K, Tsianakas A, Wagner N, Fischer J, Weller K, Metz M, et al. Efficacy and safety of canakinumab in Schnitzler syndrome: a multicenter randomized placebo-controlled study. J Allergy Clin Immunol. 2017;139:1311–20.
36. Krause K, Weller K, Stefaniak R, Wittkowski H, Altrichter S, Siebenhaar F, et al. Efficacy and safety of the interleukin-1 antagonist rilonacept in Schnitzler syndrome: an open-label study. Allergy. 2012;67:943–50.
37. Krause K, Feist E, Fiene M, Kallinich T, Maurer M. Complete remission in 3 of 3 anti-IL-6-treated patients with Schnitzler syndrome. J Allergy Clin Immunol. 2012;129:848–50.

Chapter 16
Periodic Fever, Aphthous Stomatitis, Pharyngitis, and Cervical Adenitis (PFAPA) Syndrome

Ezgi Deniz Batu and Fatma Dedeoglu

Introduction

PFAPA (periodic fever, aphthous stomatitis, pharyngitis, and cervical adenitis) syndrome is characterized by repeated episodes of high fever associated with the core features of the disease – aphthous stomatitis, pharyngitis, and adenitis [1]. Regular interval between episodes is the cardinal feature. PFAPA is considered to be the most common periodic fever syndrome in children [2–4]. It usually starts before the age of 5 years and tends to resolve spontaneously before adulthood [5]. The patients are often asymptomatic between attacks, and their growth and development are within normal range [4, 6]. Although different factors such as infectious agents, immune dysregulation, and aberrant cytokine levels were investigated, the etiopathogenesis of PFAPA remains unclear. However, previous studies indicate a polygenic background and environmental triggers. Furthermore, inflammasome-related genes and proteins and pro-inflammatory cytokines, such as interleukin-1 (IL-1), IL-6, and IL-18, likely play central roles in the disease pathogenesis [7–10].

PFAPA has a favorable course with a high rate of spontaneous resolution and no evidence of long-term sequela [6, 11, 12]. The pharmacological treatment of PFAPA includes different options such as nonsteroidal anti-inflammatory drugs (NSAIDs), colchicine, corticosteroids, cimetidine, and anti-IL-1 drugs [13]. Prompt response to one or two doses of corticosteroids in aborting an episode is very common. Tonsillectomy is also efficacious in inducing remission; however, it is important to

E. D. Batu
Department of Pediatrics, Division of Rheumatology, Ankara Training and Research Hospital, University of Health Sciences, Ankara, Turkey

F. Dedeoglu (✉)
Rheumatology Program/Division of Immunology, Department of Medicine, Boston Children's Hospital, Harvard Medical School, Boston, MA, USA
e-mail: fatma.dedeoglu@childrens.harvard.edu

P. Efthimiou (ed.), *Auto-Inflammatory Syndromes*,
https://doi.org/10.1007/978-3-319-96929-9_16

balance the risks and benefits for each patient when deciding to pursue surgical options [14]. At present, there is no consensus for the optimal treatment of PFAPA.

History and Epidemiology

PFAPA syndrome was first described in 1987 by Marshall et al. in 12 children [4]. In 1989, the PFAPA acronym was proposed to designate the Marshall syndrome [15].

PFAPA syndrome represents the most common periodic fever syndrome in children, especially among non-Mediterranean patients [2, 3, 16, 17]. The estimated annual incidence of PFAPA is approximately 2–3 cases per 10,000 children up to 5 years of age [1, 16, 18].

Most of the studies describe a slight predominance of PFAPA in boys [5, 6, 19, 20]. There is no predilection for specific ethnic groups [11].

In most cases, the disease onset occurs before 5 years of age, while it generally resolves by adolescence [5, 6, 15, 21, 22]. However, an increasing number of adult patients is being reported in the literature [12, 23].

Clinical Findings

The syndrome is characterized by intermittent episodes of high fever with clockwork regularity, usually accompanied by exudative pharyngitis (present in up to 90% of patients), swollen and tender cervical lymph nodes (in up to 75% of patients), and oral aphthosis (in up to 50% of patients) in the absence of respiratory tract infection [24]. Abdominal pain, nausea/vomiting, malaise, myalgia, arthralgia, and headache can also be seen during attacks [6, 25]. There is often a sudden rise of temperature up to 40.5 °C [24], and the duration of fever episodes is typically 3–7 days (mostly 4–5) with an interval of 2–8 weeks (mostly 3–6) [1, 5, 6, 15, 18, 20]. Clockwork regularity of episodes may disappear over time and when on corticosteroid treatment [1, 26, 27]. Nonspecific symptoms such as fatigue, malaise, and irritability as prodromes may occur during days before PFAPA episodes [20, 28].

The patients are usually asymptomatic between attacks and have normal growth and development [19]. Some symptoms such as oral aphthosis and malaise can be seen outside the flares [11, 22].

Laboratory Findings

There are no specific laboratory findings for PFAPA syndrome. Mild leukocytosis with monocytosis and neutrophilia, decrease in lymphocytes, eosinophils, thrombocytosis, increased erythrocyte sedimentation rate, C-reactive protein (CRP), serum amyloid-A, S100A8/A9, and S100A12 proteins can be observed during PFAPA episodes [7, 9, 28–31]. Since procalcitonin levels generally do not increase during PFAPA episodes, checking its level may be helpful in differentiating PFAPA episodes from infection [7, 30, 32]. Serum immunoglobulin (Ig) levels are usually within normal range, while serum IgD can be slightly elevated during attacks [33].

Diagnosis

The diagnosis of PFAPA is primarily based on clinical characteristics (history and physical examination), and there is no definitive diagnostic test available. The diagnostic criteria for PFAPA syndrome was proposed by Marshall et al. [4] and modified by Thomas et al. [6] (Table 16.1). However, due to the heterogeneity in the phenotype of PFAPA, no specific confirmatory tests, and the lack of consensus in the definition of PFAPA, these criteria may not work in some clinical settings (Figs. 16.1 and 16.2).

Table 16.1 The diagnostic criteria for PFAPA (periodic fever, aphthous stomatitis, pharyngitis, and cervical adenitis) syndrome

I	Regularly recurring fevers with an early age of onset (<5 years of age)
II	Constitutional symptoms in the absence of upper respiratory infection with at least one of the following clinical signs: (a) Aphthous stomatitis (b) Cervical lymphadenitis (c) Pharyngitis
III	Exclusion of cyclic neutropenia
IV	Completely asymptomatic interval between episodes
V	Normal growth and development

Adapted from Ref. [6]

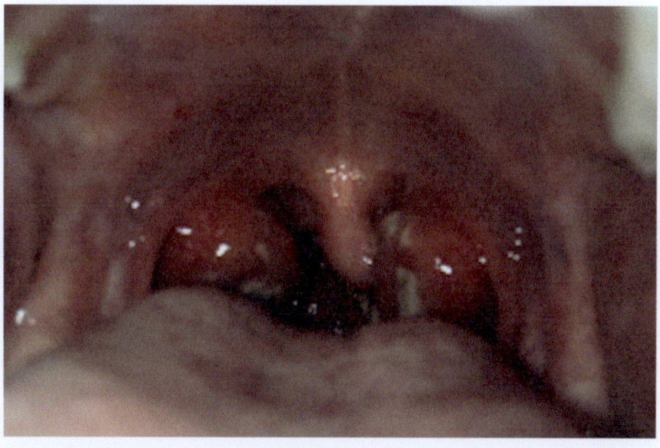

Fig. 16.1 Exudative tonsillitis. (Courtesy of Dr. Sivia Lapidus)

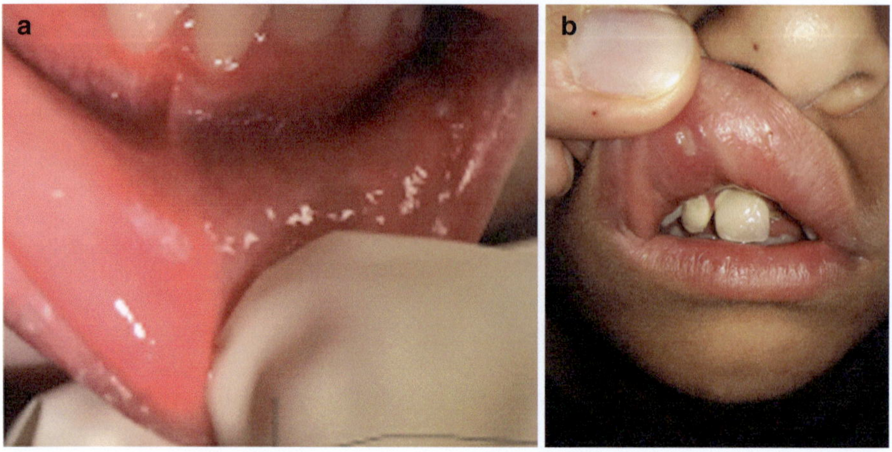

Fig. 16.2 Typical shallow aphthous ulcers in the mucosa of lower lip (**a**) and upper lip (**b**) in different PFAPA patients (Courtesy of Dr. Sivia Lapidus)

Gattorno et al. have shown that 83% of mevalonate kinase deficiency (MKD), 57% of tumor necrosis factor (TNF) receptor-associated syndrome (TRAPS), and 8% of familial Mediterranean fever (FMF) patients met the diagnostic criteria of PFAPA [34]. In 2009, they proposed a diagnostic score (Gaslini score) to help distinguish PFAPA-like patients at higher risk of carrying mutations of genes associated with monogenic periodic fever syndromes [2]. In 2015, evidence-based provisional clinical classification criteria were developed for patients with inherited periodic fever syndromes, and approximately 200 PFAPA patients were included as controls in this study [35]. Within these criteria, the age of onset, the characteristics and duration of episodes, and the ethnicity were included as differentiating features. These may also be used to differentiate PFAPA from monogenic autoinflammatory diseases, such as FMF, MKD, cryopyrin-associated periodic syndrome (CAPS), and TRAPS. Of note, MKD has the highest degree of clinical overlap with PFAPA syndrome [2].

Recently, Manthiram et al. performed an online survey assessing the diagnostic and treatment approaches of CARRA (Childhood Arthritis and Rheumatology Research Alliance) (n = 123) and PIDS (Pediatric Infectious Disease Society) (n = 154) members with PFAPA syndrome [36]. Most respondents agreed on the following diagnostic criteria to diagnose PFAPA as essential: stereotypical fever episodes, asymptomatic intervals between episodes, and normal growth and development. However, 71% of the respondents did not require "the age of onset before 5 years" criterion; 79% did not require the concomitant signs of aphthous stomatitis, adenitis, or pharyngitis during episodes in the presence of regularly occurring attacks, while 33% did not require regular attack-free intervals. Of note, 58% considered episode resolution with corticosteroids to be diagnostic of PFAPA. Interestingly, in a recent study by Lantto et al., tonsillectomy was also shown to be an effective therapy for patients who failed to meet the diagnostic criteria for PFAPA but suffered from regularly occurring fever attacks [37]. The diversity of approaches in diagnosing PFAPA underscores the need to develop consensus diagnostic criteria in well-characterized larger patient populations.

The differential diagnosis of PFAPA mainly includes cyclic neutropenia, infections, and monogenic autoinflammatory diseases [38].

In cyclic neutropenia, fever is usually accompanied by a decrease in neutrophils with a nadir of $<500/mm^3$ and by the presence of infections. Furthermore, the fever episodes do not respond to corticosteroids. Finally, the genetic test for mutations in the *ELANE* gene could confirm the diagnosis of cyclic neutropenia in the vast majority of these patients [39].

It is crucial to differentiate a PFAPA attack from an infection, especially to prevent the unnecessary use of antibiotics. High CRP is uncommon during viral respiratory tract infections, and a throat culture may be performed to exclude streptococcal infection [11, 40].

The main challenge is to differentiate PFAPA from monogenic periodic fever syndromes. The Gaslini score and the classification criteria for monogenic periodic fever syndromes (discussed above) could help with the differential. In addition, for patients with symptoms (mainly oral aphthosis) outside of flares, excluding diseases such as Behçet's disease are also important.

An updated classification system for PFAPA syndrome is needed to better verify these patients.

Pathogenesis

The exact pathogenesis or genetic background of PFAPA remains unclear. However, many possible etiologic factors such as infectious agents, immunological dysregulation, and genetic predisposition have been explored thus far. PFAPA is most likely an immune-mediated disease stemming from cytokine dysfunction to possible environmental triggers [41].

Infectious Agents At present, no single infectious agent has been identified as a cause of PFAPA syndrome. Several characteristics of PFAPA make an infectious etiology unlikely, such as clockwork episodes, lack of response to antibiotic therapy, negative throat cultures during episodes, lack of second cases in close contact, lack of clustering in season or geographic areas, and the dramatic response to corticosteroids [1].

Lantto et al. demonstrated that the microbes found in the tonsils of PFAPA patients showed significant differences from those of controls, while there was no difference in routine histology findings [42]. In PFAPA tonsils compared to controls, *C. albicans*, pneumococci, and abundant biofilm formation were found to be more common. Freeman et al. found no difference between the overall composition and diversity of tonsillar microbiota in PFAPA patients ($n = 6$) and controls ($n = 8$)

[43]. Most recently, Tejesvi et al. showed that tonsillar microbiota differed significantly in PFAPA patients ($n = 30$) from those of the controls ($n = 24$) in the largest cohort [44]. Cyanobacteria, potential producers of microcystins, and other toxins were higher, and streptococci were lower in PFAPA cases than in the controls. Studying the tonsils outside of the flares is an important limitation of all these studies.

It is likely that an overall change in the tonsillar microbiota, rather than a single microorganism or the interactions between the microbiome and the underlying immune tissue, plays a role in the activation of inflammatory response [44].

Immune Dysregulation IL-1-dependent, abnormal innate immune response to environmental triggers with recruitment of T cells to tonsils may be the major issue in PFAPA [10]. A recent study by Manthiram et al. showed that tonsils from PFAPA cases had significantly smaller germinal centers and wider squamous epithelia than those of obstructive sleep apnea patients [45]. In addition, the farther away from the last febrile episode, the larger was the germinal center area in PFAPA cases [45]. These results suggest that tonsils of PFAPA patients change histologically over time with enlarging germinal centers, possibly as a result of the local changes in the immune system.

Neutrophilia develops during PFAPA episodes [1], as well as several altered neutrophil functions including apoptosis, priming, and generation of an intracellular oxidative burst [31]. Lymphopenia is often observed during PFAPA attacks, which may be due to either decreased lymphopoiesis, as a result of increased myelopoiesis, or homing of lymphocytes to lymphatic tissues, such as tonsils and cervical lymph nodes [31].

The cytokine pattern (discussed below) supports T helper 1 (Th1) differentiation of CD4+ T cells. Furthermore, the increased numbers of T lymphocytes at early developmental stages and T cell chemoattractants, such as CXCL9, CXCL10, and CCL19, were shown in PFAPA tonsils [46]. These changes may be due to IL-18, which induces interferon γ (IFN-γ) and promotes Th1 response in the presence of IL-12 [47].

These findings indicate the involvement of both innate and adaptive immune systems in the disease pathogenesis.

Cytokines Previous studies demonstrated rapid rise and fall of certain pro-inflammatory cytokines, such as IL-1β, IL-18, and TNF-α and increase in IFN-γ in the early hours and IL-6 in the later stages of an episode with normalization in the afebrile state [7]. On the other hand, IL-7, IL-17, and anti-inflammatory cytokines, such as IL-4 and IL-10, decreased during PFAPA episodes [7, 47].

Inflammasomes control the activation of caspase-1, which cleaves pro-IL-1 and pro-IL-18 to their biologically active forms [48]. Stimulated neutrophils and monocytes have been shown to secrete significantly higher levels of IL-1β during PFAPA attacks. This reaction is inhibited by a caspase inhibitor, which emphasizes the central role of caspase and active IL-1β in PFAPA pathogenesis [9]. Along the same lines, serum levels of caspase-1 were shown to increase during PFAPA flares [9]. These findings suggest an inflammasome-mediated dysregulation in PFAPA.

Genetics

No unique genetic marker has been discovered explaining the etiopathogenesis of PFAPA, which is generally considered a sporadic disease. However, a significant number of PFAPA patients have a positive family history of recurrent febrile episodes which strongly suggests a potential genetic background for the disease [8, 9, 19, 49–51].

Variants in the genes that are known to cause monogenic autoinflammatory syndromes (mostly inflammasome-related genes) have been found in PFAPA patients in several studies [8, 10, 49, 52]; however, the impact of these variants is still unclear.

The presence of *MEFV* mutations may be causing a transient inflammatory phenotype similar to PFAPA in the presence of additional modifiers [8, 52]. Some authors suggest that *MEFV* gene could be a modifier of PFAPA phenotype in a favorable manner [49, 53]. Berkun et al. demonstrated that PFAPA patients carrying heterozygote *MEFV* variants had shorter attacks, more irregular attack intervals, and less aphthae and required a lower dose of corticosteroid to abort attacks compared to patients without a *MEFV* variant [49]. Perko et al. showed that patients with *MEFV* or *NLRP3* variants had an earlier disease onset, shorter fever attacks, and longer attack intervals than patients without these variants [19]. Phenotype of PFAPA did not differ significantly between carriers and non-carriers in other studies [8, 52].

It is important to note that some patients with R92Q variant in the *TNFRSF1A* gene (usually present in milder forms of TRAPS) express a quite similar phenotype with PFAPA patients [54, 55].

In a recent study, next-generation sequencing was performed in 82 unrelated PFAPA patients and a significant association was found between a frameshift variant in the *CARD8* gene and risk for PFAPA syndrome [56]. Moreover, the PFAPA patients with *CARD8* variant were more likely to have symptoms out of flares and oral aphthosis. *CARD8* encodes a protein component of NLRP3 inflammasome, which again underscores the role of inflammasomes in PFAPA pathogenesis.

Treatment

There are medical and surgical therapy options; however, the optimal treatment still remains debatable, emphasizing the need to develop clinical practice guidelines in PFAPA.

Medical Treatment The pharmacological treatment of PFAPA is summarized in Table 16.2.

The use of antibiotics have shown poor efficacy in resolving PFAPA episodes, while antipyretics (acetaminophen, NSAIDs) work partially, with slightly better response to NSAIDs in reducing fever in PFAPA episodes [22].

Several preventive therapies, such as cimetidine and montelukast [6, 28, 57], have been suggested by some physicians; however, these have not been confirmed by others [58]. In recent years, these therapies are prescribed less often, and there are no randomized controlled trials supporting their benefits in PFAPA. Of note, none of the patients from the EUROFEVER and Norwegian cohorts were treated with these therapies [18, 22].

Corticosteroid treatment (single dose of prednisolone [1–2 mg/kg] or betamethasone [0.1–0.2 mg/kg]) aborts the attacks (especially fever) within a few hours in most of the cases [13, 59]. Oral aphthosis can take longer to resolve. Corticosteroid therapy may be given for different indications – in some countries given during every episode, while in others, to abort a febrile episode occurring at an unsuitable time for the child/parents or only to confirm PFAPA diagnosis [1, 60]. However, corticosteroid therapy is not effective in preventing subsequent attacks, and the attack frequency may increase in 25–50% of cases [18, 61, 62]. In a randomized clinical trial, the children were divided into two groups to receive 0.5 mg/kg/day (first group) or 2 mg/kg/day (second group) prednisolone [32]. The fever ceased in 8–12 h in the first group and in 6–8 h in the second group. The other symptoms

Table 16.2 The medical treatment of PFAPA (periodic fever, aphthous stomatitis, pharyngitis, and cervical adenitis) syndrome

Drug	Statement
Antibiotics	Ineffective
Paracetamol/NSAID	Could be used as antipyretics Poor efficacy
Montelukast	Poor efficacy Insufficient data
Cimetidine	Works in some patients (about 1/4 of the patients in several studies)
Vitamin D	Efficacy? Insufficient data
Corticosteroid	Prompt resolution of attacks Less effective in adults Could increase attack frequency
Colchicine	Efficacy? More effective in patients with *MEFV* mutation Duration of therapy?
Anti-IL-1 drugs (anakinra, canakinumab)	Cost-effectiveness Insufficient data

IL-1 interleukin 1, *NSAID* nonsteroidal anti-inflammatory drugs

disappeared after 24 h in both groups, and there was no increase in episode frequency. If one dose is not effective, a second dose of corticosteroid could be given on the following day [13]. It is important to note that attacks of hereditary periodic fevers, except for MKD, do not show a dramatic response to corticosteroid treatment which may be helpful to differentiate PFAPA episodes from those of FMF or other hereditary periodic fever syndromes [28, 63]. Some experts think that the prompt response to corticosteroids could be an additional diagnostic criterion for PFAPA [11].

Previous retrospective studies have demonstrated that colchicine might be an effective preventive therapy in PFAPA [5, 57]. Some clinical and laboratory similarities between PFAPA and FMF and the long-term experience with colchicine form the basis for the rationale to use this drug in prophylaxis [13]. Butbul Aviel et al. evaluated the effect of colchicine on PFAPA in the first open-label, randomized, controlled study and found that it is effective in reducing the frequency of PFAPA attacks [64]. In another recent study, Dusser et al. showed that colchicine treatment appeared more effective in patients with less complete PFAPA phenotype and *MEFV* heterozygosity [16].

PFAPA and vitamin D deficiency were found to be correlated in a few studies [29, 65]. Furthermore, Stagi et al. demonstrated a significant reduction in the number and duration of PFAPA episodes after vitamin D supplementation (400 IU 25-hydroxyvitamin D per day during winter time) [65]. However, there is no consensus on testing and supplementing vitamin D in PFAPA cases, and randomized controlled trials are needed to prove efficacy.

IL-1 plays a central role in PFAPA pathogenesis [47]. Few patients were treated with anakinra or canakinumab, and they all showed prompt clinical response [66–68]. However, there is no consensus on the use of anti-IL-1 biologics since randomized clinical trials are lacking, and these are expensive drugs that should be considered only in patients who continue to have breakthrough episodes or cannot tolerate other treatment modalities.

Surgical Treatment Adenotonsillectomy is considered an effective solution for refractory cases. In the Cochrane database review, Burton et al. demonstrated that the evidence for the effectiveness of tonsillectomy was derived from two small randomized controlled trials which reported significant beneficial effects of surgery [14]. However, the evidence was of moderate quality due to the relatively small sample size in these studies. Recently, Erdogan et al. demonstrated that surgery was superior to medical treatment for PFAPA in their comparative trial in 105 PFAPA patients [69]. However, tonsillectomy is an invasive procedure, as there are potential surgical/anesthesia risks, and its success varies among different series [70–72]. Furthermore, PFAPA is a benign disease that can spontaneously resolve. Thus, the place of surgical treatment should be individually evaluated and discussed with the families in accordance with the rheumatologist's and otolaryngologist's indications, balancing the risks and benefits for each child. Of note, it is uncertain whether adenoidectomy adds any additional benefit to tonsillectomy alone [14].

Outcome

PFAPA syndrome is generally considered a benign disease, resolving spontaneously in most of the cases without any long-term sequela, such as secondary amyloidosis [5]. However, frequent attacks could interfere with the quality of the patients'/families' lives. The symptoms usually disappear within 3–5 years after the disease onset or in adolescence [5, 6, 15, 21, 22]. Occasionally, late relapses of the disease can be seen [1, 20]. Current studies on adult PFAPA cases have also shown that PFAPA syndrome may relapse in adulthood after a temporary remission during childhood [24, 73].

Pediatric Versus Adult Patients

An increasing number of adult PFAPA patients have been reported in recent years, and the studies underscore certain differences between pediatric and adult PFAPA cases [23, 24, 73].

In reported cases of adult PFAPA, no gender predominance can be detected, though in younger populations, boys outnumbered girls [11, 24]. The clinical characteristics of PFAPA syndrome are similar in adults and children with the exception that aphthae and chills are more frequent in children, while arthralgia and myalgia are more frequent in adults [24, 63]. In the most recent study by Rigante et al., clockwork periodicity and recurrent pharyngitis were more frequently observed in children, while joint symptoms, myalgia, headache, fatigue, ocular signs, and rashes were more common in adults [23]. A single dose of corticosteroid achieves complete resolution of the episode more frequently in children than adults, while NSAIDs have been considered significantly more effective in adults than children [12, 23, 24]. The available data suggests that tonsillectomy is not very effective in adult patients [24]. Moreover, PFAPA syndrome in adults does not seem to be a self-limited disease; however, long-term outcome data is missing [24].

Acknowledgements The authors thank Aiyana Ryan for taking time for proof-reading and providing assistance in formatting the drafts.

References

1. Wekell P, Karlsson A, Berg S, et al. Review of autoinflammatory diseases, with a special focus on periodic fever, aphthous stomatitis, pharyngitis and cervical adenitis syndrome. Acta Paediatr. 2016;105(10):1140–51.
2. Gattorno M, Caorsi R, Meini A, et al. Differentiating PFAPA syndrome from monogenic periodic fevers. Pediatrics. 2009;124(4):e721–8.
3. Krol P, Bohm M, Sula V, et al. PFAPA syndrome: clinical characteristics and treatment outcomes in a large single-centre cohort. Clin Exp Rheumatol. 2013;31(6):980–7.

4. Marshall GS, Edwards KM, Butler J, et al. Syndrome of periodic fever, pharyngitis, and aphthous stomatitis. J Pediatr. 1987;110(1):43–6.
5. Padeh S, Brezniak N, Zemer D, et al. Periodic fever, aphthous stomatitis, pharyngitis, and adenopathy syndrome: clinical characteristics and outcome. J Pediatr. 1999;135(1): 98–101.
6. Thomas KT, Feder HM Jr, Lawton AR, et al. Periodic fever syndrome in children. J Pediatr. 1999;135(1):15–21.
7. Brown KL, Wekell P, Osla V, et al. Profile of blood cells and inflammatory mediators in periodic fever, aphthous stomatitis, pharyngitis and adenitis (PFAPA) syndrome. BMC Pediatr. 2010;10:65.
8. Dagan E, Gershoni-Baruch R, Khatib I, et al. MEFV, TNF1rA, CARD15 and NLRP3 mutation analysis in PFAPA. Rheumatol Int. 2010;30(5):633–6.
9. Kolly L, Busso N, von Scheven-Gete A, et al. Periodic fever, aphthous stomatitis, pharyngitis, cervical adenitis syndrome is linked to dysregulated monocyte IL-1beta production. J Allergy Clin Immunol. 2013;131(6):1635–43.
10. Kraszewska-Glomba B, Matkowska-Kocjan A, Szenborn L. The pathogenesis of periodic fever, aphthous stomatitis, pharyngitis, and cervical adenitis syndrome: a review of current research. Mediat Inflamm. 2015;2015:563876.
11. Hofer M, Pillet P, Cochard MM, et al. International periodic fever, aphthous stomatitis, pharyngitis, cervical adenitis syndrome cohort: description of distinct phenotypes in 301 patients. Rheumatology (Oxford). 2014;53(6):1125–9.
12. Wurster VM, Carlucci JG, Feder HM Jr, et al. Long-term follow-up of children with periodic fever, aphthous stomatitis, pharyngitis, and cervical adenitis syndrome. J Pediatr. 2011;159(6):958–64.
13. Vanoni F, Theodoropoulou K, Hofer M. PFAPA syndrome: a review on treatment and outcome. Pediatr Rheumatol Online J. 2016;14(1):38.
14. Burton MJ, Pollard AJ, Ramsden JD, et al. Tonsillectomy for periodic fever, aphthous stomatitis, pharyngitis and cervical adenitis syndrome (PFAPA). Cochrane Database Syst Rev. 2014;9:CD008669.
15. Marshall GS, Edwards KM, Lawton AR. PFAPA syndrome. Pediatr Infect Dis J. 1989;8(9): 658–9.
16. Dusser P, Hentgen V, Neven B, et al. Is colchicine an effective treatment in periodic fever, aphthous stomatitis, pharyngitis, cervical adenitis (PFAPA) syndrome? Joint Bone Spine. 2016;83(4):406–11.
17. Akpolat T, Ozkaya O, Ozen S. Homozygous M694V as a risk factor for amyloidosis in Turkish FMF patients. Gene. 2012;492(1):285–9.
18. Forsvoll J, Kristoffersen EK, Oymar K. Incidence, clinical characteristics and outcome in Norwegian children with periodic fever, aphthous stomatitis, pharyngitis and cervical adenitis syndrome; a population-based study. Acta Paediatr. 2013;102(2):187–92.
19. Perko D, Debeljak M, Toplak N, et al. Clinical features and genetic background of the periodic fever syndrome with aphthous stomatitis, pharyngitis, and adenitis: a single center longitudinal study of 81 patients. Mediat Inflamm. 2015;2015:293417.
20. Tasher D, Somekh E, Dalal I. PFAPA syndrome: new clinical aspects disclosed. Arch Dis Child. 2006;91(12):981–4.
21. Kastner DL, Aksentijevich I, Goldbach-Mansky R. Autoinflammatory disease reloaded: a clinical perspective. Cell. 2010;140(6):784–90.
22. Ter Haar N, Lachmann H, Ozen S, et al. Treatment of autoinflammatory diseases: results from the Eurofever registry and a literature review. Ann Rheum Dis. 2013;72(5):678–85.
23. Rigante D, Vitale A, Natale MF, et al. A comprehensive comparison between pediatric and adult patients with periodic fever, aphthous stomatitis, pharyngitis, and cervical adenopathy (PFAPA) syndrome. Clin Rheumatol. 2017;36(2):463–8.
24. Cattalini M, Soliani M, Rigante D, et al. Basic characteristics of adults with periodic fever, aphthous stomatitis, pharyngitis, and adenopathy syndrome in comparison with the typical pediatric expression of disease. Mediat Inflamm. 2015;2015:570418.

25. Frenkel J, Kuis W. Overt and occult rheumatic diseases: the child with chronic fever. Best Pract Res Clin Rheumatol. 2002;16(3):443–69.
26. Ozen S, Bilginer Y. A clinical guide to autoinflammatory diseases: familial Mediterranean fever and next-of-kin. Nat Rev Rheumatol. 2014;10(3):135–47.
27. Federici S, Gattorno M. A practical approach to the diagnosis of autoinflammatory diseases in childhood. Best Pract Res Clin Rheumatol. 2014;28(2):263–76.
28. Feder HM, Salazar JC. A clinical review of 105 patients with PFAPA (a periodic fever syndrome). Acta Paediatr. 2010;99(2):178–84.
29. Mahamid M, Agbaria K, Mahamid A, et al. Vitamin D linked to PFAPA syndrome. Int J Pediatr Otorhinolaryngol. 2013;77(3):362–4.
30. Gunes M, Cekic S, Kilic SS. Is colchicine more effective to prevent periodic fever, aphthous stomatitis, pharyngitis and cervical adenitis episodes in Mediterranean fever gene variants? Pediatr Int. 2017;59(6):655–60.
31. Sundqvist M, Wekell P, Osla V, et al. Increased intracellular oxygen radical production in neutrophils during febrile episodes of periodic fever, aphthous stomatitis, pharyngitis, and cervical adenitis syndrome. Arthritis Rheum. 2013;65(11):2971–83.
32. Yazgan H, Keles E, Yazgan Z, et al. C-reactive protein and procalcitonin during febril attacks in PFAPA syndrome. Int J Pediatr Otorhinolaryngol. 2012;76(8):1145–7.
33. Kovacs L, Hlavata A, Baldovic M, et al. Elevated immunoglobulin D levels in children with PFAPA syndrome. Neuro Endocrinol Lett. 2010;31(6):743–6.
34. Gattorno M, Sormani MP, D'Osualdo A, et al. A diagnostic score for molecular analysis of hereditary autoinflammatory syndromes with periodic fever in children. Arthritis Rheum. 2008;58(6):1823–32.
35. Federici S, Sormani MP, Ozen S, et al. Evidence-based provisional clinical classification criteria for autoinflammatory periodic fevers. Ann Rheum Dis. 2015;74(5):799–805.
36. Manthiram K, Nesbitt E, Morgan T, et al. Family history in periodic fever, aphthous stomatitis, pharyngitis, adenitis (PFAPA) syndrome. Pediatrics. 2016;138(3):e20154572.
37. Lantto U, Koivunen P, Tapiainen T, et al. Long-term outcome of classic and incomplete PFAPA (periodic fever, aphthous stomatitis, pharyngitis, and adenitis) syndrome after tonsillectomy. J Pediatr. 2016;179:172–7. e171.
38. Esposito S, Bianchini S, Fattizzo M, et al. The enigma of periodic fever, aphthous stomatitis, pharyngitis and adenitis syndrome. Pediatr Infect Dis J. 2014;33(6):650–2.
39. Horwitz MS, Duan Z, Korkmaz B, et al. Neutrophil elastase in cyclic and severe congenital neutropenia. Blood. 2007;109(5):1817–24.
40. Feder HM Jr. Periodic fever, aphthous stomatitis, pharyngitis, adenitis: a clinical review of a new syndrome. Curr Opin Pediatr. 2000;12(3):253–6.
41. Theodoropoulou K, Vanoni F, Hofer M. Periodic fever, aphthous stomatitis, pharyngitis, and cervical adenitis (PFAPA) syndrome: a review of the pathogenesis. Curr Rheumatol Rep. 2016;18(4):18.
42. Lantto U, Koivunen P, Tapiainen T, et al. Microbes of the tonsils in PFAPA (periodic fever, aphthous stomatitis, pharyngitis and adenitis) syndrome – a possible trigger of febrile episodes. APMIS. 2015;123(6):523–9.
43. Freeman S, Bhatt A, Pedamallu C, et al. A121: in search of infectious triggers of periodic fever, aphthous stomatitis, pharyngitis and adenitis syndrome. Arthritis & Rheumatology. 2014;66:S158.
44. Tejesvi MV, Uhari M, Tapiainen T, et al. Tonsillar microbiota in children with PFAPA (periodic fever, aphthous stomatitis, pharyngitis, and adenitis) syndrome. Eur J Clin Microbiol Infect Dis. 2016;35(6):963–70.
45. Manthiram K, Correa H, Boyd K, et al. Unique histologic features of tonsils from patients with periodic fever, aphthous stomatitis, pharyngitis, and cervical adenitis (PFAPA) syndrome. Clin Rheumatol. 2018;37(5):1309–17.
46. Dytrych P, Krol P, Kotrova M, et al. Polyclonal, newly derived T cells with low expression of inhibitory molecule PD-1 in tonsils define the phenotype of lymphocytes in children

with periodic fever, aphthous stomatitis, pharyngitis and adenitis (PFAPA) syndrome. Mol Immunol. 2015;65(1):139–47.
47. Stojanov S, Hoffmann F, Kery A, et al. Cytokine profile in PFAPA syndrome suggests continuous inflammation and reduced anti-inflammatory response. Eur Cytokine Netw. 2006;17(2):90–7.
48. Palomo J, Dietrich D, Martin P, et al. The interleukin (IL)-1 cytokine family–balance between agonists and antagonists in inflammatory diseases. Cytokine. 2015;76(1): 25–37.
49. Berkun Y, Levy R, Hurwitz A, et al. The familial Mediterranean fever gene as a modifier of periodic fever, aphthous stomatitis, pharyngitis, and adenopathy syndrome. Semin Arthritis Rheum. 2011;40(5):467–72.
50. Cochard M, Clet J, Le L, et al. PFAPA syndrome is not a sporadic disease. Rheumatology (Oxford). 2010;49(10):1984–7.
51. Celiksoy MH, Ogur G, Yaman E, et al. Could familial Mediterranean fever gene mutations be related to PFAPA syndrome? Pediatr Allergy Immunol. 2016;27(1):78–82.
52. Batu ED, Kara Eroglu F, Tsoukas P, et al. Periodic fever, aphthosis, pharyngitis, and adenitis syndrome: analysis of patients from two geographic areas. Arthritis Care Res (Hoboken). 2016;68(12):1859–65.
53. Taniuchi S, Nishikomori R, Iharada A, et al. MEFV variants in patients with PFAPA syndrome in Japan. Open Rheumatol J. 2013;7:22–5.
54. Di Gioia SA, Bedoni N, von Scheven-Gete A, et al. Analysis of the genetic basis of periodic fever with aphthous stomatitis, pharyngitis, and cervical adenitis (PFAPA) syndrome. Sci Rep. 2015;5:10200.
55. Pelagatti MA, Meini A, Caorsi R, et al. Long-term clinical profile of children with the low-penetrance R92Q mutation of the TNFRSF1A gene. Arthritis Rheum. 2011;63(4): 1141–50.
56. Cheung MS, Theodoropoulou K, Lugrin J, et al. Periodic fever with aphthous stomatitis, pharyngitis, and cervical adenitis syndrome is associated with a CARD8 variant unable to bind the NLRP3 inflammasome. J Immunol. 2017;198(5):2063–9.
57. Tasher D, Stein M, Dalal I, et al. Colchicine prophylaxis for frequent periodic fever, aphthous stomatitis, pharyngitis and adenitis episodes. Acta Paediatr. 2008;97(8):1090–2.
58. Feder HM Jr. Cimetidine treatment for periodic fever associated with aphthous stomatitis, pharyngitis and cervical adenitis. Pediatr Infect Dis J. 1992;11(4):318–21.
59. Kyvsgaard N, Mikkelsen T, Korsholm J, et al. Periodic fever associated with aphthous stomatitis, pharyngitis and cervical adenitis. Dan Med J. 2012;59(7):A4452.
60. ter Haar NM, Oswald M, Jeyaratnam J, et al. Recommendations for the management of autoinflammatory diseases. Ann Rheum Dis. 2015;74(9):1636–44.
61. Licameli G, Jeffrey J, Luz J, et al. Effect of adenotonsillectomy in PFAPA syndrome. Arch Otolaryngol Head Neck Surg. 2008;134(2):136–40.
62. Peridis S, Pilgrim G, Koudoumnakis E, et al. PFAPA syndrome in children: a meta-analysis on surgical versus medical treatment. Int J Pediatr Otorhinolaryngol. 2010;74(11):1203–8.
63. Padeh S, Stoffman N, Berkun Y. Periodic fever accompanied by aphthous stomatitis, pharyngitis and cervical adenitis syndrome (PFAPA syndrome) in adults. Isr Med Assoc J. 2008;10(5):358–60.
64. Butbul Aviel Y, Tatour S, Gershoni Baruch R, et al. Colchicine as a therapeutic option in periodic fever, aphthous stomatitis, pharyngitis, cervical adenitis (PFAPA) syndrome. Semin Arthritis Rheum. 2016;45(4):471–4.
65. Stagi S, Bertini F, Rigante D, et al. Vitamin D levels and effects of vitamin D replacement in children with periodic fever, aphthous stomatitis, pharyngitis, and cervical adenitis (PFAPA) syndrome. Int J Pediatr Otorhinolaryngol. 2014;78(6):964–8.
66. Stojanov S, Lapidus S, Chitkara P, et al. Periodic fever, aphthous stomatitis, pharyngitis, and adenitis (PFAPA) is a disorder of innate immunity and Th1 activation responsive to IL-1 blockade. Proc Natl Acad Sci U S A. 2011;108(17):7148–53.

67. Cantarini L, Vitale A, Galeazzi M, et al. A case of resistant adult-onset periodic fever, aphthous stomatitis, pharyngitis and cervical adenitis (PFAPA) syndrome responsive to anakinra. Clin Exp Rheumatol. 2012;30(4):593.
68. Lopalco G, Rigante D, Vitale A, et al. Canakinumab efficacy in refractory adult-onset PFAPA syndrome. Int J Rheum Dis. 2015;20(8):1050–1.
69. Erdogan F, Kulak K, Ozturk O, et al. Surgery vs medical treatment in the management of PFAPA syndrome: a comparative trial. Paediatr Int Child Health. 2016;36(4):270–4.
70. Licameli G, Lawton M, Kenna M, et al. Long-term surgical outcomes of adenotonsillectomy for PFAPA syndrome. Arch Otolaryngol Head Neck Surg. 2012;138(10):902–6.
71. Pignataro L, Torretta S, Pietrogrande MC, et al. Outcome of tonsillectomy in selected patients with PFAPA syndrome. Arch Otolaryngol Head Neck Surg. 2009;135(6):548–53.
72. Garavello W, Romagnoli M, Gaini RM. Effectiveness of adenotonsillectomy in PFAPA syndrome: a randomized study. J Pediatr. 2009;155(2):250–3.
73. Vitale A, Orlando I, Lopalco G, et al. Demographic, clinical and therapeutic findings in a monocentric cohort of adult patients with suspected PFAPA syndrome. Clin Exp Rheumatol. 2016;34(6 Suppl 102):77–81.

Chapter 17
Chronic Nonbacterial Osteomyelitis

Liza McCann, Michael W. Beresford, Gabriele Hahn, and Christian M. Hedrich

Introduction

Chronic nonbacterial osteomyelitis (CNO) is an autoinflammatory bone disorder that covers a wide clinical spectrum with single-site involvement and/or a short course at one end and chronically active and/or recurring multifocal disease at the other end. Severe multifocal and chronically active or recurrent forms are referred to as chronic recurrent multifocal osteomyelitis (CRMO) [1–7]. Chronic nonbacterial osteomyelitis most commonly occurs in children and adolescents and can cause severe sequelae and complications, such as fractures, hyperostosis, growth anomalies, neurological symptoms, pain amplification, and others [7–10]. Psychosocial concerns are relatively common in CNO in a vulnerable age group.

The exact molecular pathophysiology of CNO remains largely unknown. Chronic nonbacterial osteomyelitis is likely to be a genetically complex disorder with variable pathomechanisms resulting in clinical phenotypes summarized as CNO. In the absence of validated diagnostic criteria and disease biomarkers, CNO remains a diagnosis of exclusion. To date, treatment is empiric but effective in at least a proportion of patients [6]. However, complications can occur during the search for sufficient treatment options, and some patients do not respond to currently available therapies. Thus, there is significant need for advances in understanding the molecular

L. McCann · M. W. Beresford · C. M. Hedrich (✉)
Department of Women's & Children's Health, Institute of Translational Medicine, University of Liverpool, Liverpool, UK

Department of Paediatric Rheumatology, Alder Hey Children's NHS Foundation Trust Hospital, Liverpool, UK
e-mail: Christian.hedrich@liverpool.ac.uk

G. Hahn
Institute of Radiology, Faculty of Medicine Carl Gustav Carus, University of Technology Dresden, Dresden, Germany

P. Efthimiou (ed.), *Auto-Inflammatory Syndromes*,
https://doi.org/10.1007/978-3-319-96929-9_17

pathophysiology of CNO, the identification and evaluation of diagnostic biomarkers, the introduction of diagnostic criteria, and prospective evaluation of available treatment options working toward personalized medicine.

In this chapter, the clinical presentation of CNO, differential diagnoses, our understanding of the molecular pathophysiology, and available treatment options will be discussed.

Definition, Nomenclature, and Epidemiology

Chronic nonbacterial osteomyelitis was first described by Giedion et al. in 1972 [11]. Sometime later, two groups (Probst et al. and Bjorksten et al.) reported the recurrent nature in a subset of patients and introduced the term "chronic recurrent multifocal osteomyelitis" (CRMO) [12, 13]. Since not all patients with noninfectious osteomyelitis develop multiple bone lesions or exhibit recurrent disease, more recently, the term CNO has been introduced and suggested for all forms of noninfectious osteomyelitis, including CRMO (Fig. 17.1).

Historically, various terms have been used to describe CNO, including chronic multifocal symmetrical osteomyelitis, nonbacterial osteomyelitis (NBO), sternoclavicular hyperostosis, chronic sclerosing osteitis, sternoclavicular pustulotic osteitis, and many others. Inconsistent nomenclature complicates literature reviews and data interpretation [9]. In adolescents and adults, CNO can be associated with joint and skin manifestations, which are usually described as SAPHO (synovitis, acne, pustulosis, hyperostosis, and osteitis) syndrome [14]. Individual symptoms of SAPHO can also occur in pediatric CNO patients with a lower frequency. Thus, CNO and SAPHO are usually considered the same disorder with slightly different presentations in different age groups [6] (Fig. 17.1).

Based on several key features, including "spontaneous" and seemingly untriggered inflammation in the absence of high-titer autoantibodies, lacking involvement of autoreactive lymphocyte populations (at least initially), CNO is considered to be an autoinflammatory condition. Furthermore, noninfectious osteomyelitis is a key symptom of other well-defined monogenic autoinflammatory conditions, including Majeed syndrome, DIRA (deficiency of the interleukin-1 receptor antagonist), and PAPA (pyogenic arthritis, pyoderma gangrenosum, and acne) [5, 15].

Though reports on incidence and prevalence are sparse and somewhat inconclusive, CNO is a rare disorder. To date, several hundred cases from almost all geographical regions and ethnicities have been reported, and recent observations suggest that the incidence of CNO and bacterial osteomyelitis may be almost equal in Central Europe [7, 16]. Though generally present in all age groups, CNO mostly affects children and adolescents with a peak onset between 7 and 12 years. It is unusual for CNO to present in children younger than 3 years of age; thus monogenic autoinflammatory conditions should be considered in this age group [7, 16–18].

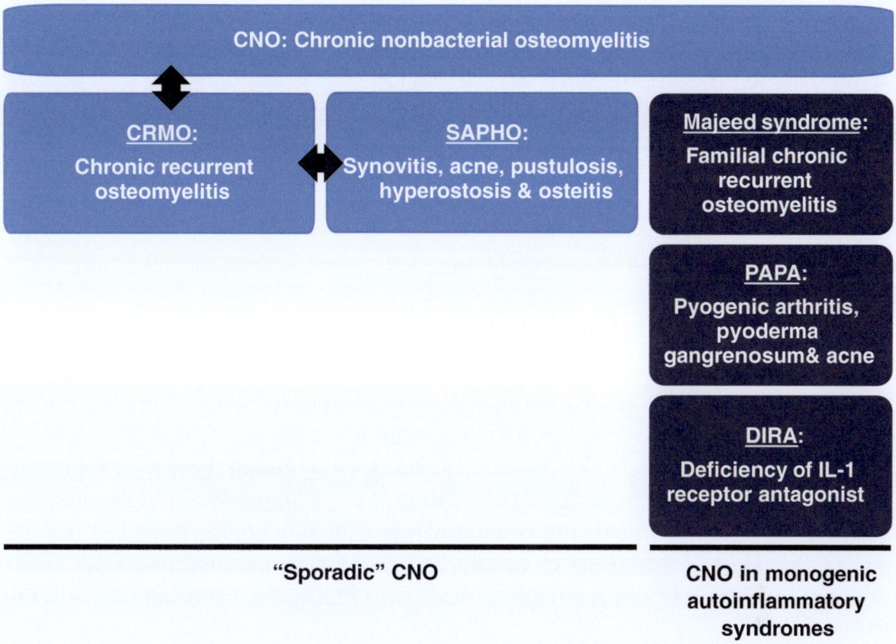

Fig. 17.1 Nomenclature of CNO. Nonbacterial osteomyelitis can be a symptom of monogenic autoinflammatory bone disorders or the key feature of CNO. Thus, discerning "sporadic" CNO (describing forms that are to our current knowledge not caused by monogenic variants and do not follow Mendelian inheritance) from CNO as a symptom of monogenic autoinflammatory disorders (Majeed syndrome, PAPA, and DIRA) appears beneficial. Though sometimes used synonymously (arrows), the terms CNO, CRMO, and SAPHO should be used with caution. In the group of "sporadic" CNO, chronic recurrent multifocal osteomyelitis (CRMO) should be limited to chronically recurrent and multifocal disease presentations, and SAPHO (synovitis, acne, pustulosis, hyperostosis, osteitis) should only be used for (usually adolescent or adult) patients with skin and joint involvement

Clinical Manifestations

As mentioned above, clinical presentation and severity of CNO can vary significantly between affected individuals [7–9]. Classical symptoms of osteitis include pain, rarely redness, swelling, and local heat and may initially be rather mild. Thus, many patients have a long delay in diagnosis or may even be missed. A subset of CNO patients exhibit inflammatory organ involvement, including psoriasis and palmoplantar pustulosis (~8%), inflammatory bowel disease (~10%), and severe acne (~10%). Indeed, a subset of CNO patients develop arthritis (up to ~40%) [7–9], and some patients may progress from childhood CNO to spondyloarthropathies [7, 19, 20]. This is of special interest, since all of these manifestations are pathophysiologically related and may represent a clinical spectrum that may include inflammatory bowel disease, psoriatic skin inflammation, arthritis, enthesiopathy, and bone inflammation. However, compared to adolescents and adult patients, extraosseous symptoms are less prevalent in younger patients [14]. Furthermore, generalized pustulosis [21], Sweet syndrome [22–24], pyoderma gangrenosum [18, 25, 26], celiac disease [18, 27, 28], Takayasu arteritis [29–31], granulomatosis with polyangiitis (GPA) [18, 32], sclerosing cholangitis [18, 33], parenchymal lung disease [34, 35], and some others have been reported in individual CNO patients.

Pathogenesis of CNO

Cytokine Dysregulation and Osteoclast Activation

As noted above, CNO is an autoinflammatory condition [5, 15]. Microbiological cultures of bone tissue remain sterile, and antibiotic treatment fails to induce long-term remission [10, 18, 27, 32, 36–42]. However, while initial reports on the detection of *Propionibacterium acnes*, *Mycoplasma* spp., or *Staphylococcus* spp. in bone biopsies most likely were due to contamination with skin commensals [10, 19, 28, 33, 37, 38, 41–43], the ability of certain bacteria to alter immune responses raises the question of whether pathogens may still indirectly contribute to disease expression.

Altered cytokine and chemokine expression patterns from innate immune cells contribute to the pathophysiology of CNO. Monocytes isolated from peripheral blood of CRMO patients fail to express the immune-regulatory cytokines IL-10 and IL-19. Conversely, monocytes from CNO patients express increased amounts of pro-inflammatory cytokines (IL-1ß, IL-6, TNF-α) and chemokines (IL-8, IP-10, MCP-1, MIP-1a, MIP-1b) [44–47]. Reduced expression of the immune-regulatory cytokines IL-10 and IL-19 has been linked with impaired activation of the mitogen-activated protein kinases (MAPK) extracellular signal-regulated kinases (ERK1 and ERK2) resulting in altered phosphorylation of the transcription factor signaling protein 1 (SP-1) and impaired recruitment to regulatory elements within the *IL-10* and the *IL-19* promoters [46, 47]. Furthermore, MAP kinases ERK1 and ERK2 are involved in the phosphorylation of histone proteins. Reduced ERK activation therefore also results in altered histone H3S10 phosphorylation at the *IL-10* promotor [46, 47]. Histone 3S10 phosphorylation is an activating epigenetic mark, mediating "opening" of chromatin and allowing transcription factor-DNA interactions [48, 49]. Thus, also reduced H3S10 phosphorylation contributes to reduced Sp-1 recruitment to *IL-10* [44, 46, 47] (Fig. 17.2a).

Another interesting finding in the search for molecular pathomechanisms in CNO is the observation of increased NLRP3 inflammasome activation in IL-10-deficient animals that has been linked with inflammatory bone loss [50]. More recently, Scianaro et al. [51] suggested that increased expression of NLRP3 inflammasome components (ASC, NLRP3, caspase-1) and increased IL-1β mRNA expression and protein release from PBMCs may be involved in bone inflammation. in human CNO. Hofmann et al. linked reduced expression of IL-10 and IL-19 with increased IL-1β mRNA expression and protein release in monocytes from CRMO

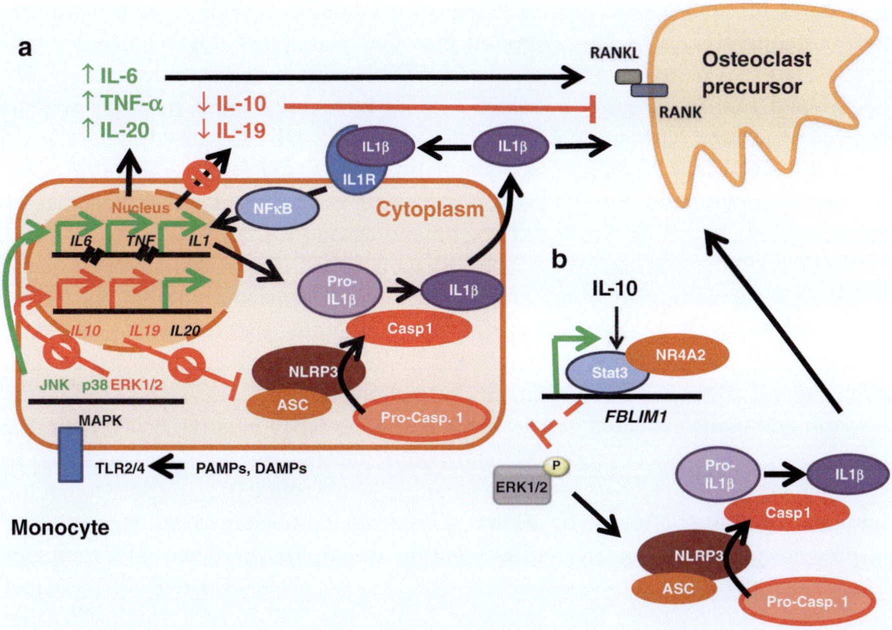

Fig. 17.2 Molecular pathophysiology of CNO. (**a**) Danger signals are sensed by pattern recognition receptors (PRRs), such as the membrane-associated Toll-like receptors (TLRs) and the cytoplasmic NOD-like receptors (NLRs). In response to contact of monocytes/macrophages to danger signals, inflammasomes are activated. The NLRP3 inflammasome comprises NLRP3, ASC, and procaspase-1. Inflammasomes mediate caspase-1 activation, which results in cleavage and activation of pro-IL-1β. In monocytes from CNO patients, MAP kinases Erk1 and Erk2 signaling is impaired, resulting in reduced expression of the immune-regulatory cytokines IL-10 and IL-19. The JNK and p38 MAP kinases, however, are unaffected, resulting in the expression of pro-inflammatory cytokines. Reduced IL-10 and IL-19 expression results in increased inflammasome activation and release of mature IL-1β. (**b**) Pro-inflammatory cytokines TNFα, IL-6, IL-20, and IL-1β increase the interaction between RANK receptors on osteoclast precursor cells and their soluble ligand (RANKL) inducing osteoclast differentiation and activation. (**b**) Filamin-binding LIM protein (FBLIM)1 is an anti-inflammatory molecule controlling bone remodeling through regulation of RANKL activation. The *FBLIM1* gene is *trans*-regulated by the transcription factor Stat3. Interleukin-10 mediates activation of Stat3, and reduced IL-10 expression in CNO patients may be linked with the involvement of FBLIM1 in disease pathology

patients [44] that was reversible by the addition of recombinant IL-10 or IL-19 to cell culture supernatants [44] (Fig. 17.2a).

Taken together, recent observations in mice and primary human cells suggest that imbalanced expression of pro- (IL-1β, IL-6, TNF-α, IL-20) and anti-inflammatory cytokines (IL-10 and IL-19) may result in bone inflammation.. A tight balance between pro- and anti-inflammatory cytokines regulates osteoclast differentiation and activation through the fine-tuning of interactions between receptor activator of nuclear factor-κB (RANK) and its soluble ligand (RANKL) on osteoclast precursor cells [6, 52–54]. Thus, imbalanced expression and release of cytokines in CNO may be very central to disease pathogenesis (Fig. 17.2a).

Studies in well-defined genetically inherited familial disorders with noninfectious osteomyelitis as a key symptom provided pathophysiological insights that contributed to a better understanding of CNO. There are at least three genetically determined human diseases in which aseptic bone inflammation. is prominent: Majeed syndrome (caused by *LPIN2* mutations) [23], DIRA (caused by mutations in *IL-1RN*) [55], and PAPA (caused by mutations in *PSTPIP1*) [56, 57]. Indeed, also in these autoinflammatory syndromes, increased activation of inflammasomes or increased IL-1 signaling results in bone inflammation [52].

Genetic predisposition (as opposed to monogenic inheritance) appears to be involved in the pathophysiology of sporadic CNO. Occasional familial clusters of CNO and relatively high incidences of other inflammatory conditions (including psoriasis, inflammatory bowel disease, etc.) in CNO patients and first-degree relatives suggest a genetic component in the pathophysiology [1, 7, 16, 27, 58–62]. Several studies investigated genetic associations in CNO cohorts. Since there are overlapping features between CNO and DIRA, the *IL-1RN* gene was screened in CNO patients, but no CNO-associated mutations were found [63]. Expression of the immune-regulatory cytokine IL-10 that is involved in the pathophysiology of CNO is predetermined by genetic variants within the *IL-10* promoter. Three single-nucleotide polymorphisms rs1800896 (−1082A > G), rs1800871 (−819T > C), and rs1800872 (−592A > C) form promoter haplotypes (GCC, ACC, and ATA) that influence transcription factor recruitment [64, 65]. Quite unexpectedly, considering the aforementioned failure to produce IL-10 in monocytes from CNO patients, enrichment of *IL-10* promoter haplotypes that encode for "high" IL-10 expression (GCC) was observed in a German cohort of CNO/CRMO patients [65, 66]. However, data may suggest that individuals with CNO-associated molecular disturbances and *IL-10* promoter haplotypes encoding for "low" IL-10 expression develop more severe disease that includes CNO as a symptom among others. Such combinations may result in phenotypes that may not be identified as CNO (e.g., IBD with CNO, etc.) [47, 67]. However, this explanation currently remains speculation.

Using whole-exome sequencing, a CRMO susceptibility gene was recently identified in two unrelated CNO patients from South Asia. One patient carried a homozygous and the other patient a compound heterozygous mutation in the filamin-binding domain of the *FBLIM1* gene [68, 69]. Though incompletely understood, filamin-binding LIM protein (FBLIM)1 happens to act as an anti-inflammatory molecule controlling bone remodeling through the regulation of RANKL activation through ERK1/ERK2 phosphorylation [68, 69]. This indicates that *FBLIM1* mutations may cause disruptions in pathways previously reported to be altered in European CNO patients [46, 47] (Fig. 17.2b). Furthermore, *trans*-activation of the *FBLIM1* gene is regulated by the transcription factor signal transducer and activator of transcription (STAT)3 [68, 69]. The immune-regulatory cytokine IL-10 positively regulates STAT3 activation. Both individuals carried such *IL-10* promoter haplotypes that code for "low" IL-10 expression, which (in conjunction with the reported mutations) may result in reduced STAT3 activation and downstream effects on FBLIM1 expression in the reported individuals (Fig. 17.2b) [69]. Since CNO-associated *FBLIM1* mutations rarely occur in healthy individuals, these observations suggest that the combination of *FBLIM1* variants together with *IL-10* promoter haplotypes encoding for "low" gene expression may result in CNO [47, 67].

Nonbacterial Osteomyelitis in Mice

Currently, three well-defined murine models are available to study nonbacterial osteomyelitis. Mice carrying loss-of-function mutations in the *Pstpip2* gene, encoding proline-serine-threonine phosphatase-interacting protein 2, develop a clinical picture equivalent to severe CRMO. *Lupo* mice were generated by chemical induction of homozygous mutations (c.Y180C; p.I282N) [70, 71], while chronic multifocal osteomyelitis (*cmo*) mice carry spontaneously acquired homozygous mutations (c.T293C, p.L98P). Recently, targeted knockout of exons 3 and 4 of *Pstpip2* delivered another murine system to study CNO that is characterized by paw swelling, synovitis, hyperostosis, and osteitis, resembling SAPHO syndrome [72]. To date, the exact contribution of *Pstpip2* mutations to sterile bone inflammation. remains somewhat unclear [72]. Proline-serine-threonine phosphatase-interacting protein 2 is a member of the F-BAR (Fes/CIP4 homology-Bin/Amphiphysin/Rvs) domain containing protein superfamily that links membrane remodeling with actin dynamics associated to endocytic pathways and filopodium formation [73]. In the absence of Pstpip2, actin polymerization is increased, and Pstpip2-deficient macrophages exhibit abnormal podosome formation, leading to a more invasive phenotype [74].

As recently suggested in human CNO, the pro-inflammatory cytokine IL-1β also plays a central role in the pathophysiology of osteomyelitis in *cmo* mice [75, 76]. Animals deficient of the IL-1 receptor inhibitor (IL-1RI) or IL-1β itself are protected from the development of osteomyelitis [75, 76]. However, NLRP3, ASC, or caspase-1-deficient *cmo* mice developed CNO. These observations at first appeared somewhat surprising and suggest the involvement of alternative kinases or proteases other than caspase-1 in the activation of IL-1β [77]. This hypothesis is supported by the observation that *cmo* mice deficient of caspase-1 or caspase-8 develop CNO, while animals deficient of both are protected from disease [78], suggesting redundant roles of caspases in vivo. Though *pstpip2*-deficient animals resemble severe CRMO and represent an interesting model for bone inflammation, it needs to be mentioned that mutations in the human equivalent *PSTPIP2* have not been reported in CNO patients. Furthermore, mutations in *cmo* and *Lupo* mice are located in a region of the *Pstpip2* gene that is not present in humans. Together with the diverse clinical picture in CNO patients, and the aforementioned finding from studies targeting molecular pathomechanisms in human disease, this indicates that variable molecular mechanisms may result in aseptic bone inflammation..

A relatively new concept links host interactions with microbiota to immune homeostasis and the onset of inflammatory disease [79]. Indeed, disturbances to microbiomes can result in inflammation. Recently, Lukens et al. [78] suggested that dietary manipulation of the microbiome in osteomyelitis-prone *cmo* mice can prevent osteomyelitis. Since CNO patients exhibit associations with disorders that also correlate with disturbed microbiomes (such as acne, inflammatory bowel disease, etc.) [7], these observations may promise future applications in disease prevention and treatment [79]. Furthermore, the potential involvement of altered microbiomes in the molecular pathophysiology of CNO may (at least partially) explain the observation that antibiotic treatment can be somewhat effective in individual CNO patients (at least during treatment administration) [36, 37].

Taken together, our current understanding of the pathophysiology is based on the assumption that CNO is a complex genetic disorder. Variable pathomechanisms may affect closely related TLR/MAPK/NLRP3 inflammasome-related molecular pathways that subsequently result in a clinical picture summarized as CNO. Further studies are necessary and warranted and will provide additional molecular pathomechanisms, disease biomarkers, and individualized therapeutic targets.

Diagnostic Approach

To date, validated diagnostic criteria and biomarkers are lacking for CNO, which leaves it a diagnosis of exclusion [1, 3–6]. Common clinical symptoms include bone pain, local swelling, and heat. Sometimes low-grade fever, redness, and fractures (usually of vertebral bodies) may occur. Arthritis is reported in up to 40% of CNO patients [7–9]. Routine laboratory inflammatory parameters (WBC, CRP, erythrocyte sedimentation rate) usually remain within normal limits or are mildly elevated [7, 45]. Genetic associations in CNO are currently unclear. While some authors reported high incidences of HLA B27 positivity, others did not see higher frequencies in CNO cohorts when compared to regional healthy controls [3, 7, 10, 19].

The diagnosis of CNO is dependent on exclusion of other bone pathologies, as summarized in Table 17.1. Some guidance in diagnosing CNO can be provided by diagnostic pathways that have been proposed by several groups [27, 80, 81]. However, suggested diagnostic criteria have not been evaluated in unrelated cohorts and are not internationally accepted.

Imaging techniques are probably the most important tools for the diagnosis of CNO and the exclusion of other diagnoses [7]. In some patients, bone lesions may be detected in plain radiographs as radiolucent, osteolytic, or sclerotic lesions [13, 40, 82, 83]. In early stages, however, radiographs usually remain normal. Magnetic resonance imaging (MRI) is particularly sensitive in early stages (Figs. 17.3, 17.4, and 17.5). In MRI studies, bone edema can be detected, even before bone erosions and sclerosis develop, and surrounding soft tissues can be assessed. Strongly T2-weighted sequences (turbo inversion recovery measurement, TIRM) and gadolinium-enhanced T1 sequences with fat saturation are usually used at the time of diagnosis to identify inflammatory bone lesions and periosseous involvement and to exclude differential diagnoses [83–87]. At least initially, whole-body imaging, usually whole-body MRI (TIRM), should be performed to identify clinically unapparent lesions [86]. If whole-body MRI is not available, regional MRIs can be combined to cover the entire body. Technical limitations in the growing skeleton

Table 17.1 Differential diagnosis of CNO (non-exhaustive)

Infections	Malignant bone tumors	Benign bone tumors	Hematological malignancies/infiltrative disease	Metabolic bone disorders	Genetic disorders	Miscellaneous
Bacterial osteomyelitis	Osteosarcoma	Osteoid osteoma	Lymphoma	Hypophosphatasia	DIRA	Osteonecrosis (vascular necrosis)
Mycobacteriosis	Ewing's sarcoma	Osteoblastoma	Leukemia	Hypertrophic osteoarthropathy	PAPA	
Fungal infections	Bony metastases	Fibrous dysplasia	Langerhans cell histiocytosis		Majeed syndrome	
		Enchondromatosis			Cherubism	
		Hemangiomatosis				
		Bone cysts				

From Refs. [1, 3–6, 10, 41, 52]

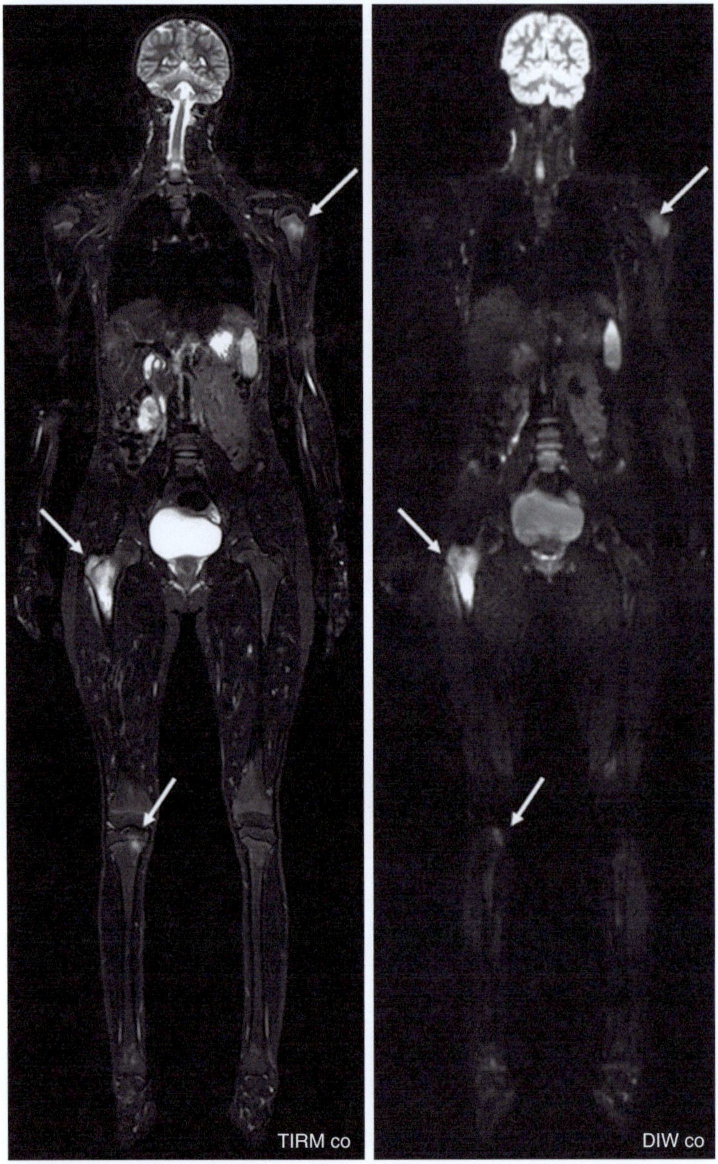

Fig. 17.3 MRI findings in CRMO. Coronary whole-body MRI of a 12-year-old girl showing hyperintense lesions in her left humerus, right femur, and right tibia in TIRM-sequence and diffusion-weighted images as a reflection of CNO

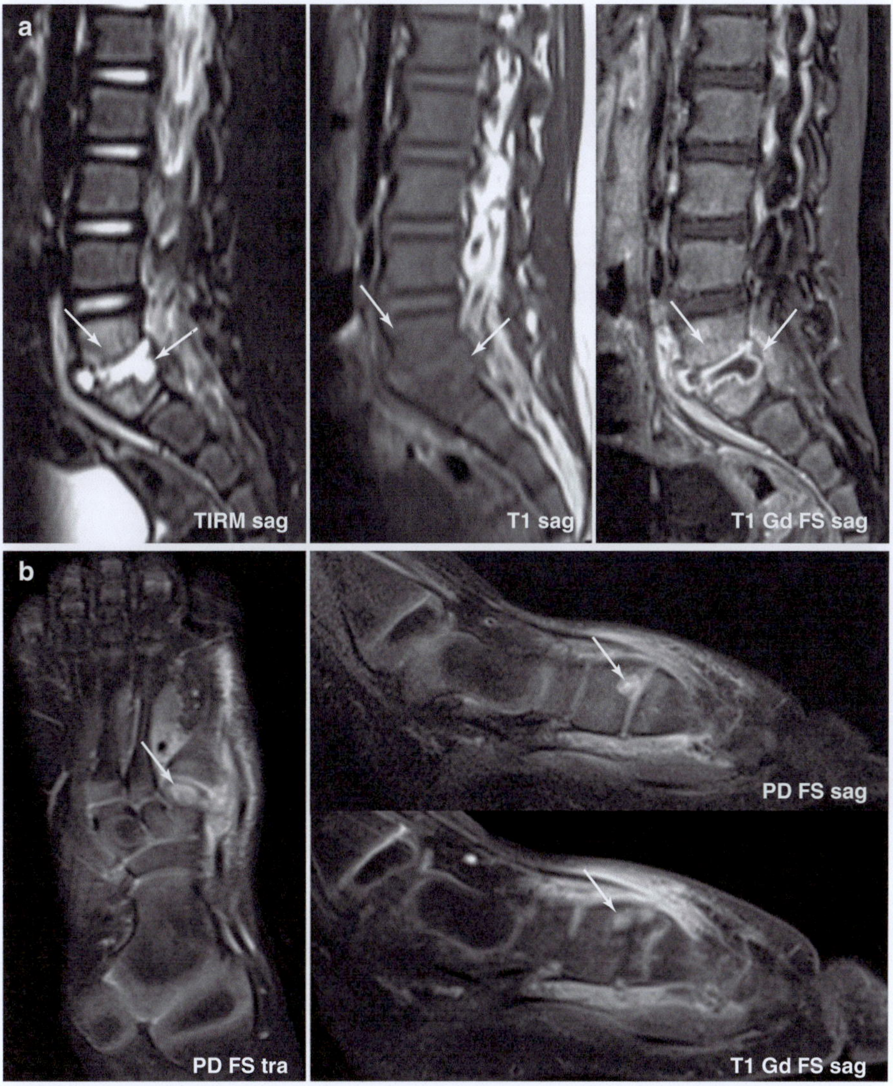

Fig. 17.4 Infectious osteomyelitis as differential diagnosis to CNO. (**a**) MRI of the spine with spondylodiscitis in L5/S1 (1½-year-old boy): hyperintense bone edema and destruction of the endplates of L5/S1 in TIRM, gadolinium enhancement of L5/S1, and the fluid-filled intervertebral disc in T1 sequences with fat saturation (T1 Gd FS) (arrows). (**b**) MRI of the foot (1½-year-old girl) showing chondritis of os cuneiforme with hyperintense round destruction in PD with fat saturation (FS) and gadolinium enhancement in T1 (T1 Gd FS) (arrows), inflammatory soft tissue of the tarsus

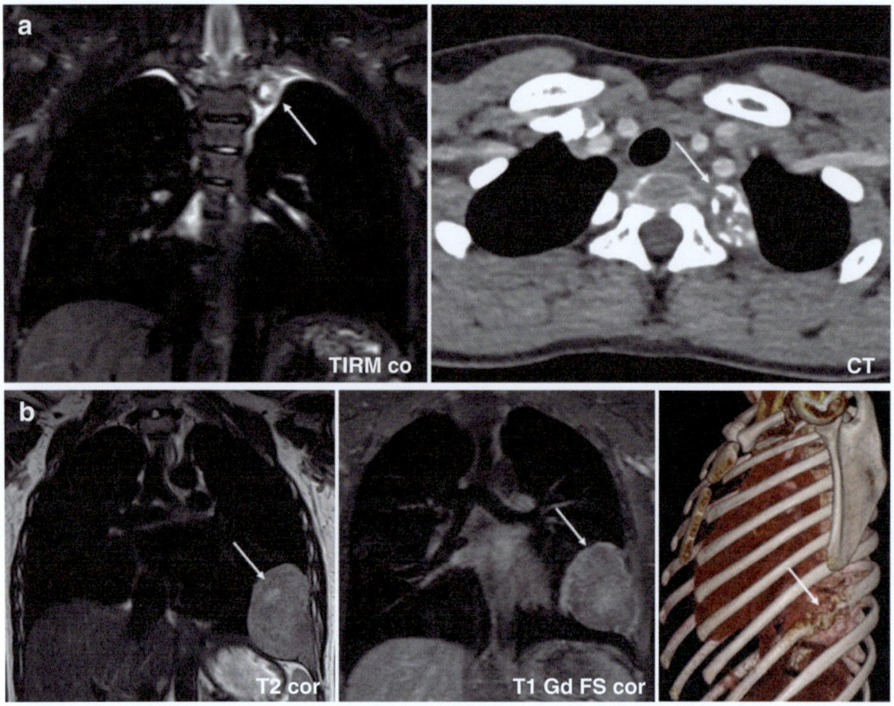

Fig. 17.5 Bone tumors as differential diagnoses to CNO. (**a**) MRI of the thorax (10-year-old girl): osteoblastoma of the second left rib with intermediate signal intensity (arrow) and fluid accumulation in the surrounding tissue in TIRM sequences. CT of the thorax with popcorn-like calcifications in the paravertebral tumor of the second left rib (arrow). (**b**) MRI of the thorax (11 year-old girl): Ewing's sarcoma of the eighth left rib with intermediate signal intensity in T2 and minimal enhancement in gadolinium-enhanced T1 sequence with fat saturation (T1 Gd FS). CT of the thorax with severe destruction of the lateral left eighth rib

(signal from growth plates, etc.) and high scintigraphy-associated radiation [85] make MRI the modality of choice. Thus, bone scintigraphy should only be considered when MRI is not available.

If the diagnosis remains unclear, *bone biopsies* should be performed to exclude malignancy, infection, or other systemic disorders (Table 17.1) [41]. However, histologic findings vary significantly between affected individuals, partially depending on the age of the lesions (Fig. 17.6). Generally, neutrophilic granulocytes and monocytes/macrophages are the predominant cell types in early CNO. Later during disease, infiltrates of lymphocytes and plasma cells can be seen, indicating secondary activation of the adaptive immune system. After months or years of inflammation, bone fibrosis in the absence of immune cells may be the predominant feature [5, 39, 41, 42, 88]. However, various stages can also coexist in the same patient, which is likely caused by the "waxing and waning" character of CNO. Furthermore, cellular infiltrates are not disease specific. Thus, microbiological cultures and/or

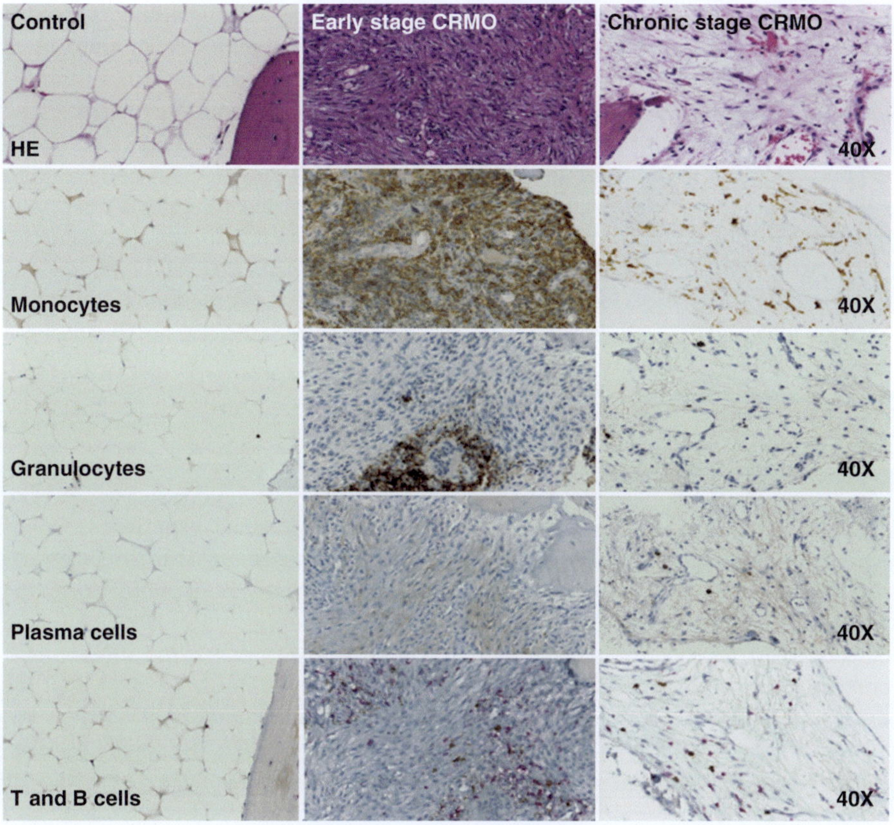

Fig. 17.6 Histological features of CNO. Early-phase CRMO (center column) is characterized by dense infiltrates of inflammatory cells as compared to the healthy bone (left column). Predominantly neutrophilic granulocytes and monocytes, increased osteoblast activity, and bone remodeling can be observed. Bone biopsies from patients with chronic-phase CRMO (right column) show infiltrates of inflammatory cells, predominantly plasma cells and mononuclear cells. Furthermore, bone remodeling, marrow fibrosis, and an increased number of blood vessels with endothelial cell proliferation can be seen. In late or fibrosing stage, CRMO is characterized by bone fibrosis and only few inflammatory mononuclear cells (not shown). Top lane, HE staining of healthy bone, early and chronic stage CRMO as indicated; middle three lanes, immunohistochemistry (IHC) staining for monocytes, neutrophils, or plasma cells as indicated (target cells are stained brown); bottom lane, IHC staining for T (brown) and B (pink) cells

nucleic acid workup should be performed, and histologic exams mainly allow the exclusion of differential diagnoses.

Preliminary data from two studies suggest that *serum biomarkers* may also be used to diagnose CNO [45, 89]. Studies delivered potential biomarkers that may allow differentiating between treatment-naïve patients with CNO, Crohn's disease, hematologic malignancies, osteoarticular infections, and healthy controls. Proposed biomarkers include monocyte-derived chemokines MCP-1 and MIP-1b, pro-inflammatory cytokines IL-6 and IL-12, mast cell-derived chemokine CCL-11/eotaxin, RANTES, and soluble IL-2 receptor. Indeed, the minimal set of biomarkers may even be reduced to CCL11/eotaxin and IL-6 [89]. In addition to serum biomarkers, cytokine and chemokine expression from isolated immune cells may be used to support the diagnosis of CNO [45]. Monocytes from CRMO patients fail to express GM-CSF and anti-inflammatory molecules IL-10 and IL-1RA under resting conditions and/or in response to TLR4 stimulation with LPS [15]. Conversely, monocytes from CRMO patients express increased amounts of pro-inflammatory IL-1β, IL-6, TNF-α, IL-8, IP-10, MCP-1, MIG, MIP-1a, and MIP-1b. Though interesting and promising, available observations require confirmation in unrelated cohorts, investigation of additional parameters, and further differential diagnoses.

Treatment

Treatment of CNO is largely empiric and based on personal experience, expert opinion, case reports, and small case series. However, consensus treatment plans (based on the very limited evidence available) have recently been published by the North American Childhood Arthritis and *Rheumatology* Research Alliance (CARRA) to prospectively collect data on treatment responses and disease outcomes (Fig. 17.6). Currently, nonsteroidal anti-inflammatory drugs (NSAIDs) are usually used as first-line agents. They provide symptomatic relief [9, 27, 29, 38, 45, 90–92] and are effective in a subset of patients within the first 18 months of treatment. However, a recent retrospective analyses reported flares in over 50% of patients after 2 years, underscoring the chronic character of CNO [7] and implying that NSAIDS alone may not be sufficient to induce disease remission. Therapeutic effects of NSAIDs are mediated through inhibition of cyclooxygenase and variable suppressive effects on inflammasomes [93]. The observations that prostaglandins are involved in osteoclast activation and that inflammasome activation is a hallmark of pro-inflammatory monocytes in CNO may explain therapeutic effects of NSAIDs [6]. However, NSAIDs alone are most likely not sufficiently effective in CNO/CRMO patients presenting with arthritis and/or spinal involvement [92]. For these patients and individuals who failed to respond to NSAIDs, additional treatments are required.

In individual case reports, small case series, and retrospective case collections, corticosteroids, disease-modifying anti-rheumatic drugs (DMARDs) including sulfasalazine and methotrexate (MTX), biologic treatments (anti-TNF agents), and bisphosphonates have all been reported to be effective in CNO [1, 3–6, 10, 45, 67]. Through the inhibition of phospholipase A1, corticosteroids reduce prostaglandin production. Furthermore, they alter expression of NFκB-mediated pro-inflammatory cytokines, including IL-1, IL-6, and TNF-α [6]. Usually, short "oral bursts" of 2 mg/kg/day prednisone equivalent are administered over 5–10 days. Others may use low-dose prednisone equivalent (0.1–0.2 mg/kg/day) as "bridging therapy" until concomitantly introduced DMARDs develop full efficacy. Indeed, corticosteroids quickly and effectively control bone inflammation. in most cases (79%) but rarely induce long-term remission [7]. However, since a significant proportion of patients flare after discontinuation and corticosteroid-associated side effects can be debilitating, long-term use should be avoided [6, 9, 29, 90].

The pro-inflammatory cytokine TNF-α contributes to bone inflammation in CNO (Fig. 17.2). Several case collections report the induction of clinical and radiological remission in CNO in response to TNF blockade. In particular, patients with CNO-associated extra-osseous manifestations (including arthritis, psoriasis, or IBD) may benefit from cytokine blockade. Due to the off-label character and relatively high associated costs, cytokine-blocking strategies should only be considered for cases refractory to other treatment [6, 8, 10, 27, 90, 94].

Bisphosphonates inhibit osteoclast activity, and pamidronate furthermore exerts dampening effects on pro-inflammatory cytokine expression [6]. Since osteoclasts are likely involved in bone inflammation. in CNO, and pro-inflammatory monocytes are a hallmark in CNO patients, bisphosphonates promise to be efficacious in the treatment of CNO. Pamidronate in particular has been reported to induce rapid and long-lasting remission in most CNO patients [6, 10, 95–98]. Two alternative treatment regimens have been reported: 1 mg/kg/dose (max. 60 mg/dose) every month and 1 mg/kg/dose (max. 60 mg/dose) on 3 consecutive days every 3 months for 9–12 months. Furthermore, Zhao et al. reported rapid response to treatment with zoledronic acid plus infliximab. However, the combination with the TNF-inhibitor infliximab does not allow an assessment of the exact contribution of each therapeutic agent [99]. Because of potential side effects and the fact that bisphosphonates remain in the system for many years, they should only be considered in otherwise treatment refractory cases or in individuals with primary vertebral involvement and structural damage [6, 10].

Reports on DMARD treatment (MTX, sulfasalazine) in CNO are limited and delivered conflicting data [3, 6, 8, 10, 19, 27].

Because of increased assembly of NLRP3 inflammasomes in monocytes from CNO patients, resulting in IL-1β activation and release (Fig. 17.2), IL-1 blocking strategies may be a promising therapeutic strategy. In light of this, surprisingly few cases of anti-IL-1 treatment with recombinant IL-1 receptor antagonist anakinra have been reported in CNO and showed mixed response with variable outcomes [100]. Potential explanations for mixed and rather poor responses may include low tissue concentrations of anakinra and pathophysiological heterogeneity in CNO/CRMO.

To date, the required duration of treatment remains unclear. Recent reports suggest CNO to be a chronic disease with flares even years after first "remission." However, patients are frequently treated for 6–12 months past the induction of clinical and radiological remission. Current routine is empiric, based on expert opinion, and not backed by studies targeting treatment durations and outcomes [1, 2, 4–6, 10, 18, 67, 90]. To aid treatment decisions and prospectively assess efficacy of frequently applied treatment options and optimal treatment duration, consensus treat-

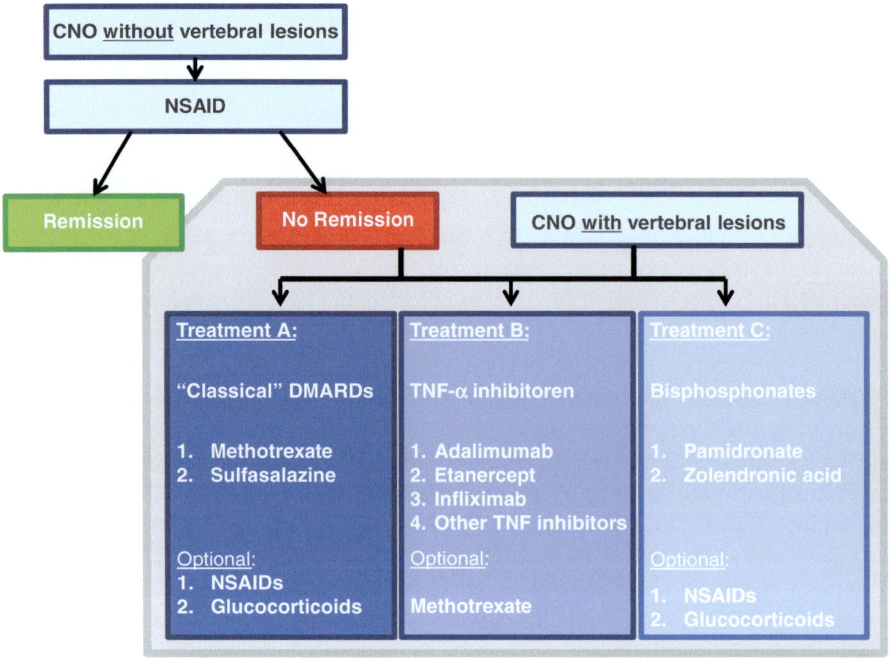

Fig. 17.7 Treatment protocols for CNO. In the absence of vertebral involvement, CNO patients are usually treated with NSAIDs. Patients who fail to respond to NSAIDs or individuals with primary involvement of the vertebral column can be treated according to the recently published CARRA consensus treatment plans [102] (Grey box; plans A–C)

ment plans (CTPs) have been released by CARRA [101] (Fig. 17.7). The concept of CTPs is to limit treatment practice variation to allow comparative effectiveness studies; they should not be confused with treatment recommendations or even guidelines. Furthermore, treatment decisions must be taken with caution, since (i) findings on MRI may be overinterpreted in clinically asymptomatic patients, (ii) lesions may resolve without becoming clinically apparent or causing sequelae, and (iii) therapeutic agents may cause side effects or generate significant cost. On the other hand, vertebral involvement holds the risk of fractures and associated sequelae, and long-lasting uncontrolled disease activity contributes to unfavorable long-term outcomes with polyarthritis/spondyloarthropathy, pain amplification, and others [3, 6, 10].

Disease Monitoring and Outcomes

Treatment decisions can be particularly difficult in the absence of accepted tools to measure disease activity. Thus, treatment regimens and duration largely depend on the experience of the individual healthcare provider. Various activity measures have been suggested, including the PedCNO score (consisting of pain Visual Analogue

Scale (VAS) scores, disease activity VAS scores by physician, number of lesions on MRI, and erythrocyte sedimentation rates) [92], signs of inflammation on MRI [99], childhood health assessment questionnaire (CHAQ), and others [8, 17, 27]. Imaging techniques are essential for the assessment of disease activity and the identification and monitoring of disease-associated sequelae, such as fractures, inflammatory involvement, and tissue damage to surrounding anatomical structures [86]. Though for most questions MRI is the gold standard, plain radiographs may be used to follow up on fractures or sclerotic bone lesions. While radiographic response to treatment should usually be assessed no sooner than 3 months after its initiation, CNO patients with involvement of the vertebral column may be exempt from this. In those patients, treatment responses should be assessed after 4–6 weeks by MRI, and treatment escalation should be discussed at such early time points, since compression fractures are a considerable threat [90, 101].

Since MRI techniques are time consuming, relatively expensive, and difficult to perform in young children, biomarkers reflecting disease activity would be considered particularly beneficial. Some of the aforementioned recently proposed serum biomarkers promise potential as a measure of disease activity after treatment initiation. Interleukin-12, MCP-1, and sIL-2R can act as markers for treatment response, since they remained elevated in individuals who did not reach clinical and radiographical remission in response to the introduction of NSAID treatment [45]. However, reported findings require confirmation in unrelated cohorts.

Not uncommonly, disease activity is "waxing and waning" in CNO with periods of remission and disease activity. Individual disease courses are highly variable with occasional spontaneous resolution after several weeks or months but more frequently prolonged courses. While initial studies suggested that CNO may be benign and spontaneously resolve in most patients [9, 38], more recent evidence indicates that CNO is a chronic disease with disease-related sequelae in a subset of patients, particularly those with prolonged and insufficiently controlled inflammatory activity [18, 90] and spinal involvement. Pathologic fractures can occur in up to 50% of patients with vertebral involvement [27, 90]. Other sequelae include bone sclerosis and hyperostosis, leg-length discrepancies, muscle atrophy, polyarthritis and spondyloarthropathies, psychosocial problems, and pain amplification syndromes [9, 18, 27, 32, 82, 90].

Conclusions

Chronic nonbacterial osteomyelitis is an autoinflammatory bone disorder. Associations with other autoimmune/inflammatory disorders have been reported. Complex pathophysiology with several genetic factors contributes to distinct molecular disturbances resulting in cytokine dysregulation and bone inflammation.. Imbalanced expression of pro- and anti-inflammatory cytokines and osteoclast activation can be therapeutically targeted with NSAIDs, corticosteroids, TNF inhibitors, bisphosphonates, and classical DMARDs. Early and sufficient treatment, particularly in individuals with spinal involvement, should be considered to prevent prolonged disease and severe complications.

References

1. Ferguson PJ, El-Shanti HI. Autoinflammatory bone disorders. Curr Opin Rheumatol. 2007;19:492–8.
2. Ferguson PJ, Sandu M. Current understanding of the pathogenesis and management of chronic recurrent multifocal osteomyelitis. Curr Rheumatol Rep. 2012;14:130–41.
3. Girschick HJ, Zimmer C, Klaus G, Darge K, Dick A, Morbach H. Chronic recurrent multifocal osteomyelitis: what is it and how should it be treated? Nat Clin Pract Rheumatol. 2007;3:733–8.
4. Hedrich CM, Hahn G, Girschick HJ, Morbach H. A clinical and pathomechanistic profile of chronic nonbacterial osteomyelitis/chronic recurrent multifocal osteomyelitis and challenges facing the field. Expert Rev Clin Immunol. 2013;9:845–54.
5. Hedrich CM, Hofmann SR, Pablik J, Morbach H, Girschick HJ. Autoinflammatory bone disorders with special focus on chronic recurrent multifocal osteomyelitis (CRMO). Pediatr Rheumatol Online J. 2013;11:47.
6. Hofmann SR, Schnabel A, Rosen-Wolff A, Morbach H, Girschick HJ, Hedrich CM. Chronic nonbacterial osteomyelitis: pathophysiological concepts and current treatment strategies. J Rheumatol. 2016;43:1956–64.
7. Schnabel A, Range U, Hahn G, Siepmann T, Berner R, Hedrich CM. Unexpectedly high incidences of chronic non-bacterial as compared to bacterial osteomyelitis in children. Rheumatol Int. 2016;36:1737–45.
8. Borzutzky A, Stern S, Reiff A, Zurakowski D, Steinberg EA, Dedeoglu F, et al. Pediatric chronic nonbacterial osteomyelitis. Pediatrics. 2012;130:e1190–e7.
9. Girschick HJ, Raab P, Surbaum S, Trusen A, Kirschner S, Schneider P, et al. Chronic non-bacterial osteomyelitis in children. Ann Rheum Dis. 2005;64:279–85.
10. Ferguson PJL, Laxer RM. Autoinflammatory bone disorders. In: Petty L, Lindsley W, editors. Textbook of pediatric rheumatology. 7th ed. Philadelphia, PA: Elsevier; 2016. p. 627–41.
11. Giedion A, Holthusen W, Masel LF, Vischer D. Subacute and chronic "symmetrical" osteomyelitis. Ann Radiol (Paris). 1972;15:329–42.
12. Bjorksten B, Gustavson KH, Eriksson B, Lindholm A, Nordstrom S. Chronic recurrent multifocal osteomyelitis and pustulosis palmoplantaris. J Pediatr. 1978;93:227–31.
13. Probst FP, Bjorksten B, Gustavson KH. Radiological aspect of chronic recurrent multifocal osteomyelitis. Ann Radiol (Paris). 1978;21:115–25.
14. Hayem G, Bouchaud-Chabot A, Benali K, Roux S, Palazzo E, Silbermann-Hoffman O, et al. SAPHO syndrome: a long-term follow-up study of 120 cases. Semin Arthritis Rheum. 1999;29:159–71.
15. Hofmann SR, Kapplusch F, Girschick HJ, Morbach H, Pablik J, Ferguson PJ, Hedrich CM. Chronic recurrent multi-focal osteomyelitis (CRMO): presentation, pathogenesis and treatment. Curr Osteoporos Rep. 2017;15(6):542–54.
16. Jansson AF, Grote V, Group ES. Nonbacterial osteitis in children: data of a German incidence surveillance study. Acta Paediatr. 2011;100:1150–7.
17. Wipff J, Costantino F, Lemelle I, Pajot C, Duquesne A, Lorrot M, et al. A large national cohort of French patients with chronic recurrent multifocal osteitis. Arthritis Rheumatol. 2015;67:1128–37.
18. Huber AM, Lam PY, Duffy CM, Yeung RS, Ditchfield M, Laxer D, et al. Chronic recurrent multifocal osteomyelitis: clinical outcomes after more than five years of follow-up. J Pediatr. 2002;141:198–203.
19. Vittecoq O, Said LA, Michot C, Mejjad O, Thomine JM, Mitrofanoff P, et al. Evolution of chronic recurrent multifocal osteitis toward spondyloarthropathy over the long term. Arthritis Rheum. 2000;43:109–19.
20. Rohekar G, Inman RD. Conundrums in nosology: synovitis, acne, pustulosis, hyperostosis, and osteitis syndrome and spondylarthritis. Arthritis Rheum. 2006;55:665–9.

21. Prose NS, Fahrner LJ, Miller CR, Layfield L. Pustular psoriasis with chronic recurrent multifocal osteomyelitis and spontaneous fractures. J Am Acad Dermatol. 1994;31:376–9.
22. Edwards TC, Stapleton FB, Bond MJ, Barrett FF. Sweet's syndrome with multifocal sterile osteomyelitis. Am J Dis Child. 1986;140:817–8.
23. Majeed HA, Kalaawi M, Mohanty D, Teebi AS, Tunjekar MF, al-Gharbawy F, et al. Congenital dyserythropoietic anemia and chronic recurrent multifocal osteomyelitis in three related children and the association with sweet syndrome in two siblings. J Pediatr. 1989;115:730–4.
24. Arndt JH. Sweet's syndrome and chronic recurrent multifocal osteomyelitis. Am J Dis Child. 1987;141:721.
25. Omidi CJ, Siegfried EC. Chronic recurrent multifocal osteomyelitis preceding pyoderma gangrenosum and occult ulcerative colitis in a pediatric patient. Pediatr Dermatol. 1998;15:435–8.
26. Koturoglu G, Vardar F, Ozkinay F, Kurugol Z, Akalin T, Ozkinay C. Pyoderma gangrenosum in a six-month-old boy. Turk J Pediatr. 2006;48:159–61.
27. Jansson A, Renner ED, Ramser J, Mayer A, Haban M, Meindl A, et al. Classification of nonbacterial osteitis: retrospective study of clinical, immunological and genetic aspects in 89 patients. Rheumatology (Oxford). 2007;46:154–60.
28. Schilling F, Marker-Hermann E. Chronic recurrent multifocal osteomyelitis in association with chronic inflammatory bowel disease: entheropathic CRMO. Z Rheumatol. 2003;62:527–38.
29. Job-Deslandre C, Krebs S, Kahan A. Chronic recurrent multifocal osteomyelitis: five-year outcomes in 14 pediatric cases. Joint Bone Spine. 2001;68:245–51.
30. Kim JE, Kolh EM, Kim DK. Takayasu's arteritis presenting with focal periostitis affecting two limbs. Int J Cardiol. 1998;67:267–70.
31. McConachie NS, Morley KD, Jones MC. Case report: periosteal new bone formation in Takayasu arteritis. Clin Radiol. 1995;50:578–80.
32. Pelkonen P, Ryoppy S, Jaaskelainen J, Rapola J, Repo H, Kaitila I. Chronic osteomyelitislike disease with negative bacterial cultures. Am J Dis Child. 1988;142:1167–73.
33. Bousvaros A, Marcon M, Treem W, Waters P, Issenman R, Couper R, et al. Chronic recurrent multifocal osteomyelitis associated with chronic inflammatory bowel disease in children. Dig Dis Sci. 1999;44:2500–7.
34. Kerem E, Manson D, Laxer RM, Levison H, Reilly BJ. Pulmonary association in a case of chronic recurrent multifocal osteomyelitis. Pediatr Pulmonol. 1989;7:55–8.
35. Ravelli A, Marseglia GL, Viola S, Ruperto N, Martini A. Chronic recurrent multifocal osteomyelitis with unusual features. Acta Paediatr. 1995;84:222–5.
36. Assmann G, Kueck O, Kirchhoff T, Rosenthal H, Voswinkel J, Pfreundschuh M, et al. Efficacy of antibiotic therapy for SAPHO syndrome is lost after its discontinuation: an interventional study. Arthritis Res Ther. 2009;11:R140.
37. Schilling F, Wagner AD. Azithromycin: an anti-inflammatory effect in chronic recurrent multifocal osteomyelitis? A preliminary report. Z Rheumatol. 2000;59:352–3.
38. Schultz C, Holterhus PM, Seidel A, Jonas S, Barthel M, Kruse K, et al. Chronic recurrent multifocal osteomyelitis in children. Pediatr Infect Dis J. 1999;18:1008–13.
39. Bj0rksten B, Boquist L. Histopathological aspects of chronic recurrent multifocal osteomyelitis. J Bone Joint Surg Br. 1980;62:376–80.
40. Jurik AG. Chronic recurrent multifocal osteomyelitis. Semin Musculoskelet Radiol. 2004;8:243–53.
41. Girschick HJ, Huppertz HI, Harmsen D, Krauspe R, Muller-Hermelink HK, Papadopoulos T. Chronic recurrent multifocal osteomyelitis in children: diagnostic value of histopathology and microbial testing. Hum Pathol. 1999;30:59–65.
42. King SM, Laxer RM, Manson D, Gold R. Chronic recurrent multifocal osteomyelitis: a noninfectious inflammatory process. Pediatr Infect Dis J. 1987;6:907–11.
43. Carr AJ, Cole WG, Roberton DM, Chow CW. Chronic multifocal osteomyelitis. J Bone Joint Surg Br. 1993;75:582–91.

44. Hofmann SR, Kubasch AS, Ioannidis C, Rosen-Wolff A, Girschick HJ, Morbach H, et al. Altered expression of IL-10 family cytokines in monocytes from CRMO patients result in enhanced IL-1beta expression and release. Clin Immunol. 2015;161:300–7.
45. Hofmann SR, Kubasch AS, Range U, Laass MW, Morbach H, Girschick HJ, et al. Serum biomarkers for the diagnosis and monitoring of chronic recurrent multifocal osteomyelitis (CRMO). Rheumatol Int. 2016;36:769–79.
46. Hofmann SR, Morbach H, Schwarz T, Rosen-Wolff A, Girschick HJ, Hedrich CM. Attenuated TLR4/MAPK signaling in monocytes from patients with CRMO results in impaired IL-10 expression. Clin Immunol. 2012;145:69–76.
47. Hofmann SR, Schwarz T, Moller JC, Morbach H, Schnabel A, Rosen-Wolff A, et al. Chronic non-bacterial osteomyelitis is associated with impaired Sp1 signaling, reduced IL10 promoter phosphorylation, and reduced myeloid IL-10 expression. Clin Immunol. 2011;141:317–27.
48. Lucas M, Zhang X, Prasanna V, Mosser DM. ERK activation following macrophage FcgammaR ligation leads to chromatin modifications at the IL-10 locus. J Immunol. 2005;175:469–77.
49. Zhang X, Edwards JP, Mosser DM. Dynamic and transient remodeling of the macrophage IL-10 promoter during transcription. J Immunol. 2006;177:1282–8.
50. Greenhill CJ, Jones GW, Nowell MA, Newton Z, Harvey AK, Moideen AN, et al. Interleukin-10 regulates the inflammasome-driven augmentation of inflammatory arthritis and joint destruction. Arthritis Res Ther. 2014;16:419.
51. Scianaro R, Insalaco A, Bracci Laudiero L, De Vito R, Pezzullo M, Teti A, et al. Deregulation of the IL-1beta axis in chronic recurrent multifocal osteomyelitis. Pediatr Rheumatol Online J. 2014;12:30.
52. Morbach H, Hedrich CM, Beer M, Girschick HJ. Autoinflammatory bone disorders. Clin Immunol. 2013;147:185–96.
53. Nakashima T, Takayanagi H. Osteoimmunology: crosstalk between the immune and bone systems. J Clin Immunol. 2009;29:555–67.
54. Nakashima T, Takayanagi H. Osteoclasts and the immune system. J Bone Miner Metab. 2009;27:519–29.
55. Aksentijevich I, Masters SL, Ferguson PJ, Dancey P, Frenkel J, van Royen-Kerkhoff A, et al. An autoinflammatory disease with deficiency of the interleukin-1-receptor antagonist. N Engl J Med. 2009;360:2426–37.
56. Lindor NM, Arsenault TM, Solomon H, Seidman CE, McEvoy MT. A new autosomal dominant disorder of pyogenic sterile arthritis, pyoderma gangrenosum, and acne: PAPA syndrome. Mayo Clin Proc. 1997;72:611–5.
57. Smith EJ, Allantaz F, Bennett L, Zhang D, Gao X, Wood G, et al. Clinical, molecular, and genetic characteristics of PAPA syndrome: a review. Curr Genomics. 2010;11:519–27.
58. Paller AS, Pachman L, Rich K, Esterly NB, Gonzalez-Crussi F. Pustulosis palmaris et plantaris: its association with chronic recurrent multifocal osteomyelitis. J Am Acad Dermatol. 1985;12:927–30.
59. Festen JJ, Kuipers FC, Schaars AH. Multifocal recurrent periostitis responsive to colchicine. Scand J Rheumatol. 1985;14:8–14.
60. Ben Becher S, Essaddam H, Nahali N, Ben Hamadi F, Mouelhi MH, Hammou A, et al. Recurrent multifocal periostosis in children. Report of a familial form. Ann Pediatr (Paris). 1991;38:345–9.
61. Ferguson PJ, Lokuta MA, El-Shanti HI, Muhle L, Bing X, Huttenlocher A. Neutrophil dysfunction in a family with a SAPHO syndrome-like phenotype. Arthritis Rheum. 2008;58:3264–9.
62. Golla A, Jansson A, Ramser J, Hellebrand H, Zahn R, Meitinger T, et al. Chronic recurrent multifocal osteomyelitis (CRMO): evidence for a susceptibility gene located on chromosome 18q21.3-18q22. Eur J Hum Genet. 2002;10:217–21.
63. Beck C, Girschick HJ, Morbach H, Schwarz T, Yimam T, Frenkel J, et al. Mutation screening of the IL-1 receptor antagonist gene in chronic non-bacterial osteomyelitis of childhood and adolescence. Clin Exp Rheumatol. 2011;29:1040–3.

64. Hedrich CM, Bream JH. Cell type-specific regulation of IL-10 expression in inflammation and disease. Immunol Res. 2010;47:185–206.
65. Hofmann SR, Rosen-Wolff A, Tsokos GC, Hedrich CM. Biological properties and regulation of IL-10 related cytokines and their contribution to autoimmune disease and tissue injury. Clin Immunol. 2012;143:116–27.
66. Hamel J, Paul D, Gahr M, Hedrich CM. Pilot study: possible association of IL10 promoter polymorphisms with CRMO. Rheumatol Int. 2012;32:555–6.
67. Hofmann SR, Roesen-Wolff A, Hahn G, Hedrich CM. Update: cytokine dysregulation in chronic nonbacterial osteomyelitis (CNO). Int J Rheumatol. 2012;2012:310206.
68. Cox ADB, Laxer R, Bing X, Finer A, Erives A, Mahajan V, Bassuk AG, Ferguson P. Recessive coding and regulatory mutations in FBLIM1 underlie the pathogenesis of sterile osteomyelitis [abstract]. Arthritis Rheumatol. 2016;68(suppl 10) http://acrabstracts.org/abstract/recessive-coding-and-regulatory-mutations-in-fblim1-underlie-the-pathogenesis-of-sterile-osteomyelitis/.
69. Cox AJ, Darbro BW, Laxer RM, Velez G, Bing X, Finer AL, Erives A, Mahajan VB, Bassuk AG, Ferguson PJ. Recessive coding and regulatory mutations in FBLIM1 underlie the pathogenesis of chronic recurrent multifocal osteomyelitis (CRMO). PLoS One. 2017;12(3):e0169687.
70. Chitu V, Nacu V, Charles JF, Henne WM, McMahon HT, Nandi S, et al. PSTPIP2 deficiency in mice causes osteopenia and increased differentiation of multipotent myeloid precursors into osteoclasts. Blood. 2012;120:3126–35.
71. Grosse J, Chitu V, Marquardt A, Hanke P, Schmittwolf C, Zeitlmann L, et al. Mutation of mouse Mayp/Pstpip2 causes a macrophage autoinflammatory disease. Blood. 2006;107:3350–8.
72. Liao HJ, Chyuan IT, Wu CS, Lin SW, Chen KH, Tsai HF, et al. Increased neutrophil infiltration, IL-1 production and a SAPHO syndrome-like phenotype in PSTPIP2-deficient mice. Rheumatology (Oxford). 2015;54:1317–26.
73. Ahmed S, Bu W, Lee RT, Maurer-Stroh S, Goh WI. F-BAR domain proteins: families and function. Commun Integr Biol. 2010;3:116–21.
74. Tsujita K, Kondo A, Kurisu S, Hasegawa J, Itoh T, Takenawa T. Antagonistic regulation of F-BAR protein assemblies controls actin polymerization during podosome formation. J Cell Sci. 2013;126:2267–78.
75. Cassel SL, Janczy JR, Bing X, Wilson SP, Olivier AK, Otero JE, et al. Inflammasome-independent IL-1beta mediates autoinflammatory disease in Pstpip2-deficient mice. Proc Natl Acad Sci U S A. 2014;111:1072–7.
76. Lukens JR, Gross JM, Calabrese C, Iwakura Y, Lamkanfi M, Vogel P, et al. Critical role for inflammasome-independent IL-1beta production in osteomyelitis. Proc Natl Acad Sci U S A. 2014;111:1066–71.
77. Netea MG, van de Veerdonk FL, van der Meer JW, Dinarello CA, Joosten LA. Inflammasome-independent regulation of IL-1-family cytokines. Annu Rev Immunol. 2015;33:49–77.
78. Lukens JR, Gurung P, Vogel P, Johnson GR, Carter RA, McGoldrick DJ, et al. Dietary modulation of the microbiome affects autoinflammatory disease. Nature. 2014;516:246–9.
79. Ter Horst R, Jaeger M, Smeekens SP, Oosting M, Swertz MA, Li Y, et al. Host and environmental factors influencing individual human cytokine responses. Cell. 2016;167(1111–24):e13.
80. Jansson AF, Muller TH, Gliera L, Ankerst DP, Wintergerst U, Belohradsky BH, et al. Clinical score for nonbacterial osteitis in children and adults. Arthritis Rheum. 2009;60:1152–9.
81. Roderick MR, Shah R, Rogers V, Finn A, Ramanan AV. Chronic recurrent multifocal osteomyelitis (CRMO) – advancing the diagnosis. Pediatr Rheumatol Online J. 2016;14:47.
82. Duffy CM, Lam PY, Ditchfield M, Allen R, Graham HK. Chronic recurrent multifocal osteomyelitis: review of orthopaedic complications at maturity. J Pediatr Orthop. 2002;22:501–5.
83. Ferguson PJ, Sykelyk A, Figueredo R, Koropatnick J. Synergistic cytotoxicity against human tumor cell lines by oncolytic adenovirus dl1520 (ONYX-015) and melphalan. Tumori. 2016;102:31–9.
84. Jurik AG, Egund N. MRI in chronic recurrent multifocal osteomyelitis. Skelet Radiol. 1997;26:230–8.

85. Morbach H, Schneider P, Schwarz T, Hofmann C, Raab P, Neubauer H, et al. Comparison of magnetic resonance imaging and 99mTechnetium-labelled methylene diphosphonate bone scintigraphy in the initial assessment of chronic non-bacterial osteomyelitis of childhood and adolescents. Clin Exp Rheumatol. 2012;30:578–82.
86. Hofmann C, Wurm M, Schwarz T, Neubauer H, Beer M, Girschick H, et al. A standardized clinical and radiological follow-up of patients with chronic non-bacterial osteomyelitis treated with pamidronate. Clin Exp Rheumatol. 2014;32:604–9.
87. Khanna G, Sato TS, Ferguson P. Imaging of chronic recurrent multifocal osteomyelitis. Radiographics. 2009;29:1159–77.
88. Jurik AG, Helmig O, Ternowitz T, Moller BN. Chronic recurrent multifocal osteomyelitis: a follow-up study. J Pediatr Orthop. 1988;8:49–58.
89. Hofmann SR, Böttger F, Range U, Lück C, Morbach H, Girschick HJ, Suttorp M, Hedrich CM. Serum IL-6 and CCL11/eotaxin may be suitable biomarkers for the diagnosis of chronic nonbacterial osteomyelitis. Front Pediatr. 2017;5:256.
90. Schnabel A, Range U, Hahn G, Berner R, Hedrich CM. Treatment response and long-term outcomes in children with chronic non-bacterial osteomyelitis (CNO). J Rheum. 2016;36(12):1737–45.
91. Girschick HJ, Krauspe R, Tschammler A, Huppertz HI. Chronic recurrent osteomyelitis with clavicular involvement in children: diagnostic value of different imaging techniques and therapy with non-steroidal anti-inflammatory drugs. Eur J Pediatr. 1998;157:28–33.
92. Beck C, Morbach H, Beer M, Stenzel M, Tappe D, Gattenlohner S, et al. Chronic nonbacterial osteomyelitis in childhood: prospective follow-up during the first year of anti-inflammatory treatment. Arthritis Res Ther. 2010;12:R74.
93. Daniels MJ, Rivers-Auty J, Schilling T, Spencer NG, Watremez W, Fasolino V, et al. Fenamate NSAIDs inhibit the NLRP3 inflammasome and protect against Alzheimer's disease in rodent models. Nat Commun. 2016;7:12504.
94. Carpenter E, Jackson MA, Friesen CA, Scarbrough M, Roberts CC. Crohn's-associated chronic recurrent multifocal osteomyelitis responsive to infliximab. J Pediatr. 2004;144:541–4.
95. Twilt M, Laxer RM. Clinical care of children with sterile bone inflammation. Curr Opin Rheumatol. 2011;23:424–31.
96. Hospach T, Langendoerfer M, von KT MJ, Dannecker GE. Spinal involvement in chronic recurrent multifocal osteomyelitis (CRMO) in childhood and effect of pamidronate. Eur J Pediatr. 2010;169:1105–11.
97. Tlougan BE, Podjasek JO, O'Haver J, Cordova KB, Nguyen XH, Tee R, et al. Chronic recurrent multifocal osteomyelitis (CRMO) and synovitis, acne, pustulosis, hyperostosis, and osteitis (SAPHO) syndrome with associated neutrophilic dermatoses: a report of seven cases and review of the literature. Pediatr Dermatol. 2009;26:497–505.
98. Miettunen PM, Wei X, Kaura D, Reslan WA, Aguirre AN, Kellner JD. Dramatic pain relief and resolution of bone inflammation following pamidronate in 9 pediatric patients with persistent chronic recurrent multifocal osteomyelitis (CRMO). Pediatr Rheumatol Online J. 2009;7:2.
99. Zhao Y, Chauvin NA, Jaramillo D, Burnham JM. Aggressive therapy reduces disease activity without skeletal damage progression in chronic nonbacterial osteomyelitis. J Rheumatol. 2015;42:1245–51.
100. Pardeo M, Pires Marafon D, Messia V, Garganese MC, De Benedetti F, Insalaco A. Anakinra in a cohort of children with chronic nonbacterial osteomyelitis. J Rheumatol. 2017;44:1231–8.
101. Zhao Y, Wu EY, Oliver MS, Cooper AM, Basiaga ML, Vora SS, Lee TC, Fox E, Amarilyo G, Stern SM, Dvergsten JA, Haines KA, Rouster-Stevens KA, Onel KB, Cherian J, Hausmann JS, Miettunen P, Cellucci T, Nuruzzaman F, Taneja A, Barron KS, Hollander MC, Lapidus SK, Li SC, Ozen S, Girschick H, Laxer RM, Dedeoglu F, Hedrich CM, Ferguson PJ, The CRMO study group and the CARRA SVARD subcommittee. Consensus treatment plans for chronic nonbacterial osteomyelitis refractory to nonsteroidal anti inflammatory drugs and/or with active spinal lesions. In preparation; 2017.
102. Zhao Y, Wu EY, Oliver MS, Cooper AM, Basiaga ML, Vora SS, et al. Consensus treatment plans for chronic nonbacterial osteomyelitis refractory to nonsteroidal anti-inflammatory drugs and/or with active spinal lesions. Arthritis Care Res (Hoboken). 2018;70(8):1228–37. https://doi.org/10.1002/acr.23462. Epub 2018 Jul 12. PMID: 29112802. [Epub ahead to print].

Chapter 18
Improving the Transition from Pediatric to Adult Care for Adolescents and Young Adults with Autoinflammatory Diseases

Jonathan S. Hausmann and Kitty O'Hare

Introduction

The genetic basis for most autoinflammatory diseases (AIDs) makes them unique in rheumatology because most patients will be diagnosed during childhood and will continue to have active disease during adulthood [10]. Improvements in the management of children with AIDs have permitted most to reach adulthood and lead productive lives. As a result, adolescents and young adults (AYAs) will need to transition to an adult rheumatologist at some point during their medical care.

While a successful transition provides an opportunity for increased patient engagement and education, it is fraught with multiple challenges, including those that arise from the patient as she gains independence, from the family as they forego their role as managers of the patient's care, and from the pediatric and adult rheumatologist, who must exchange information, often using electronic health records that are not interoperable. Patients with AIDs face similar challenges in transitioning as those with other chronic health conditions, but the rarity of AIDs, their episodic nature, and the frequent use of immunosuppressive drugs impose unique obstacles that must be overcome. We will first discuss the importance of transition and will then address factors that will facilitate this process, including the acquisition of self-

J. S. Hausmann, MD (✉)
Autoinflammatory Diseases Clinic, Boston Children's Hospital, Boston, MA, USA

Autoinflammatory Disease Center, Beth Israel Deaconess Medical Center, Boston, MA, USA

Harvard Medical School, Boston, MA, USA
e-mail: jonathan.hausmann@childrens.harvard.edu

K. O'Hare, MD
Harvard Medical School, Boston, MA, USA

Transition Medicine for Primary Care, Weitzman Family BRIDGES Adult Transition Program, Boston Children's Hospital, Boston, MA, USA

Pediatric Population Health, Brigham and Women's Hospital, Boston, MA, USA

P. Efthimiou (ed.), *Auto-Inflammatory Syndromes*,
https://doi.org/10.1007/978-3-319-96929-9_18

management skills and supportive decision-making. Finally, we will address critical aspects of the medical care for patients with AIDs including long-term sequelae, issues related to pregnancy, primary care, stress management, attending college, and the development of a transition plan for pediatric and adult rheumatology practices.

The Need for Transition

Transitioning pediatric rheumatology patients to adult care requires patients to be able to care for and manage their chronic disease; to become aware of their medical histories, treatments, and complications; as well as to manage their future care, including making appointments, obtaining medication refills, and addressing health insurance issues. The time for transition typically occurs at a particularly vulnerable time, as AYAs usually have worse health than younger adolescents and older adults [21]. Unfortunately, most pediatric patients receive little or no preparation for transitioning into adult care [20], and few pediatrics practices are prepared to manage the transition process for their young adult patients [24]. AYAs transitioning their care to adult providers frequently miss their scheduled visits with adult providers; one study showed that the transfer time between the last pediatric rheumatology visit to the first adult rheumatology visit within the same hospital was over seven months [11].

Transitioning pediatric patients to adult providers should not be a onetime event; instead, it should be a process of education, planning, and skills development that starts at a very young age to prepare patients to transition into the adult world. Various transition interventions have been shown to improve adherence to care [7]. Within rheumatology, transition interventions have been most often studied in patients with juvenile idiopathic arthritis. These transition programs have shown improvement in the perceived health and quality of life [12, 18], as well as parent's ability to foster autonomy and independence [12]. Transition interventions also improve the success of establishing care with adult rheumatologists [13].

Self-Management Skills

A large part of the transition process involves educating patients about their own health conditions. This includes teaching patients to understand the cause of their illness and its genetic basis (if applicable), clinical manifestations, treatment options, and complications. At the same time, physicians should strive to provide patients with self-management skills, that is, problem-solving skills to help them identify issues with their condition, make decisions, take appropriate action, and reflect on the results of their actions to guide future behavior [2]. Adolescents with chronic rheumatic diseases do not naturally possess self-management skills to successfully manage their conditions into adulthood [15], but these skills can be taught. Studies have shown that teaching self-management improves clinical outcomes and reduces costs [2]. Table 18.1 provides examples of self-management skills required for patients with AIDs.

Table 18.1 Self-management skills that should be developed and mastered by patients with autoinflammatory diseases prior to transitioning to adult care

Healthcare skill	Age to begin development (years)	Age of mastery (years)
Understanding diagnosis, clinical features, and potential complications	5	15
Owning and knowing how to use a thermometer	8	13
Learning to identify and prevent disease triggers (emotional stress, medication nonadherence, strenuous activities)	8	16
Learning to identify sources of pain and acquiring pain management skills	8	16
Understanding the timing of medication administration (e.g., daily medications versus abortive medications)	11	16
Recognizing medication side effects	11	18
Differentiating disease flares from infections	14	18
Scheduling medical appointments	14	18
Obtaining medication refills; knowing who to call for prescriptions, who dispenses medications, and how to get medications delivered	14	18
Recognizing signs/symptoms that require medical attention	14	18
Understand how pregnancy can affect symptoms and make an informed choice about pregnancy prevention	14	21
Understand how substance use (alcohol, marijuana, illicits) can affect symptoms and disease progression	14	21
Having a health insurance card and knowing how to navigate it	16	18

Supportive Decision-Making

As children with AIDs progress through adolescence and into adulthood, they should increasingly participate in decisions regarding management of their disease, including the types of treatment they will receive (subcutaneous versus oral medications, frequency of administration, etc.), especially since they are the ones who will receive all the benefits and harms of treatment. In medicine, and especially in AIDs, decisions must often be made under uncertainty. Uncertainties may include the specific diagnosis, the utility of genetic testing, the optimal treatment strategy, long-term sequela of the disease, and/or potential complications from the treatment. Physicians should openly discuss these inherent uncertainties in the management of AIDs with patients and their families.

Supportive decision-making can be practiced from a very early age. A first step could be allowing a preschool-aged child to decide in which arm they want to receive an injection. The school-aged child can be coached to ask questions about the effects of medications on daily activities, for example, the impact of medications on sports or school. Adolescents should be allowed to have one-on-one time with the clinician for at least part of the visit, to better allow development of confidentiality as well as to improve confidence in decision-making. Adolescents can also cosign consents for treatments.

In most parts of the United States, patients become legal adults as of the 18th birthday. Achieving legal adulthood adds a new layer of complexity to decision-making. All adults should be encouraged to document a health care proxy, that is, another adult who is designated to make treatment decisions if the patient is unable to do so. If the disease course is severe, then young adults should be encouraged to consider advanced directives as well. For patients who may be unable to make their own medical decisions, perhaps secondary to neurologic compromise from aseptic meningitis (NOMID) or recurrent stroke (DADA2), it will be essential to discuss pathways for legal guardianship. The pathway to legal guardianship varies from state to state. If legal guardianship is advisable, the patient's potential guardian should begin the process well in advance of the age of majority. Neurocognitive testing can be beneficial for discerning how much support a young adult requires for making complex medical decisions.

It is also essential for transitioning patients to be aware of their health insurance benefits. Under the current law in the United States, young adults may continue enrollment on their parents' insurance until they turn 26 years of age. Patients on Medicaid should reapply to receive Medicaid as adults once they turn 18 [5].

Long-Term Sequelae

As children with AIDs grow into adulthood, they may continue to experience disease flares and may also face long-term complications from their chronic disease (or its treatment). Long-term data on patients with AIDs are scant, and the risks of biologic use throughout the lifespan are still largely unknown. Below, we will briefly discuss outcomes from some of the better-known AIDs, which may help to inform the management of patients with other syndromes.

Long-term outcomes in patients with familial Mediterranean fever (FMF), the most common and well-known AID, are excellent in patients treated with colchicine. A study of children with FMF followed through adulthood found that those who take colchicine do not develop amyloidosis, and most (64%) have complete remission of their attacks, while the rest have partial remission [33]. Children with FMF do not have abnormal growth or development, and adults reach normal heights.

Patients with mevalonate kinase deficiency (MKD, or hyper IgD syndrome [HIDS]) have some relief of their symptoms as they grow, with decreased frequency of attacks, although patients will continue to have intermittent attacks during adulthood [29]. In one study, almost half of adult patients with MKD reported that their disease delayed their education, and a third stated their disease contributed to being fired from a job; one-quarter were unemployed as adults [29]. Health-related quality-of-life measures were lower in patients with MKD than in healthy controls. Patients with MKD experienced limitations in their activities of daily living and scored slightly lower on autonomy and social development skills than controls.

In TRAPS, there is no spontaneous improvement in the frequency or severity of the episodes over time [22], although long-term outcomes are not well known.

In patients with periodic fevers, aphthous stomatitis, pharyngitis, and adenitis (PFAPA), the most common AID in childhood, 85% of patients have complete symptom resolution without sequelae after an average duration of 6 years [31]. Of those that continued to have symptoms, the duration of fever and the frequency of flares decreased significantly [31], and the vast majority were well when they reach adulthood.

Pregnancy and Genetic Counseling

The effects of AIDs on fertility are unclear. FMF patients who are treated with colchicine have been shown to have normal fertility [33]. However, studies of patients with cryopyrin-associated periodic syndrome (CAPS) showed reduced fertility in males and females with this condition [17, 28], although most had not received regular treatment with biologics from an early age. Fertility with the other AIDs is mostly unknown.

Nevertheless, the need for contraception should be addressed in patients with AIDs. Most of the drugs used to treat autoinflammatory conditions are not considered teratogenic, although there is limited data as to their effect on the fetus if taken during pregnancy. The little data that exists regarding the safety of IL-1 blockade does not seem to be concerning for women who become pregnant while on these drugs, or for males who take these medications at the time of conception [32].

Given the genetic basis of most AIDs, patients should be educated as to the risk of transmitting their disease to future offspring; genetic counseling may be beneficial.

Primary Care

Many patients with autoinflammatory and other rheumatic illness have close follow-up with their rheumatologists, and as a result, may forego routine primary care with potential adverse sequelae. Adolescents with other chronic medical conditions, such as those with cystic fibrosis and sickle cell disease, have fewer rates of preventive health counseling [3]. Adults with congenital heart disease have lower rates of cancer screening (Pap smears, mammography) than an otherwise healthy population [6]. As a result, it is essential for patients with AIDs to establish a primary care medical home and to receive all of the appropriate primary care counseling and screening appropriate for their age, in addition to the specialized care required for their condition.

Age-appropriate killed vaccines should be given to all patients, including the yearly influenza vaccine. Patients with MKD traditionally report febrile episodes occurring after childhood vaccinations [8], although it is not considered a contraindication to vaccinate these patients; in one case, anakinra given 72 hours after vaccine administration was successful in aborting the febrile episode without affecting immunogenicity [1].

According to the Centers for Disease Control and Prevention (CDC), patients on chronic immunosuppressive drugs should also receive pneumococcal vaccinations, including PCV13 and PPSV23. PCV13 is now routinely given to children, but it should also be given to those on chronic immunosuppression if it has not already been given. Patients on immunosuppression should also receive PPSV23 at least eight weeks after PCV13 immunization [4]. A second PPSV23 dose is recommended five years after the first dose. However, there are reports of patients with CAPS developing severe local and systemic reactions after the pneumococcal polysaccharide vaccine (PPSV23) [30], so the benefits and risks of this vaccine should be carefully weighed for this group.

Stress Management

Patients with rheumatic illnesses, and especially those with AIDs, are particularly vulnerable to stress. In those with AIDs, many types of stress, including emotional and physical, may provoke fever flares [10, 14, 25]. Thus, the occurrence of a flare may be a useful indicator that the patient is under stress. In AYAs, we often see flares triggered by starting college, final exams, lack of sleep, and travel. It is essential for patients to be mindful of the effect of these stressors on their disease. Patients should be encouraged to employ stress reduction techniques such as exercise, mindful meditation, yoga, biofeedback, acupuncture, massage, and cognitive behavioral therapy as methods to prevent flares. Many colleges now provide Wellness services to their students that offer several of these practices. Clinicians should also consider routine screening of their young adult patients for depression and anxiety using standardized instruments such as the PHQ9 and GAD7.

Going to College

For patients that plan to attend college, we find that it is easier to transition them to adult providers after they graduate from college. College brings multiple challenges to the care of patients with AIDs, especially if they require biologic medications, and continuation with their pediatric rheumatologist can facilitate their medical care during this time. If patients encounter disease complications while in college, they often reach out to their parents first rather than to their rheumatologist. By continuing with their pediatric providers, the parent is more familiar with the pediatric practice and may feel more comfortable helping to coordinate their care. We realize that some pediatric practices and hospitals have strict guidelines about when the transition of care should occur. However, the American Academy of Pediatrics argues against the establishment of arbitrary age limits on when the transition should be made; instead they recommend that the timing of this decision should be individualized and should take into account the patient and family's needs, as well as the availability of providers able to meet the patient's needs [9].

The availability of on-site medical care at colleges and universities is inconsistent at best [16]. For the safest and optimal college experience, students should be prepared to manage their health while away from home. Most students will benefit from having a written care plan which outlines what to do in certain situations, such as when developing an infection or a fever flare. The student should keep a copy of this care plan, and one should be filed with the Student Health Center. Students requiring reasonable accommodations, due to mobility problems or test-taking concerns, should identify themselves to their school's office of disability services. Unlike at the high school level, most colleges and universities do not actively seek out students in need of accommodation; students must identify themselves as being in need of these services.

If the patient is going to college far away from home, it is often useful to identify a (likely adult) rheumatologist who may be able to evaluate the patient in the case of an emergency. Patients can continue visiting their pediatric rheumatologist when they are home during vacations. AYAs should be encouraged to sign up for their pediatric rheumatologist's patient portal, if available, as a means of accessing their health information remotely, and to communicate with their home providers.

Although colleges and universities often provide health insurance, most of our patients stay on their parents' insurance throughout college, as this avoids having to obtain new prior authorization (PA) by different insurance companies, often ones with fewer prescription benefits.

If a patient is on a biologic medication, it will be necessary to coordinate drug delivery. If they go to school near their home, parents can deliver the drug to the patient, or the patient can pick it up from home. However, if the patient goes to school away from home, it is typically best to send the medications directly to the Student Health Center rather than to the student, as most medications require special handling to maintain them refrigerated. For other prescription drugs, they can be sent directly to a pharmacy near the school.

For students that receive infusions, it will be essential to coordinate their administration in a hospital close to the college. A PA will need to be rewritten for that hospital, and the family will need to find a provider with affiliation to the hospital who is willing to write the orders. When students are home for the summer, a new PA will need to be written to allow them to receive the medication at home.

Once patients graduate from college, we find that this is the best time for transition. They may move away from home and obtain their own insurance. They are typically more mature and better able to visit an adult rheumatologist on their own.

A Plan for Transition

The Center for Healthcare Transition Improvement created a structured model called the Six Core Elements of Healthcare Transition to facilitate the establishment of transition programs. Initial testing of this approach into several practices showed improvements in quality indicators [19]. They later refined their process based on feedback from this project, in addition to expert consensus, which they released as version 2.0.

The Six Core Elements of Healthcare Transition 2.0 contains advice for pediatric practices transitioning their patients to adult providers, for adult providers who are receiving adolescent and young adults from pediatric practices, as well as for physicians who provide a continuum of care (e.g., Med-Peds providers, family medicine physicians). It provides a structured framework that can be adapted and instituted in a wide variety of practice settings, including for patients with AIDs (Table 18.2).

Table 18.2 Transitioning AYAs with AIDs to adult healthcare providers, modeled after The Six Core Elements of Healthcare Transition 2.0

1. Transition policy • Develop a transition policy/statement with input from youth and families that describes the practice's approach to transition, including privacy and consent information • Educate all staff about the practice's approach to transition, the policy/statement, the Six Core Elements, and distinct roles of the youth, family, and pediatric and adult rheumatology teams in the transition process, taking into account cultural preferences • Post policy and share/discuss with youth and families, beginning at ages 12–14, and regularly review as part of ongoing care	**4. Transition planning** • Develop and regularly update a medical summary, including plans for response to a fever or other emergencies • Prepare youth and parent/caregiver for the adult approach to care at age 18, including legal changes in decision-making and privacy and consent, self-advocacy, and access to information • Determine the level of need for decision-making supports for youth with intellectual challenges, and make referrals to legal resources • Assist youth in identifying an adult rheumatologist, obtain consent from the youth/guardian for the release of medical information, and communicate with the selected provider about pending transfer of care • Provide linkages to insurance resources, self-care management information, and culturally appropriate community supports
2. Transition tracking and monitoring • Identify all youth with AIDs ages 12 or older in your practice • Utilize individual flow sheet or registry to track youth's transition progress with the Six Core Elements • Build electronic health record (EHR) tools to help support transition processes	**5. Transfer of care** • Confirm date of first adult rheumatology appointment • Complete transfer package, including final transition readiness assessment, plan of care with transition goals and pending actions, medical summary and emergency care plan, any legal documents, condition fact sheet, and additional provider records • Prepare a letter with transfer package, send to adult rheumatology practice, and confirm adult practice's receipt of transfer package
3. Transition readiness • Create an AID-specific fact sheet to educate the youth and their future adult health team about their condition • Conduct regular transition readiness assessments to identify and discuss with youth and parent/caregiver their needs and goals in self-care • Jointly develop goals and prioritized actions with youth and parent/caregiver, and document regularly in a plan of care	**6. Transition completion** • Contact young adult 3–6 months after last pediatric rheumatology visit to confirm the transfer of responsibilities to adult practice and elicit feedback on experience with the transition process • Communicate with adult practice confirming completion of transfer and offer consultation assistance, as needed • Build ongoing and collaborative partnerships with adult rheumatologists

Adapted from Got Transition [26]

Conclusions

There are many unmet needs in transitioning youth with AIDs to adult providers. A better understanding of long-term outcomes of patients with AIDs, perhaps from large international registries such as Eurofever Project [27], may provide us with more specific recommendations in managing these patients during the transition period. The establishment of specialized, comprehensive transition programs for patients with AIDs could significantly improve patient satisfaction and health outcomes. Finally, improving the education of health professionals on the importance of establishing transition services and recommendations on how to do this most effectively could also enhance care [23].

The transition of youth with AIDs to adult providers should not be viewed as a onetime event; rather, it is a process that should begin many years before the transfer of care to adult providers. It requires patients to learn self-management skills, recognize disease flares and complications, develop the ability to make decisions concerning their AIDs, and understand how their illness has the potential to affect other parts of their lives. The process of transition requires a team effort with the patient at the center, with open and active communication between all involved, including pediatric and adult rheumatologists, primary care providers, nurses, school officials, and hospital systems. A good transition has the potential to bring significant health benefits for AYAs with AIDs that may last a lifetime.

References

1. Bodar EJ, van der Hilst JCH, Drenth JPH, et al. Effect of etanercept and anakinra on inflammatory attacks in the hyper-IgD syndrome: introducing a vaccination provocation model. Neth J Med. 2005;63:260–4.
2. Bodenheimer T, Lorig K, Holman H, Grumbach K. Patient self-management of chronic disease in primary care. JAMA. 2002;288:2469–75. https://doi.org/10.1080/13814788.2017.1306516.
3. Britto MT, Garrett JM, Dugliss MAJ, et al. Preventive services received by adolescents with cystic fibrosis and sickle cell disease. Arch Pediatr Adolesc Med. 1999;153:27–32. https://doi.org/10.1001/archpedi.153.1.27.
4. Centers for Disease Control and Prevention. Use of 13-valent pneumococcal conjugate vaccine and 23-valent pneumococcal polysaccharide vaccine for adults with immunocompromising conditions: recommendations of the Advisory Committee on Immunization Practices (ACIP). MMWR Morb Mortal Wkly Rep. 2012;61:816–9.
5. Centers for Medicare Medicaid Services (2017) Young Adults and the Affordable Care Act: protecting young adults and eliminating burdens on families and businesses – Centers for Medicare & Medicaid Services. In: www.cms.govCCIIOResourcesFilesadultchildfactsheet.html. Accessed 25 Dec 2017.
6. Christman MP, Castro-Zarraga M, DeFaria Yeh D, et al. Adequacy of cancer screening in adult women with congenital heart disease. ISRN Cardiol. 2013;2013:827696. https://doi.org/10.1155/2013/827696.
7. Gabriel P, McManus M, Rogers K, White P. Outcome evidence for structured pediatric to adult health care transition interventions: a systematic review. J Pediatr. 2017;188:263–269.e15. https://doi.org/10.1016/j.jpeds.2017.05.066.

8. ter Haar NM, Jeyaratnam J, Lachmann HJ, et al. The phenotype and genotype of mevalonate kinase deficiency: a series of 114 cases from the Eurofever registry. Arthritis & Rheumatology. 2016;68:2795–805. https://doi.org/10.1002/art.39763.
9. Hardin AP, Hackell JM, Committee on Practice and Ambulatory Medicine. Age limit of pediatrics. Pediatrics. 2017. https://doi.org/10.1542/peds.2017-2151
10. Hausmann JS, Dedeoglu F. Autoinflammatory diseases in pediatrics. Dermatol Clin. 2013;31:481–94. https://doi.org/10.1016/j.det.2013.04.003.
11. Hersh AO, Pang S, Curran ML, et al. The challenges of transferring chronic illness patients to adult care: reflections from pediatric and adult rheumatology at a US academic center. Pediatr Rheumatol. 2009;7:13. https://doi.org/10.1186/1546-0096-7-13.
12. Hilderson D, Moons P, Van der Elst K, et al. The clinical impact of a brief transition programme for young people with juvenile idiopathic arthritis: results of the DON'T RETARD project. Rheumatology (Oxford). 2016;55:133–42. https://doi.org/10.1093/rheumatology/kev284.
13. Jensen PT, Karnes J, Jones K, et al. Quantitative evaluation of a pediatric rheumatology transition program. Pediatr Rheumatol. 2015;13:17. https://doi.org/10.1186/s12969-015-0013-0.
14. Lachmann HJ, Papa R, Gerhold K, et al. The phenotype of TNF receptor-associated autoinflammatory syndrome (TRAPS) at presentation: a series of 158 cases from the Eurofever/EUROTRAPS international registry. Ann Rheum Dis. 2014;73:2160–7. https://doi.org/10.1136/annrheumdis-2013-204184.
15. Lawson EF, Hersh AO, Applebaum MA, et al. Self-management skills in adolescents with chronic rheumatic disease: a cross-sectional survey. Pediatr Rheumatol. 2011;9:35. https://doi.org/10.1186/1546-0096-9-35.
16. Lemly DC, Lawlor K, Scherer EA, et al. College health service capacity to support youth with chronic medical conditions. Pediatrics. 2014;134:885–91. https://doi.org/10.1542/peds.2014-1304.
17. Leslie KS, Lachmann HJ, Bruning E, et al. Phenotype, genotype, and sustained response to anakinra in 22 patients with autoinflammatory disease associated with CIAS-1/NALP3 mutations. Arch Dermatol. 2006;142:1591–7. https://doi.org/10.1001/archderm.142.12.1591.
18. McDonagh JE, Southwood TR, Shaw KL, British Society of Paediatric and Adolescent Rheumatology. The impact of a coordinated transitional care programme on adolescents with juvenile idiopathic arthritis. Rheumatology. 2007;46:161–8. https://doi.org/10.1093/rheumatology/kel198.
19. McManus M, White P, Barbour A, et al. Pediatric to adult transition: a quality improvement model for primary care. J Adolesc Health. 2015;56:73–8. https://doi.org/10.1016/j.jadohealth.2014.08.006.
20. McManus MA, Pollack LR, Cooley WC, et al. Current status of transition preparation among youth with special needs in the United States. Pediatrics. 2013;131:1090–7. https://doi.org/10.1542/peds.2012-3050.
21. Park MJ, Scott JT, Adams SH, et al. Adolescent and young adult health in the United States in the past decade: little improvement and young adults remain worse off than adolescents. J Adolesc Health. 2014;55:3–16. https://doi.org/10.1016/j.jadohealth.2014.04.003.
22. Pelagatti MA, Meini A, Caorsi R, et al. Long-term clinical profile of children with the low-penetrance R92Q mutation of the TNFRSF1A gene. Arthritis Rheum. 2011;63:1141–50. https://doi.org/10.1002/art.30237.
23. Sharma N, O'Hare K, Antonelli RC, Sawicki GS. Transition care: future directions in education, health policy, and outcomes research. Acad Pediatr. 2014;14:120–7. https://doi.org/10.1016/j.acap.2013.11.007.
24. Sharma N, O'Hare K, O'Connor KG, et al. Care coordination and comprehensive electronic health records are associated with increased transition planning activities. Acad Pediatr. 2017. https://doi.org/10.1016/j.acap.2017.04.005.
25. Sohar E, Gafni J, Pras M, Heller H. Familial Mediterranean fever. A survey of 470 cases and review of the literature. Am J Med. 1967;43:227–53.

26. The Six Core Elements of Health Care Transition. URL: http://www.gottransition.org/resourceGet.cfm?id=206. Accessed 30 Dec 2017.
27. Toplak N, Frenkel J, Ozen S, et al. An international registry on autoinflammatory diseases: the Eurofever experience. Ann Rheum Dis. 2012;71:1177–82. https://doi.org/10.1136/annrheumdis-2011-200549.
28. Tran T-A, Koné-Paut I, Marie I, et al. Muckle-Wells syndrome and male hypofertility: a case series. Semin Arthritis Rheum. 2012;42:327–31. https://doi.org/10.1016/j.semarthrit.2012.03.005.
29. van der Hilst JCH, Bodar EJ, Barron KS, et al. Long-term follow-up, clinical Features, and quality of life in a series of 103 patients with hyperimmunoglobulinemia D syndrome. Medicine. 2008;87:301–10. https://doi.org/10.1097/MD.0b013e318190cfb7.
30. Walker UA, Hoffman HM, Williams R, et al. Brief report: severe inflammation following vaccination against streptococcus pneumoniae in patients with cryopyrin-associated periodic syndromes. Arthritis Rheumatol. 2016;68:516–20. https://doi.org/10.1002/art.39482.
31. Wurster VM, Carlucci JG, Feder HM, Edwards KM. Long-term follow-up of children with periodic fever, aphthous stomatitis, pharyngitis, and cervical adenitis syndrome. J Pediatr. 2011;159:958–64. https://doi.org/10.1016/j.jpeds.2011.06.004.
32. Youngstein T, Hoffmann P, Lane T, et al. International experience of pregnancy outcomes in auto-inflammatory syndromes treated with Interleukin-1 inhibitors. Pediatr Rheumatol. 2015;13:O67.
33. Zemer D, Livneh A, Danon YL, et al. Long-term colchicine treatment in children with familial mediterranean fever. Arthritis Rheum. 1991;34:973–7. https://doi.org/10.1002/art.1780340806.

Additional Resources

American College of Rheumatology Pediatric to Adult Rheumatology Care Transition Toolkit. https://www.rheumatology.org/Practice-Quality/Pediatric-to-Adult-Rheumatology-Care-Transition.

Arthritis Foundation Transition Toolkit. http://www.jiatransition.org.

Autoinflammatory Diseases Transition Tools and Templates. http://autoinflammatorydiseases.org/transition.

BC Children's Hospital ON TRAC, Transitioning Responsibly to Adult Care. http://ontracbc.ca.

George Washington University Directory of Transition Websites. https://www.heath.gwu.edu/directory-of-transition-websites.

Got Transition. http://gottransition.org.

National Collaborative on Workforce and Disability A Young Person's Guide to Health Care Transition. http://www.ncwd-youth.info/sites/default/files/Young-Persons-Guide-to-Health-Care-Transition.pdf.

Transition Readiness Assessment Questionnaire. www.etsu.edu/com/pediatrics/traq/.

University of Washington Adolescent Health Transition Project. http://depts.washington.edu/healthtr.

Chapter 19
Adult-Onset Still's Disease

Petros Efthimiou and Sujani Yadlapati

Introduction

Adult-onset Still's disease (AOSD) is a rare, idiopathic, systemic, autoinflammatory disorder. Patients can present with the "Still's triad", arthritis, evanescent salmon-colored rash, and quotidian or double quotidian fevers, although atypical cases abound. Described as early as 1896 by George Still in children and further characterized in 1971 by Eric Bywaters who an adult onset of symptoms, "Still's disease" has come to define a disease spectrum with systemic juvenile idiopathic arthritis (SJIA) at one end and AOSD at the other, based on age of symptom onset [1]. Clinical manifestations may include hepatosplenomegaly, lymphadenopathy, serositis, and aseptic meningitis. Severe disease complications include endocarditis, myocarditis, and pericarditis, coagulation abnormalities, and, especially, macrophage activation syndrome (MAS). The precise etiology of AOSD remains unclear; however, activation of the innate immunity via an unknown trigger has been described as the key inciting factor. Establishing the diagnosis of AOSD is often difficult due to the protean nature of the disease; the presence of non-specific symptoms, especially in the early phases of the disease; and the absence of characteristic serological diagnostic markers. Importantly, albeit inconsistent, laboratory findings include neutrophil-predominant leukocytosis, negative rheumatoid factor (RF), and antinuclear antibodies (ANA) as well as frequently elevated serum ferritin levels with a low-glycosylated fraction [2].

P. Efthimiou (✉)
New York University School of Medicine, New York, NY, USA

NYU/Langone Health, New York, NY, USA
e-mail: petros.efthimiou@nyumc.org

S. Yadlapati
Department of Internal Medicine, Albert Einstein Medical Center, Philadelphia, PA, USA

P. Efthimiou (ed.), *Auto-Inflammatory Syndromes*,
https://doi.org/10.1007/978-3-319-96929-9_19

AOSD remains a diagnosis of exclusion, since more common illnesses can present with very similar symptoms. Definitive diagnosis should only be made after ruling out infectious, malignant, and other autoimmune and autoinflammatory diseases. Yamaguchi criteria are often used to aid in diagnosis and, especially, classification [3, 4]. Patients frequently have a favorable prognosis with timely diagnosis, unless life-threatening complications such as macrophage activation syndrome (MAS) ensue.

Epidemiology

Prevalence of AOSD is estimated to be less than one case per 100,000 people. AOSD is rare, and hence there are currently no consensus on its incidence and prevalence in different populations. Based on larger reviews from the 1980s, it appears that AOSD occurs worldwide and may affect slightly more women than men. This disease characteristically affects younger people between the age of 16 and 35 years of age [5, 6]. A bimodal peak at ages 15–25 and 36–46 without a sex bias has been described in a retrospective study of 62 patients from western France [7]. However, an epidemiological survey from Japan described that 67% of the cases presented after the age of 35, the majority (65–70%) being women [8]. AOSD affects all ages, and stress has been suggested as an important risk factor for all ages [9]. No familial trend has been reported in the recent literature; however, an association with certain HLA alleles has been observed in certain populations. These HLA subtypes include HLA DR4, B17, B18, B35, DR2, DR5, and DQ1.

Etiopathogenesis

Pathophysiology of AOSD was largely obscure until the recent past. A myriad of factors such as genetics, infectious (bacterial and viral) agents, and environmental factors have been thought to play a causative role. Concurrent elevations of serologic markers of infectious agents have been noted in some patients with Still's disease. These infectious triggers include EBV; parvovirus B19; CMV; HHV; HIV; Coxsackievirus; mumps; rubella; echovirus; hepatitis A, B, and C viruses; *Campylobacter jejuni*; *Chlamydia pneumoniae*; adenovirus; influenza virus; parainfluenza virus; and *Mycoplasma* [5, 10]. However, to date definite insight in to precise role of infection in AOSD is lacking.

Several associations with distinct HLA alleles and AOSD have been described thus far. Pouchot et al. described a strong association between HLA-B17, B18, B35, and DR2 and AOSD [11]. In a small study of 25 AOSD patients, HLA-Bw35 was associated with disease susceptibility conferring a favorable prognosis [12]. Wouters et al. noted an increased frequency of the HLA-DR4 allele in 29 patients with AOSD compared to normal controls, with the presence of HLA-DRw6 being linked to root joint involvement [13]. An association between a chronic articular form of AOSD and HLA-DRB1*1501 (DR2), DRB1*1201 (DR5), and DQB1*0602 (DQ1) was previously reported, while HLA-DQB1*0602 (DQ1) have been also associated with the systemic form of the disease in Japanese population [14]. Statistics from a Korean report supported an association between HLA-DRB1*12 and DRB1*15 and AOSD, while HLA-DRB1*04 seemed to be protective. Conversely, HLA-DRB1*14 alleles were more frequently present in patients with the monocyclic systemic type of AOSD [15].

Hallmark of AOSD involves neutrophil and macrophage activation triggered by the pro-inflammatory cytokine IL-18. Neutrophil (PMN) CD64, a marker of neutrophil activation, has been found to be upregulated in patients with active AOSD. Calprotectin (calcium-binding protein) secreted by neutrophils and macrophages and macrophage migration inhibitory factor (MIF) have been found to be useful markers of disease activity [13]. Intercellular adhesion molecule (ICAM-1) upregulated by IL-18 has been implicated as a useful clinical marker whose expression typically reflects the level of disease activity. Macrophage colony-stimulating factor, a cytokine which orchestrates proliferation and differentiation of macrophages, also appears to play a role in AOSD.

More recently, regulation of cytokine production has been noted in patients with AOSD. A predominance of Th1 subset of cytokines has been seen in peripheral blood and tissues of active untreated AOSD patients. Th1 immune cascade is characterized by elevated secretion of interferon γ (IFNγ), interleukin-2 (IL-2), and tumor necrosis factor α (TNFα) cytokines that direct B cells toward IgG2a production, activate macrophages and natural killer (NK) cells, and promote cell-mediated immunity [10]. When compared with controls, serum levels of IL6, TNFα, and IFNγ were significantly increased in 12 patients with active AOSD [16] . IL18 is a pro-inflammatory cytokine that is overproduced in the acute phase of AOSD and is believed to be the cytokine initiating the inflammatory cascade that includes IFNγ, IL6, and TNFα [17]. Genetic polymorphisms of the human IL18 gene have been described to confer disease susceptibility in a Japanese study [18]. Conversely, in another Japanese study, serum levels of soluble IL2 receptors, IL4, and IL18 correlated with chronic articular AOSD activity, whereas IFNγ and IL8 levels were found to be persistently raised, even in disease remission.

Understanding of the Still's disease was also enhanced by the description of autoinflammatory syndromes. These disorders are associated with recurrent bouts of inflammation without an instigating antigenic stimulus. Defective interleukin-1 processing, regulation of nuclear factor-B transcription factor, and possible uncharacteristic apoptosis are all anticipated mechanisms that may possibly play a role in the generation and perseverance of an inflammatory cascade. Patients with autoinflammatory syndromes, in particular, the typical hereditary periodic fever syndromes, may share certain genetic traits; MEFV gene mutation associated with familial Mediterranean fever (FMF) and IL-1 hypersecretion was seen with augmented frequency in Turkish children with SJIA. Mutation of perforin and the MUNC13–4 genes have been seen in patients with macrophage activation syndrome (MAS), a known severe, life-threatening complication of AOSD [3]. Mutations in genes encoding the tumor necrosis factor (TNF) receptor and pyrin superfamilies of molecules may result in the endurance of leukocytes that would customarily go through apoptosis [3]. As a result, relatively minor pro-inflammatory triggers may lead to an exaggerated and potentially harmful, inflammatory response.

IL-1b, the pivotal cytokine in AOSD and other autoinflammatory syndromes, activates the thermoregulatory center, resulting in fever; may activate IL-1 receptors on the endothelium, resulting in rash; and can also act on the bone marrow to increase mobilization of granulocyte progenitors and mature neutrophils, resulting in peripheral neutrophilia. IL-1 also causes an increase in platelet production, which results in thrombocytosis, and decreases the response to erythropoietin, causing anemia. IL-1 induces the production of IL-6. Circulating IL-6 stimulates the hepatocytes to synthesize several acute-phase proteins, such as CRP, ferritin, and D-dimer.

Clinical Features

In general, three types of AOSD have been described. The monocyclic pattern, which is the most benign form, is characterized by a single episode of AOSD without recurrence. In the polycyclic pattern, the patient experiences recurrent attacks, although the subsequent AOSD attacks often seem not as severe as the first one. In both the monocyclic and the polycyclic forms, systemic symptoms (rash, fever) are very prominent. The worst prognosis is carried by the chronic articular form, which is thought to be an unfortunate evolution of the polycyclic form. Often, the systemic symptoms are absent or so remotely in the past that the patient may not even remember them and the main morbidity is from a chronic articular polyarthritis that mimics RA.

Common findings of AOSD are fever, arthralgia, rash, and sore throat. Other accompanying symptoms include, but are not limited to, myalgia, pharyngitis, lymphadenopathy, splenomegaly, and serositis. Fever is usually quotidian and often precedes other manifestations. Temperature spikes of >39°C frequently occur and are associated with chills and rigors, joint pain, or rash. AOSD is one of the main causes of pyrexia of unknown origin (PUO). Temperature fluctuations can be dramatic. Fever may persist between spikes in approximately 20% of cases, and complete defervescence is not always a characteristic of the quotidian fevers [11]. High-grade temperatures, more than 39.5° C, can be associated more strongly with monophasic pattern of AOSD [19].

Skin rash associated with AOSD is a salmon-pink colored, maculopapular eruption that tends to accompany or, more frequently, be exacerbated by fever. Rash usually presents centrally at the trunk and the adjacent extremities (arms/thighs). Histopathology of the rash often reveals non-specific findings including dermal edema and mild perivascular inflammation in the superficial dermis with lymphocytes and histiocytes. Complement deposits (C3) have been described with immunofluorescence. Arthralgias and myalgias are common manifestations of AOSD. Most commonly involved joints include the wrists, ankles, knees, elbows, proximal interphalangeal joints, and shoulders. These manifestations can evolve into more severe and potentially destructive polyarthritis that can mimic other systemic inflammatory arthritides, such as rheumatoid arthritis [20]. Myalgia can be debilitating and often associated with fever spikes. The muscle involvement, when severe, may be accompanied by an elevation of serum creatinine kinase and aldolase concentrations. However, muscle biopsy and electromyographic (EMG) studies are typically normal. Sterile pharyngitis manifesting as throat pain can occasionally precede the development of fever or rash by weeks, or even months, as a prodromal symptom and can often reoccur with disease relapses.

Hepatomegaly and modest elevation of serum hepatic aminotransferases and alkaline phosphatase are not uncommon in patients with AOSD. Several cases of fulminant liver failure in association with AOSD have been described and may be associated with overexpression of IL-18 [11]. Myocarditis, pericarditis, and pleural effusions have also been observed in AOSD patients, and they seem to respond to anti-inflammatory treatment. Uncommonly, some patients may develop severe interstitial lung disease and some progress to acute respiratory distress syndrome (ARDS). Enlarged, symmetrical, cervical nodes are seen in about one half of patients with AOSD. Lymphadenopathy is often accompanied by fever, leukocytosis creating diagnostic confusion with lymphoma. Lymph node biopsy typically shows intense, paracortical immunoblastic hyperplasia [21]. Splenomegaly is also seen in up to one third of patients.

Macrophage activation syndrome (MAS) or reactive hemophagocytic syndrome (RHS) is a life-threatening complication of AOSD. Mortality rate ranges between 10% and 22% [22–25], and an incidence of 12–14% has been noted in two recent series, a rate higher than other rheumatic diseases [26, 27]. It is categorized by an uncontrollable activation of the reticuloendothelial system within the bone marrow, reticuloendothelial system, and central nervous system, with successive phagocytosis of hematopoietic cells by tissue macrophages (histiocytes) [25, 28]. Patients developing MAS present with acute high fever, lymphadenopathy, and hepatosplenomegaly. Laboratory findings include pancytopenia, elevated ferritin levels, triglycerides, and liver enzymes, often accompanied by normal erythrocyte sedimentation rate (ESR). The most commonly implicated triggers include infections, medications, and disease flares [29–31]. Patients with MAS have a decreased ability to eliminate antigen stimulation, thereby inducing T cell activation and proliferation resulting in cytokine secretion (interferon-gamma and granulocyte macrophage colony-stimulating factor) and macrophage hyperactivation. The end result is an uncontrollable increase in cytokines, specifically TNFα, interleukin-1, and interleukin-6 production resulting in severe systemic inflammatory reaction, i.e., "cytokine storm" [25]. There is also a suggestion that certain therapeutic agents, such as nonsteroidal anti-inflammatory drugs, methotrexate, sulfasalazine, penicillamine, and lately TNF-α, IL-1, and IL-6 inhibitors may be capable of provoking MAS, often complicating their therapeutic use [27]. In theory, these therapies may create a state of immunodeficiency resulting in the reactivation of latent viruses (Epstein-Barr virus or *Cytomegalovirus*) which in turn can stimulate MAS. The counter-argument would be that anti-inflammatory medications may not be able to prevent the development of MAS, at least in the dosages used in AOSD or SJIA.

Early suspicion of MAS is most commonly raised by the detection of subtle laboratory changes, whereas clinical symptoms may be delayed. A recent international effort to identify candidate markers using an expert consensus process identified nine criteria that included a falling platelet count, hyperferritinemia, evidence of macrophage hemophagocytosis in the bone marrow, increased liver enzymes, falling leukocyte count, a persistent continuous fever ≥38 °C, a falling erythrocyte sedimentation rate (ESR), hypofibrinogenemia, and hypertriglyceridemia [32]. Hemophagocytosis, seen in bone marrow aspiration and biopsy, establishes the diagnosis, even though hemophagocytosis could be seen more frequently in biopsies from the liver, spleen, and/or lymph nodes. Bone marrow aspiration is considered the gold standard and is usually required in atypical cases, causing a diagnostic dilemma. There is significant overlap between AOSD and MAS, and these two conditions are often thought to be anchoring the same disease spectrum, with AOSD representing the milder form.

Laboratory and Radiographic Findings

AOSD, unlike other systemic rheumatic diseases driven by adaptive immunity, is not typically associated with rheumatoid factor (RF) or antinuclear antibody (ANA) positivity, although several cases have been published with low-level positivity of these autoantibodies. This has been considered in various sets of classification criteria. Elevated ESR is a common finding in most patients [11, 33]. C-reactive protein (CRP) may also be found to be raised. Other laboratory abnormalities include leukocytosis, thrombocytosis, and anemia which often accompany increased disease activity. Pancytopenia is often an alarming sign of coexisting or developing MAS and necessitates prompt intervention. Abnormal coagulation testing can rarely be seen and, in extreme cases, may develop into full-blown disseminated intravascular coagulation (DIC) which can be fatal [11]. Abnormal liver and biliary function tests (increase in lactic dehydrogenase, aspartate aminotransferase, alanine aminotransferase, γ-glutamyl transferase, and bilirubin) can also be seen in up to 75% of patients and often accompany fever and exacerbation of arthritis. Mild periportal inflammation with monocyte infiltration may be seen on liver biopsy.

Serum ferritin has gained attention as both a diagnostic test for AOSD and a marker of disease activity (biomarker). In AOSD, ferritin is an acute phase reactant involved in inflammation, is linked to initiation of histiocyte-macrophage system and/or augmented release from damaged hepatocytes, and is not related to iron metabolism and storage. Ferritin production is driven by cytokines such as IL1β, IL18, TNFα, and IL6 [2]. Serum ferritin levels as high as 1000 ng/ml, five times the upper limits of normal, have been described in these patients. Levels ranging from 4000 ng/ml to 30,000 ng/ml are not uncommon. Fautrel et al. evaluated the validity of hyperferritinemia as a diagnostic tool in a retrospective analysis looking at 49 patients with Still's disease [2]. A fivefold increase in serum ferritin had 80% sensitivity and 41% specificity. Similar results were seen in a Japanese study[57] with 82% sensitivity and 46% specificity [4]. Serum ferritin levels are seen in other diseases such as hemochromatosis, Gaucher's disease, infections (sepsis, HIV), and malignancies (leukemia, lymphomas). Serum ferritin levels correlate with disease activity and often normalize when the disease flare subsides. However, the absence of elevated serum ferritin does not exclude active AOSD. Some patients with active AOSD do not have elevated serum ferritin levels at all, or the rise of serum ferritin may lag behind the symptom presentation.

Glycosylated fraction is a more specific diagnostic marker than ferritin, albeit not commercially available in the USA. In healthy subjects, 50–80% of ferritin is glycosylated. Saturation of glycosylation mechanisms results in a drop in glycosylated fraction to drop to 20–50%. This phenomenon is particularly prevalent in AOSD. Glycosylated ferritin often remains elevated for months after the disease goes into remission and hence cannot be used to monitor disease activity or response to treatment. Improved diagnostic tests are clearly desirable, and new immunological tests, such as IL18, may prove useful in the near future for diagnosis as well as monitoring disease activity and response to treatment [17]. Currently available tests: complete blood count and differential, ESR, CRP, ANA, and RF (both negative), liver function tests (LFTs) and albumin, ferritin, and glycosylated ferritin (if available) are of practical use to most clinicians.

Radiographs are often of limited significance in the early phase of the disease. Images are either normal or show soft tissue swelling, joint effusion, or mild periarticular demineralization. Bone scan and gadolinium-enhanced magnetic resonance imaging were assessed in small series and may prove to be more sensitive imaging modalities for early diagnosis and successful treatment in follow-up. In one study, distinctive pattern of intercarpal and carpometacarpal joint space narrowing was seen in 41% of the subjects (bilateral in 69%) that led to pericapitate ankylosis in 25% of the cases [11]. Other investigators have also reported a tendency for distal interphalangeal, intertarsal, and cervical zygapophyseal ankylosis. Patients who have the chronic articular disease pattern can present with joint erosions making the differential diagnosis from RA problematic, especially in the absence of systemic signs and symptoms.

Diagnosis

The differential diagnosis of AOSD is extensive, especially at presentation, when the systemic symptoms predominate. Conditions such as infections, neoplasms, and autoimmune disorders should be ruled out before the diagnosis of AOSD can be confidently made. Viral syndromes (e.g., rubella, cytomegalovirus, Epstein-Barr virus, mumps, Coxsackievirus, adenovirus) can be excluded if the symptoms persist for more than 3 months and serologies are negative. Neoplastic disorders that can mimic AOSD include leukemia and lymphoma, such as angioimmunoblastic lymphoma. However, the clinical presentation can differ substantially, with atypical rashes and/or isolated lymph node enlargement. At times bone marrow and/or lymph node biopsy may be needed to differentiate these entities. Common mimickers of AOSD include reactive arthritis and the other spondyloarthropathies, hemophagocytic syndrome, dermatomyositis, Kikuchi's syndrome, Sweet's syndrome, granulomatous disorders, and the vasculitides. Other differentials of AOSD are the periodic fever syndromes and, in particular, familial Mediterranean fever, hyper IgD syndrome (HIDS), and TNF receptor-associated periodic syndrome (TRAPS). Patients with familial Mediterranean fever often present with acute, self-limited episodes of fever accompanied by signs of peritonitis, pleuritis, synovitis, and erysipelas-like erythema. The disease commonly starts in childhood or early adolescence. A significant family history, clinical presentation, and response to colchicine can aid in making the correct diagnosis. This can be verified, in many cases, with genetic analysis for the *MEFV* gene. TRAPS and HIDS commonly start in childhood and also have strong familial distributions. However, adult-onset cases of those rare syndromes do exist, and the genetic tests that are commercially available can be helpful in excluding them, especially when atypical presentations are present.

Several classification criteria have been developed from retrospective data available on AOSD. One such study attempted to validate these classification criteria: Yamaguchi's criteria were found to be the most sensitive (93.5%), followed by Cush's (80.6%) and Calabro's (80.6%) criteria (Table 19.1) [4, 34]. Of late, a French group has proposed a new set of criteria which takes into consideration the two new disease markers: serum ferritin and its glycosylated fraction (Table 19.2). This set provided a sensitivity of 80.6% and a specificity of 98.5%, which remains to be authenticated in a different population before becoming widely accepted [35].

Table 19.1 *Yamaguchi criteria require the presence of five features, with at least two being major diagnostic criteria [4]

Major Yamaguchi criteria
Fever of at least 39 degrees C (102.2 F) last at least 1 week
Arthralgias or arthritis lasting 2 weeks or longer
A non-pruritic macular or maculopapular skin rash that is salmon-colored in appearance and usually found over the trunk or extremities during febrile episodes
Leukocytosis (10,000/microL or greater), with at least 80% granulocytes
Minor Yamaguchi criteria
Sore throat
Lymphadenopathy
Hepatomegaly or splenomegaly
Abnormal liver function studies, particularly elevations in aspartate and alanine aminotransferase and lactate dehydrogenase concentrations
Negative tests for antinuclear antibody (ANA) and rheumatoid factor (RF)

*Several classification criteria have been developed from retrospective data available on AOSD. One such study attempted to validate these classification criteria: Yamaguchi's criteria were found to be the most sensitive (93.5%)

Table 19.2 *Fautrel criteria for diagnosis of AOSD require four or more major criteria or three major and two minor criteria [35]

Fautrel criteria for diagnosis of AOSD
Major criteria
Spiking fever ≥39 °C
Arthralgia
Transient erythema
Pharyngitis
Polymorphonuclear cells ≥80%
Glycosylated ferritin ≤20%
Minor criteria
Maculopapular rash
Leukocytosis ≥10,000/mm3

*Fautrel's criteria has also been proved to be sensitive

Treatment

Therapeutic goals include controlling physical signs and symptoms of inflammation, which is typically associated with the improvement in laboratory parameters. Decisions about optimal therapy are influenced by the severity and chronicity of the disease and involve taking into consideration the adverse effect profile of the treatments, both long and short term, and the clinical response to initial therapies. The primary goal of therapy not only involves achieving control of acute symptoms but also preventing end-organ damage, including joint injury and major organ complications. The initial choice of therapy depends upon disease severity and extent of organ involvement. There has been a lack of head-to-head randomized controlled trials comparing different therapeutic modalities given the rarity of disease. Treatment options constantly keep evolving as more insight is gained into the pathogenesis of AOSD. Support for the use of biologics as first-line therapy in severe disease is based upon the published experience in AOSD and, especially, more extensive evidence supporting use of these agents in children with SJIA, since recent evidence supports that SJIA and AOSD are different chronological disease onsets of the same "Still's disease."

Mild-to-Moderate Disease

Patients with mild-to-moderate disease may present with fevers and rash, as well as with arthralgias or mild arthritis.

NSAIDs

While NSAIDs, such as naproxen or ibuprofen, were the first medications to be used in AOSD, their role today is a very limited one. Their use can be justified either as adjunct treatment or as monotherapy in mild, monocyclic cases for symptomatic relief. In addition to adverse effects that are commonly associated with NSAIDs, an association between the use of NSAIDs and macrophage activation syndrome (MAS) has been described, as well [11]. Patients responsive to NSAIDs alone, who remain asymptomatic for at least a month, could have NSAID doses gradually reduced.

Glucocorticoids

Glucocorticoids can be started immediately, as first-line treatment, or when NSAIDs are insufficient to control signs and symptoms of the disease. Glucocorticoid dose can be gradually tapered once disease activity is controlled. Oral prednisone is typically initiated at a dose of 0.5-1 mg/kg per day, depending on the severity of disease. Intravenous, high-dose steroids are reserved for those with refractory disease [2]. Approximately 70% of patients respond to glucocorticoids alone or to glucocorticoids used after a trial of NSAIDs [36]. In addition to systemic steroids, those with one or two inflamed joints despite systemic therapy may benefit from intraarticular glucocorticoid injections.

DMARDs

Disease-modifying antirheumatic drugs (DMARDs) are typically used in the event of inadequate response to corticosteroids or as steroid-sparing medications. Methotrexate remains the first-line steroid-sparing agent in AOSD and is also a useful agent to treat Still's arthritis. Methotrexate can result in complete remission in up to 70% of patients and is effective in corticosteroid weaning [37]. Sulfasalazine is contraindicated because of lack of efficacy and association with MAS development.

Moderate-to-Severe Disease

Internal organ damage and debilitating joint symptoms with radiographic are characteristic of moderate-to-severe disease. Severe disease is defined as refractory disease, especially when terminal organ and/or life-threatening involvement exists, such as MAS, severe hepatic injury, cardiac involvement with/or without tamponade, or disseminated intravascular coagulation (DIC). Biologic therapies such as IL-1 inhibitors (anakinra, canakinumab) and IL-6 receptor antagonists (tocilizumab) are used as first line or second line for SJIA often without any prior use of corticosteroids or traditional DMARDs and that practice may be justified in moderate-to-severe AOSD as well. Small series have reported some efficacy of IVIG when used early in the course of AOSD [38, 39].

IL-1 Inhibitors

Target biologic agents have been historically reserved for refractory AOSD (Fig. 19.1) [40]. These agents include a recombinant antagonist of the IL-1 receptor (IL-1Ra, anakinra), a human monoclonal antibody directed against IL-1β (canakinumab), and a soluble IL-1 trap fusion protein (rilonacept).

Anakinra is particularly efficient in the rapid relief of the systemic symptoms. Several retrospective case series and one open-labeled prospective randomized trial have evaluated the use of anakinra in AOSD patients [41, 42]. Anakinra is approved as a daily subcutaneous injection (100 mg) in RA. In AOSD, higher dose may be necessary, since anakinra has a very short half-life (4–6 h). While anakinra does not work in all AOSD cases, for the ones it does work, its onset of action is very rapid. In many cases, resolutions of systemic symptoms and normalization of inflammatory markers were reported within 2 weeks of anakinra use, allowing for rapid tapering of corticosteroids, if they were ever used in the first place. However, relapses are not uncommon with the cessation of these agents. In certain patients, gradual reduction in dose has enabled the weaning of anakinra. Daily anakinra injections are often complicated by frequent injection site reactions. If response to anakinra is incomplete or tolerability issues ensue, rilonacept and/or canakinumab can be considered. They have longer half-lives and can be administered at greater intervals, once or twice weekly for rilonacept and every 4–8 weeks for canakinumab, respectively. Additional supplemental data is available in the setting of SJIA. Swart and associates reviewed data pertaining to 140 children with SJIA treated with anakinra [43]. Systemic symptoms resolved in 98% of the patients, and fatigue and well-being improved in 93% of cases. Arthritis improved in 66% of the cases in time. Absolute disease remission was mostly detected in patients with systemic symptoms, less arthritis, and a shorter duration of disease. Similar findings were corroborated in a large, multicenter, randomized, placebo controlled trial by Quartier et al. [44]. Sample population included 24 patients with a systemic-onset JIA for duration of more than 6 months and steroid dependency. In 1 month, anakinra was effective in 8 out of 12 patients (versus one in the placebo group) who

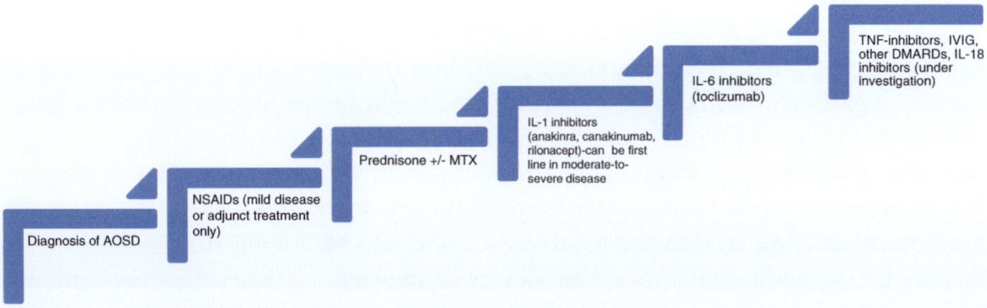

Fig. 19.1 Proposed step-up therapeutic strategies for AOSD

reached the modified American College of Rheumatology (ACR) Pediatric 30 score. After 2 months, majority of patients (9/10) who had been switched to anakinra were also responders. Nigrovic and associates studied 46 patients who received anakinra as first-line treatment. Rapid resolution of systemic symptoms was observed in about 95% of cases, along with a supplementary preventive effect on refractory arthritis in almost 90% of the patients. Based on these results, it was postulated that there could be a benefit for IL-1 blockade therapy in initial phase of the disease (i.e., within 6 months after onset) [45]. These findings were also further reinforced by Vaster et al. in 2014 [46]. In a prospective series of 20 patients who received anakinra as first-line therapy, 85% of the patients showed an American College of Rheumatology Pediatric 90 score response or had inactive disease within 3 months. Overall, 75% of the patients treated with anakinra achieved remission. These results clearly indicate that IL-1 blockade has an early place in the treatment strategy.

IL-6 Inhibitors

Tocilizumab, humanized monoclonal antibody directed against IL-6 receptor, is used in refractory AOSD. This agent has been studied with randomized placebo-controlled trials in SJIA patients but not yet in AOSD. Effects of tocilizumab have been described to persist for ≥6 months after its discontinuation. Tocilizumab appears to have a marked corticosteroid-sparing effect and has a good safety and tolerance profile [47]. Most of the early data was with tocilizumab administered intravenously (IV) at a dosage of 5–8 mg/kg body weight every 2–4 weeks. Nevertheless, larger randomized studies are still needed to further determine the optimal therapeutic scheme for tocilizumab, i.e., optimal dosing, interval, and duration of treatment for both the intravenous but also the subcutaneous route of administration.

TNF-Inhibitors

Although those agents were the first biologics to be used in refractory AOSD, these agents are no longer recommended as first-line treatment in AOSD. Anti-TNF-α agents, in particular infliximab, etanercept, and adalimumab, have been used to treat refractory AOSD, but data on adalimumab are limited to a few cases [48]. Although complete resolution of symptoms has been observed, efficacy of the TNF-inhibitors has been mostly limited to Still's arthritis. Efficacy was better with the monoclonal antibodies, as compared to the soluble receptor, and switching from one agent to another had no additional effect [19]. Moreover, in one published series, two patients who were started on etanercept and adalimumab developed MAS that could be allied with the initiation of therapy [49, 50]. Overall, TNF-α blockers should be considered for the treatment of chronic polyarticular disease, after the use of IL-1 and/or IL-6 inhibitors.

NSAIDs, Corticosteroids, and Traditional DMARDs

Non-refractory disease comprises of monocyclic and polycyclic AOSD. NSAIDs can be used in monocyclic course of AOSD without major systemic or articular involvement. Preferred NSAID is high-dose indomethacin (150–200 mg/day). Corticosteroids should be started promptly once the diagnosis is confirmed. Usually, corticosteroid therapy starts at a dosage of 0.5–1 mg/kg/day. Pulse dose methylprednisolone is used if there is severe visceral involvement or there is suspicion of MAS complicating the clinical presentation. Higher dosages seem to be more efficient in controlling the disease and lessening the number of relapses. Tapering of corticosteroids can start after 4–6 weeks, when symptoms have resolved, and biological parameters have returned to baseline. Methotrexate (MTX) could be considered early for its steroid-sparing effect. Typically, methotrexate (7.5–20 mg/week) enables complete remission of the disease (70%) and limits frequent corticosteroid use. Blood count and renal and hepatic function should be monitored before initiation of methotrexate and then at monthly intervals. Alternative DMARDs may be use in the event of methotrexate failure; however, more recent literature suggests better results with targeted biologic treatment.

Treatments Under Development

IL-18 Inhibition/Tadekinig Alpha

An open-label, multicenter, phase II study of subcutaneous Tadekinig alfa (IL-18BP) in patients with AOSD was recently published and showed promise. Tadekinig alfa is the drug name for recombinant human interleukin-18-binding protein (IL-18BP). This study was based on the principle that high levels of IL-18 were noted during active flares of AOSD. Ten patients were assigned to receive 80 mg tadekinig alfa, and 13 patients received the 160 mg dose. At week 3, 5 of 10 patients receiving 80 mg and 6 of 12 patients receiving 160 mg achieved the predefined response criteria. The agent was overall well tolerated with the exception of one case of optic neuropathy [51].

Summary

It is becoming exceedingly evident that AOSD patients fall into two distinct subsets, i.e., those presenting with systemic manifestations and those presenting with prominent articular manifestations. In addition, these findings are also reinforced by molecular evidence, cytokine profiles, clinical course, and response to therapy. Predictors for a prominent articular pattern include female sex, proximal arthritis at disease onset, thrombocytosis, and corticosteroid dependency, whereas high fever, transaminitis, or elevated acute phase reactants are more likely to be connected with a systemic pattern of AOSD [14, 52]. Alternative evidence to identify the systemic subtype of AOSD are the following: thrombocytopenia, RHL, and hyperferritinemia. IL-18, interferon-γ, IL-10, and IL-4 are typically associated with systemic AOSD, whereas IL-6, IL-17, and IL-23 are associated with arthritic AOSD [53]. This dichotomy aids in management as patients fall into one of the two categories and should benefit from different therapies.

Patients with systemic symptom predominant AOSD often benefit from systemic corticosteroid therapy. From traditional DMARDs, methotrexate has been studied the most and may continue to have a role as steroid-sparing and in the treatment of chronic articular disease. IL-1 antagonists should be considered first line in severe or refractory AOSD, either alone or in initial combination with systemic corticosteroids when necessary. Regularly reported side effects with anakinra include injection site reactions. Longer acting IL-1 inhibitors (rilonacept or canakinumab) may play a role in refractory disease or when tolerability issues exist with anakinra. Tocilizumab, the IL-6 receptor antagonist, has shown efficacy in both systemic and articular disease predominant AOSD, even in cases where IL-1 inhibition has been unsuccessful. In contrast to IL-1 and IL-6 inhibitors, anti-TNF-α agents typically have less sustained effect on systemic symptoms, but they may have a limited role for the chronic inflammatory polyarthritis.

In an effort to standardize therapeutic management and evaluate comparative efficacy in an observational setting, the Childhood Arthritis and Rheumatology Research Alliance has developed four consensus treatment plans for SJIA [54]. This includes glucocorticoid plan, a methotrexate plan, an anakinra plan, and a tocilizumab plan. Since no guidelines are available yet in AOSD, this consensus may act as a rough guide for its treatment, as it coincides with the published clinical experience. New therapeutic agents are being developed for AOSD, and future randomized, controlled trials will fill the knowledge gap that currently exists.

References

1. Still GF. On a form of chronic joint disease in children. Med Chir Trans. 1897;80:47–60. 9.
2. Fautrel B. Adult-onset Still disease. Best Pract Res Clin Rheumatol. 2008;22(5):773–92.
3. Efthimiou P, et al. Adult onset Still's disease and autoinflammation. Int J Inflam. 2012;2012:964751.
4. Yamaguchi M, et al. Preliminary criteria for classification of adult Still's disease. J Rheumatol. 1992;19(3):424–30.
5. van de Putte LB, Wouters JM. Adult-onset Still's disease. Baillieres Clin Rheumatol. 1991;5(2):263–75.
6. Ohta A, et al. Adult Still's disease: review of 228 cases from the literature. J Rheumatol. 1987;14(6):1139–46.
7. Magadur-Joly G, et al. Epidemiology of adult Still's disease: estimate of the incidence by a retrospective study in west France. Ann Rheum Dis. 1995;54(7):587–90.
8. Wakai K, et al. Estimated prevalence and incidence of adult Still's disease: findings by a nationwide epidemiological survey in Japan. J Epidemiol. 1997;7(4):221–5.
9. Sampalis JS, et al. Risk factors for adult Still's disease. J Rheumatol. 1996;23(12):2049–54.

10. Efthimiou P, Paik PK, Bielory L. Diagnosis and management of adult onset Still's disease. Ann Rheum Dis. 2006;65(5):564–72.
11. Pouchot J, et al. Adult Still's disease: manifestations, disease course, and outcome in 62 patients. Medicine (Baltimore). 1991;70(2):118–36.
12. Terkeltaub R, et al. HLA—Bw35 and prognosis in adult Still's disease. Arthritis Rheum. 1981;24(12):1469–72.
13. Wouters JMGW, Reekers P, van de Putte LBA. Adult-onset still's disease. Disease course and HLA associations. Arthritis Rheum. 1986;29(3):415–8.
14. Fujii T, et al. Cytokine and immunogenetic profiles in Japanese patients with adult Still's disease. Association with chronic articular disease. Rheumatology (Oxford). 2001;40(12):1398–404.
15. Joung CI, et al. Association between the HLA-DRB1 gene and clinical features of systemic sclerosis in Korea. Scand J Rheumatol. 2006;35(1):39–43.
16. Hoshino T, et al. Elevated serum interleukin 6, interferon-gamma, and tumor necrosis factor-alpha levels in patients with adult Still's disease. J Rheumatol. 1998;25(2):396–8.
17. Kawashima M, et al. Levels of interleukin-18 and its binding inhibitors in the blood circulation of patients with adult-onset Still's disease. Arthritis Rheum. 2001;44(3):550–60.
18. Sugiura T, et al. Association between adult-onset Still's disease and interleukin-18 gene polymorphisms. Genes Immun. 2002;3(7):394–9.
19. Gerfaud-Valentin M, et al. Adult-onset still disease: manifestations, treatment, outcome, and prognostic factors in 57 patients. Medicine (Baltimore). 2014;93(2):91–9.
20. Elkon KB, et al. Adult-onset Still's disease. Twenty-year follow up and further studies of patients with active disease. Arthritis Rheum. 1982;25(6):647–54.
21. Valente RM, Banks PM, Conn DL. Characterization of lymph node histology in adult onset Still's disease. J Rheumatol. 1989;16(3):349–54.
22. Silva CA, et al. Macrophage activation syndrome associated with systemic juvenile idiopathic arthritis. J Pediatr (Rio J). 2004;**80**(6):517–22.
23. Ramanan AV, Schneider R. Macrophage activation syndrome following initiation of etanercept in a child with systemic onset juvenile rheumatoid arthritis. J Rheumatol. 2003;30(2):401–3.
24. Sawar H, Espinoza LR, Gedalia A. Macrophage activation syndrome and etanercept in children with systemic juvenile rheumatoid arthritis. J Rheumatol. 2004;31(3):623. author reply 623-4.
25. Tristano AG. Macrophage activation syndrome: a frequent but under-diagnosed complication associated with rheumatic diseases. Med Sci Monit. 2008;14(3):RA27–36.
26. Arlet JB, et al. Reactive haemophagocytic syndrome in adult onset Still's disease: report of 6 patients and review of the literature. Ann Rheum Dis. 2006;65:1596.
27. Singh S, Samant R, Joshi VR. Adult onset Still's disease: a study of 14 cases. Clin Rheumatol. 2008;27(1):35–9.
28. Durand M, et al. Macrophage activation syndrome treated with anakinra. J Rheumatol. 2010;37(4):879–80.
29. Arlet JB, et al. Reactive haemophagocytic syndrome in adult-onset Still's disease: a report of six patients and a review of the literature. Ann Rheum Dis. 2006;65(12):1596–601.
30. Ravelli A, et al. Preliminary diagnostic guidelines for macrophage activation syndrome complicating systemic juvenile idiopathic arthritis. J Pediatr. 2005;146(5):598–604.
31. Sawhney S, Woo P, Murray KJ. Macrophage activation syndrome: a potentially fatal complication of rheumatic disorders. Arch Dis Child. 2001;85(5):421–6.
32. Davi S, et al. An international consensus survey of diagnostic criteria for macrophage activation syndrome in systemic juvenile idiopathic arthritis. J Rheumatol. 2011;38(4):764–8.
33. Wouters JM, van de Putte LB. Adult-onset Still's disease; clinical and laboratory features, treatment and progress of 45 cases. Q J Med. 1986;61(235):1055–65.
34. Cush JJ. Adult-onset Still's disease. Bull Rheum Dis. 2000;49(6):1–4.
35. Fautrel B, et al. Proposal for a new set of classification criteria for adult-onset still disease. Medicine (Baltimore). 2002;81(3):194–200.
36. Franchini S, et al. Efficacy of traditional and biologic agents in different clinical phenotypes of adult-onset Still's disease. Arthritis Rheum. 2010;62(8):2530–5.

37. Fautrel B, et al. Corticosteroid sparing effect of low dose methotrexate treatment in adult Still's disease. J Rheumatol. 1999;26(2):373–8.
38. Vignes S, et al. Intravenous immunoglobulin in adult Still's disease refractory to non-steroidal anti-inflammatory drugs. Clin Exp Rheumatol. 1998;16(3):295–8.
39. Permal S, et al. Treatment of Still disease in adults with intravenous immunoglobulins. Rev Med Interne. 1995;16(4):250–4.
40. Kadavath S, Efthimiou P. Adult-onset Still's disease-pathogenesis, clinical manifestations, and new treatment options. Ann Med. 2015;47(1):6–14.
41. Lequerre T, et al. Interleukin-1 receptor antagonist (anakinra) treatment in patients with systemic-onset juvenile idiopathic arthritis or adult onset Still disease: preliminary experience in France. Ann Rheum Dis. 2008;67(3):302–8.
42. Fitzgerald AA, et al. Rapid responses to anakinra in patients with refractory adult-onset Still's disease. Arthritis Rheum. 2005;52(6):1794–803.
43. Swart JF, et al. The efficacy and safety of interleukin-1-receptor antagonist anakinra in the treatment of systemic juvenile idiopathic arthritis. Expert Opin Biol Ther. 2010;10(12):1743–52.
44. Quartier P, et al. A multicentre, randomised, double-blind, placebo-controlled trial with the interleukin-1 receptor antagonist anakinra in patients with systemic-onset juvenile idiopathic arthritis (ANAJIS trial). Ann Rheum Dis. 2011;70(5):747–54.
45. Nigrovic PA, et al. Anakinra as first-line disease-modifying therapy in systemic juvenile idiopathic arthritis: report of forty-six patients from an international multicenter series. Arthritis Rheum. 2011;63(2):545–55.
46. Vastert SJ, et al. Effectiveness of first-line treatment with recombinant interleukin-1 receptor antagonist in steroid-naive patients with new-onset systemic juvenile idiopathic arthritis: results of a prospective cohort study. Arthritis Rheumatol. 2014;66(4):1034–43.
47. De Benedetti F, et al. Randomized trial of tocilizumab in systemic juvenile idiopathic arthritis. N Engl J Med. 2012;367(25):2385–95.
48. Benucci M, et al. Adalimumab (anti-TNF-alpha) therapy to improve the clinical course of adult-onset Still's disease: the first case report. Clin Exp Rheumatol. 2005;23(5):733.
49. Kaneko K, et al. Exacerbation of adult-onset Still's disease, possibly related to elevation of serum tumor necrosis factor-alpha after etanercept administration. Int J Rheum Dis. 2010;13(4):e67–9.
50. Agarwal S, et al. A rare trigger for macrophage activation syndrome. Rheumatol Int. 2011;31(3):405–7.
51. Gabay C, et al. Open-label, multicentre, dose-escalating phase II clinical trial on the safety and efficacy of tadekinig alfa (IL-18BP) in adult-onset Still's disease. Ann Rheum Dis. 2018;77:840–47.
52. Ichida H, et al. Clinical manifestations of adult-onset Still's disease presenting with erosive arthritis: association with low levels of ferritin and Interleukin-18. Arthritis Care Res (Hoboken). 2014;66(4):642–6.
53. Shimizu M, Nakagishi Y, Yachie A. Distinct subsets of patients with systemic juvenile idiopathic arthritis based on their cytokine profiles. Cytokine. 2013;61(2):345–8.
54. DeWitt EM, et al. Consensus treatment plans for new-onset systemic Juvenile idiopathic arthritis. Arthritis Care Res. 2012;64(7):1001–10.

Chapter 20
Idiopathic Recurrent Acute Pericarditis

Apostolos Kontzias

Definition of Pericarditis

Pericarditis is clinically diagnosed based on symptoms of precordial chest pain worse with inspiration and when supine, pericardial friction rub on exam, electrocardiogram (ECG) changes characterized by ST-segment elevation and PR deviation, and a pericardial effusion by echocardiogram. A diagnosis of pericarditis requires two of these four characteristics, usually chest pain in conjunction with either ECG changes or a pericardial effusion. High inflammatory markers and delayed enhancement on cardiac magnetic resonance imaging (MRI) are adjunct surrogate markers [1].

Pericarditis is classified as *incessant* if symptoms last more than 4–6 weeks and *chronic* if symptoms are present for more than 3 months. Symptom-free intervals of at least 4–6 weeks between flares render pericarditis as *recurrent* [2].

Etiology

The cause of recurrent pericarditis remains elusive in about 80% of the cases, hence called idiopathic recurrent acute pericarditis (IRAP) (Table 20.1). A proportion of idiopathic pericarditis may be attributed to viral infection [3]. However, there is general consensus that in clinical practice, rigorous pursuit of the viral cause is not indicated given that no change in management will be mandated [4]. Laboratory investigation for rheumatologic causes should be pursued only in high suspicion of such cases as often low titers of autoantibodies are non-specific and therefore

A. Kontzias
Division of Rheumatology, Allergy and Immunology, Stony Brook University,
Stony Brook, NY, USA
e-mail: apostolos.kontzias@stonybrookmedicine.edu

P. Efthimiou (ed.), *Auto-Inflammatory Syndromes*,
https://doi.org/10.1007/978-3-319-96929-9_20

Table 20.1 Causes of pericarditis

Infections	Viral: enteroviruses (coxsackieviruses, echoviruses), herpesviruses (EBV, CMV, HHV-6), adenoviruses, parvovirus B19 Bacterial: *Mycobacterium tuberculosis* (esp in the developing world) *Coxiella burnetii, Borrelia burgdorferi, Pneumococcus* spp., *Meningococcus* spp., *Gonococcus* spp., *Streptococcus* spp., *Staphylococcus* spp., *Haemophilus* spp., *Chlamydia* spp., *Mycoplasma* spp., *Legionella* spp. Fungal: *Histoplasma* spp. (endemic areas in immunocompetent patients), *Aspergillus* spp., *Blastomyces* spp., *Candida* spp. (in immunocompromised host)
Autoimmune	Systemic lupus erythematosus Sjögren syndrome Rheumatoid arthritis Scleroderma Vasculitis Inflammatory bowel disease
Autoinflammatory	Familial Mediterranean fever TNF receptor-associated periodic syndrome Cryopyrin-associated periodic syndrome Adamantiades-Behcet's syndrome Systemic-onset juvenile idiopathic arthritis (soJIA) Adult onset Still's disease
Malignancy	Pericardial mesothelioma Lung cancer Breast cancer Lymphoma
Metabolic	Uremia
Injury	Postmyocardial infarction syndrome Post-pericardiotomy syndrome Post-cardiac interventions, i.e., coronary percutaneous intervention, pacemaker lead insertion, and radiofrequency ablation
Medications	Drug-induced lupus related: procainamide, hydralazine, methyldopa, isoniazid, phenytoin Chemotherapy related: doxorubicin and daunorubicin, cyclophosphamide

non-diagnostic [1]. In patients with a rheumatic disease, involvement of other organs is usually apparent before the onset of pericarditis. Autoinflammatory syndromes can be associated with serositis including pericarditis. In a registry of 346 pediatric patients with FMF, pericarditis occurred in approximately 18%, although chest pain was more common (56%) [5]. In TRAPS the estimated prevalence of pericarditis is about 7% [6]. Prevalence of pericarditis in other autoinflammatory syndromes is difficult to estimate due to their rarity.

A positive family history of recurrent pericarditis should prompt further screening given that familial clustering may reveal incomplete TRAPS phenotypes with low-penetrance mutations [7]. A 10% of familial occurrence of pericarditis among the relatives of IRAP patients has been observed [8].

In a cohort of 134 patients with IRAP, 6% were found to have low-penetrance TNFRSF1 polymorphisms. These patients were found to have poor response to colchicine with frequent recurrences along with the need for immunosuppressive agents [9].

TRAPS patients with low-penetrance variants (R92Q, P46L, D12E, V95 M, and R104Q) compared to patients who have clearly pathogenic structural mutations are reported to have increased prevalence of pericarditis, but overall less severe inflammatory attacks and later disease onset present less frequently with a chronic course. Notably, they report a higher episode frequency, but remission in between attacks with normal inflammatory markers is observed [10].

Other secondary causes of pericarditis include trauma; hemorrhage; infections; metabolic, neoplastic, postmyocardial infarction; post-percutaneous coronary intervention and electrophysiology procedures; or post-pericardiotomy. Historical features suggestive of the need for more aggressive diagnostic workup include high fever, residing in countries with high prevalence of tuberculosis, constitutional symptoms such as weight loss and fever, history of malignancy, chest irradiation, and anticoagulation [2].

Risk Factors for Recurrent and Complicated Pericarditis

Acute pericarditis can be complicated by myocardial involvement in about 15% of cases (Table 20.2). Younger age, male sex, fever, arrhythmia, and ST-segment elevation on ECG should raise suspicion for myocarditis [11]. High troponin levels are diagnostically useful as they are normal in isolated pericarditis. Interestingly, myocarditis as a complication of acute pericarditis is not associated with an increased risk of recurrent pericarditis or pericardial tamponade, but it is accompanied by lower systolic function on ECHO. However, the majority of patients tend to fully recover with no cardiac sequelae [11].

IRAP occurs in up to 30% after an acute episode of acute pericarditis [12]. The recurrence rate increases up to 50% after a first episode, particularly, if the patients are treated with steroids [13]. An incomplete response to nonsteroidal anti-inflammatory agents and a persistently elevated high-sensitivity C-reactive protein (CRP) at 1 week after acute pericarditis confer a high risk of recurrence [13]. Early institution of colchicine is associated with decreased recurrence rate [12, 14]. Younger age, female sex, and presence of pericardial effusion do not increase the risk of recurrent pericarditis.

Table 20.2 Risk factors for recurrent pericarditis

Steroid use especially high doses 1 mg/kg/day
No colchicine use
High C-reactive protein
Partial response to nonsteroid anti-inflammatory medications

Constrictive pericarditis requiring pericardiectomy is not a common complication of recurrent pericarditis, and consistent epidemiologic data are lacking [1].

Proposed Pathophysiology of Recurrent Pericarditis

The pathophysiology of IRAP remains poorly understood. It is suggested to result from an interplay between environmental triggers with innate and adaptive immunity in the background of a genetically susceptible host [15].

An increased frequency of HLA-A*02, HLA-Cw07, and HLA-DQB1*0202 alleles and a decreased frequency of the HLA DQB1*0302 are detected in Greek IRAP patients compared to controls suggesting that antigen presentation to T cells may play a role in the disease pathogenesis [16]. An adaptive immunity component is suspected by the presence of antinuclear antibodies (ANA) detected in 43.3% of IRAP patients, compared to 9.8% of healthy controls, in addition to the detection of serum anti-heart and anti-intercalated-disk antibodies in about 67.5% of patients in a single cohort [17]. Nonetheless, the clinical significance of these antibodies remains to be determined.

More recently, innate immunity and its effector mechanisms are at the epicenter of IRAP pathogenesis. IRAP shares similar clinical features with other well-defined autoinflammatory syndromes in that flares are characterized by seemingly unprovoked attacks of pericardial inflammation in the absence of antigen-specific T cells and high titers of autoantibodies.

Pivotal structure to the immunopathology of autoinflammatory syndromes is the inflammasome, an assembled macromolecular intracellular platform serving as an innate immunity sensor [18] (Fig. 20.1). Among all identified inflammasomes, the best characterized inflammasome is NLR family pyrin domain-containing 3 (NALP3) after the discovery that gain of function mutations cause the cryopyrin-associated periodic syndromes (CAPS), a group of autosomal-dominant autoinflammatory diseases. NALP3 is a macromolecular structure composed of a NOD-like receptor (NLR) protein, the adaptor ASC, and caspase 1. NALP3 is activated by a wide array of pathogen and danger-associated molecular patterns leading to caspase-induced cleavage of pro-interleukin 1β to active interleukin 1β. An autoinflammatory phenotype is considered to be skewed toward an IL-1/IL-18 signature as opposed to conditions such as systemic lupus erythematosus (SLE) where type I interferon (IFN) signatures predominate [19]. Interestingly, viruses associated with pericarditis such as adenovirus, influenza A, herpesvirus, and *Cytomegalovirus*, are known to activate NALP3 and other inflammasomes [20–23].

There is a paucity of primary data concerning the implication of pro-inflammatory cytokines in the pathogenesis of pericarditis. The detection of interleukin-6, interleukin-8, and interferon-γ in the pericardial fluid of patients with IRAP supports their contributing role [24]. However, pericardial fluid cytokine levels may not reflect accurately the pathways involved at the pericardial tissue level.

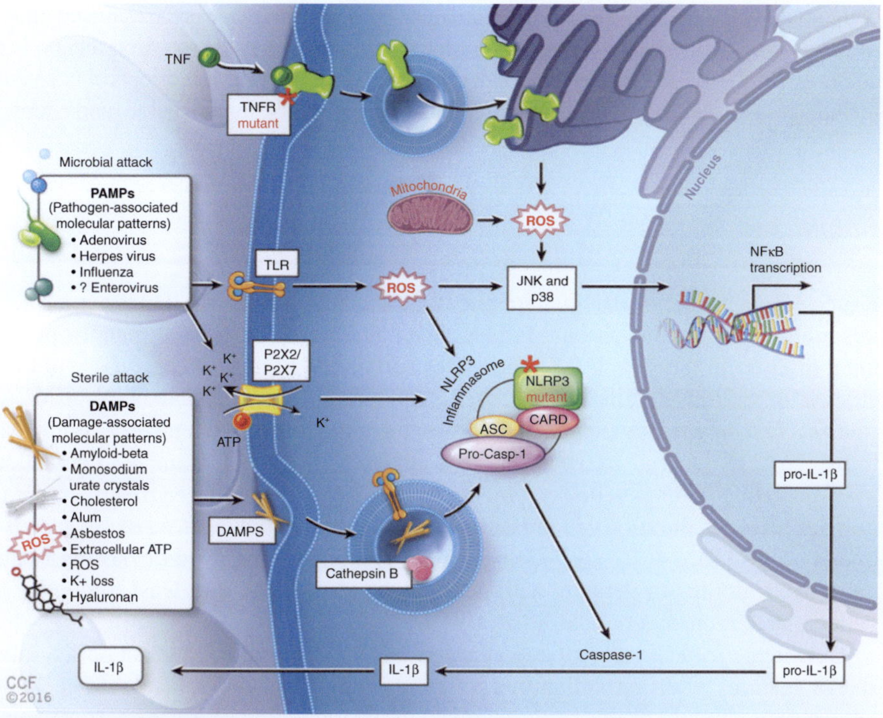

Fig. 20.1 This schematic represents the activation of NLP3 inflammasome which is speculatively implicated in IRAP pathogenesis. Pathogen-associated molecular patterns (PAMPs) and damage-associated molecular patterns (DAMPs) provide the first signal priming the inflammasome to become activated. Danger signals such as reactive oxygen species (ROS), potassium efflux, and ATP constitute a second signal. A wide array of stimuli especially certain viral species is of pathophysiologic relevance to IRAP. Inflammasome activation leads to caspase-induced cleavage of pro-interleukin 1β to interleukin 1β. It remains to be determined if polymorphisms in the genes encoding proteins regulating the inflammasome are associated with its constitutive activation

It remains to be determined whether in IRAP certain polymorphisms in regulatory components of the inflammasome may be conducive of an inflammatory phenotype in the presence of the suitable trigger (viral infection, injury, stress).

Treatment of Acute and Recurrent Pericarditis

Nonsteroid Anti-inflammatory Drugs (NSAIDs)

Acute pericarditis is treated with nonsteroid anti-inflammatory drugs (NSAIDs) based on an early randomized trial of 149 patients with post-pericardiotomy syndrome. Ibuprofen and indomethacin were efficacious compared to placebo alleviating symptoms within 48 h [25]. Ibuprofen 800 mg three times daily or indomethacin 75 mg twice daily until symptoms subside and inflammatory markers normalize is the mainstay treatment of acute pericarditis. Addition of a proton pump inhibitor for gastroprotection is a common practice given the required high dose regimen. Common side effects of NSAIDs include gastritis and peptic ulcer disease, acute kidney injury, hypertension, and edema.

Colchicine

Expectedly a subset of patients are not ideal candidates for NSAIDs if comorbidities are present such as chronic kidney disease, anticoagulation regimen, or peptic ulcer disease. In the search for alternatives and driven by the successful use of colchicine in familial Mediterranean fever (FMF), cardiologists embraced this medication as a first-line treatment based on prospective randomized open-label controlled trials [26, 27]. Overall based on a meta-analysis of eight randomized controlled trials including 1635 patients, colchicine has been proven to shorten treatment duration, increase the duration of remission, and decrease the recurrence risk by approximately 50% [12, 14, 27–29]. Colchicine is prescribed at a dose of 0.6 mg twice daily for 3 months in patients with acute pericarditis and for at least 6 months in patients with recurrent pericarditis [30].

Colchicine's mechanism of action is central to the idea that recurrent pericarditis shares features with autoinflammatory syndromes. This is because colchicine is known to be directly or indirectly involved in the regulation of inflammasomes and their cytokine signatures. It is long known that it inhibits microtubule polymerization and the release of chemotactic factors from neutrophils and therefore interferes with neutrophil chemotaxis. In a dose-dependent fashion, colchicine inhibits expression of E-selectin on endothelial cells preventing neutrophil adhesion as well as promoting the shedding of L-selectin from neutrophils abrogating further recruitment. Colchicine inhibits the activation of P2X2 and P2X7 pores which is the first signal in ATP-induced NALP3 activation. It also interferes with the NALP3 assembly and caspase 1 activation by inhibiting the Rho/RhoA effector kinase pathway. Furthermore, it directly inhibits the release of TNFα, NO, and reactive oxygen species (ROS). Interestingly, colchicine promotes maturation of dendritic cells priming them to act as antigen-presenting cells [31].

Common side effects of colchicine include gastrointestinal intolerance in up to 10% of patients, bone marrow suppression and resultant cytopenias, and neuromyotoxicity especially in older patients with chronic kidney disease.

Corticosteroids

Corticosteroids have been used in acute and recurrent pericarditis given the rapid resolution of symptoms. However, prednisone especially at high doses of 1 mg/kg/day is associated with increased risk of relapses [32] and therefore should be avoided as opposed to lower doses (0.2–0.5 mg/kg/day) which in cases where NSAIDs or colchicine is contraindicated, it may be beneficial with heightened risk. Prednisone tapering should occur at small increments every 2–4 weeks in a similar fashion to the treatment of polymyalgia rheumatica [33]. Iatrogenic Cushing's syndrome, hypertension, diabetes mellitus, early cataract, hypertension, osteoporosis, and avascular necrosis are some of the common side effects on this refractory group of patients.

Nonbiologic Steroid-Sparing Agents

A fraction of patients who are administered corticosteroids are unable to be weaned off and require steroid-sparing agents. Azathioprine has been most commonly prescribed due to its known safety profile and cost-effectiveness. Its use is based on anecdotal evidence from a single-center retrospective study of 46 patients in which azathioprine at a dose of 1.5–2.5 mg/kg/day for about 1 year resulted in stable remission allowing steroid tapering to nil in more than 50% of patients [34]. Azathioprine is overall well-tolerated, with liver function abnormalities, leukopenia, and gastrointestinal symptoms being the most common side effects. Increased risk of infections and rarely pancreatitis have been reported. Screening for thiopurine S-methyltransferase (TPMT) deficiency is advocated by some clinicians to avoid life-threatening complications as 1 in 300 individuals lack enzyme activity and 11% are heterozygous for a variant low activity allele and have an intermediate activity [35].

In refractory recurrent pericarditis cases, IVIG has been used with reportedly fast amelioration of acute flares. Clinical experience is derived from 30 patients with recurrent pericarditis [36]. IVIG is infused over 3–5 days at a dose of 400–500 mg/kg/day and can be repeated monthly. IVIG is associated with infusions reactions, aseptic meningitis, liver function abnormalities, and rash. Due to its high cost, IVIG is reserved in refractory patients especially those with an underlying autoimmune disease if other disease-modifying medications fail.

Biologics

Among all biologic medications, anakinra, an interleukin 1 (IL-1) receptor antagonist, is the most promising for the treatment of recurrent pericarditis refractory to conventional steroid-sparing agents. The effectiveness of anakinra provides the most direct evidence of IL-1's contribution in disease pathogenesis. Anakinra is administered as a daily subcutaneous injection at 1–2 mg/kg/day, up to 100 mg. It is currently unclear how long should patients be treated.

In a recent double-blind, placebo-controlled, randomized withdrawal trial (open label with anakinra followed by a double-blind withdrawal step with anakinra or placebo until recurrent pericarditis occurred) conducted among 21 steroid-dependent, colchicine-resistant patients, anakinra reduced the risk of recurrence over a median of 14 months and allowed for steroid discontinuation in all patients [37]. Larger studies are needed to validate these results and inform clinicians on the duration of treatment, tapering strategies and relapse rate after discontinuation. Anakinra results in rapid improvement of symptoms within days (as opposed to weeks in azathioprine use) normalizing markers of inflammation and pericarditis as evidenced in echocardiogram or cardiac magnetic resonance imaging (MRI) [38]. Side effects of anakinra include injection site reactions in up to 10% of patients, increased risk of infection, transaminitis, and leukopenia. Prior to anakinra initiation, screening for hepatitis B virus infection and latent tuberculosis should be performed.

References

1. Cremer PC, Kumar A, Kontzias A, Tan CD, Rodriguez ER, Imazio M, et al. Complicated pericarditis: understanding risk factors and pathophysiology to inform imaging and treatment. J Am Coll Cardiol. 2016;68(21):2311–28.
2. Imazio M, Gaita F. Diagnosis and treatment of pericarditis. Heart. 2015;101(14):1159–68.
3. Imazio M, Gaita F, LeWinter M. Evaluation and treatment of pericarditis: a systematic review. JAMA. 2015;314(14):1498–506.
4. Permanyer-Miralda G, Sagrista-Sauleda J, Soler-Soler J. Primary acute pericardial disease: a prospective series of 231 consecutive patients. Am J Cardiol. 1985;56(10):623–30.
5. Ozen S, Demirkaya E, Amaryan G, Kone-Paut I, Polat A, Woo P, et al. Results from a multicentre international registry of familial Mediterranean fever: impact of environment on the expression of a monogenic disease in children. Ann Rheum Dis. 2014;73(4):662–7.
6. Lachmann HJ, Papa R, Gerhold K, Obici L, Touitou I, Cantarini L, et al. The phenotype of TNF receptor-associated autoinflammatory syndrome (TRAPS) at presentation: a series of 158 cases from the Eurofever/EUROTRAPS international registry. Ann Rheum Dis. 2014;73(12):2160–7.
7. Cantarini L, Lucherini OM, Baldari CT, Laghi Pasini F, Galeazzi M. Familial clustering of recurrent pericarditis may disclose tumour necrosis factor receptor-associated periodic syndrome. Clin Exp Rheumatol. 2010;28(3):405–7.
8. Brucato A, Brambilla G. Recurrent idiopathic pericarditis: familial occurrence. Int J Cardiol. 2005;102(3):529.
9. Cantarini L, Lucherini OM, Brucato A, Barone L, Cumetti D, Iacoponi F, et al. Clues to detect tumor necrosis factor receptor-associated periodic syndrome (TRAPS) among patients with idiopathic recurrent acute pericarditis: results of a multicentre study. Clin Res Cardiol. 2012;101(7):525–31.
10. Cantarini L, Rigante D, Merlini G, Vitale A, Caso F, Lucherini OM, et al. The expanding spectrum of low-penetrance TNFRSF1A gene variants in adults presenting with recurrent inflammatory attacks: clinical manifestations and long-term follow-up. Semin Arthritis Rheum. 2014;43(6):818–23.
11. Imazio M, Brucato A, Barbieri A, Ferroni F, Maestroni S, Ligabue G, et al. Good prognosis for pericarditis with and without myocardial involvement. Results from a multicenter, prospective cohort study. Circulation. 2013;128(1):42–9.
12. Imazio M, Brucato A, Cemin R, Ferrua S, Belli R, Maestroni S, et al. Colchicine for recurrent pericarditis (CORP): a randomized trial. Ann Intern Med. 2011;155(7):409–14.

13. Imazio M, Cecchi E, Demichelis B, Ierna S, Demarie D, Ghisio A, et al. Indicators of poor prognosis of acute pericarditis. Circulation. 2007;115(21):2739–44.
14. Imazio M, Belli R, Brucato A, Cemin R, Ferrua S, Beqaraj F, et al. Efficacy and safety of colchicine for treatment of multiple recurrences of pericarditis (CORP-2): a multicentre, double-blind, placebo-controlled, randomised trial. Lancet. 2014;383(9936):2232–7.
15. Imazio M. Idiopathic recurrent pericarditis as an immune-mediated disease: current insights into pathogenesis and emerging treatment options. Expert Rev Clin Immunol. 2014;10(11):1487–92.
16. Lazaros G, Karavidas A, Spyropoulou M, Tsiachris D, Halapas A, Zacharoulis A, et al. The role of the immunogenetic background in the development and recurrence of acute idiopathic pericarditis. Cardiology. 2011;118(1):55–62.
17. Maestroni S, Di Corato PR, Cumetti D, Chiara DB, Ghidoni S, Prisacaru L, et al. Recurrent pericarditis: autoimmune or autoinflammatory? Autoimmun Rev. 2012;12(1):60–5.
18. Yang CA, Chiang BL. Inflammasomes and human autoimmunity: a comprehensive review. J Autoimmun. 2015;61:1–8.
19. van Kempen TS, Wenink MH, Leijten EF, Radstake TR, Boes M. Perception of self: distinguishing autoimmunity from autoinflammation. Nat Rev Rheumatol. 2015;11(8):483–92.
20. Muruve DA, Petrilli V, Zaiss AK, White LR, Clark SA, Ross PJ, et al. The inflammasome recognizes cytosolic microbial and host DNA and triggers an innate immune response. Nature. 2008;452(7183):103–7.
21. Ichinohe T, Pang IK, Iwasaki A. Influenza virus activates inflammasomes via its intracellular M2 ion channel. Nat Immunol. 2010;11(5):404–10.
22. Nour AM, Reichelt M, Ku CC, Ho MY, Heineman TC, Arvin AM. Varicella-zoster virus infection triggers formation of an interleukin-1beta (IL-1beta)-processing inflammasome complex. J Biol Chem. 2011;286(20):17921–33.
23. Rathinam VA, Jiang Z, Waggoner SN, Sharma S, Cole LE, Waggoner L, et al. The AIM2 inflammasome is essential for host defense against cytosolic bacteria and DNA viruses. Nat Immunol. 2010;11(5):395–402.
24. Karatolios K, Moosdorf R, Maisch B, Pankuweit S. Cytokines in pericardial effusion of patients with inflammatory pericardial disease. Mediat Inflamm. 2012;2012:382082.
25. Horneffer PJ, Miller RH, Pearson TA, Rykiel MF, Reitz BA, Gardner TJ. The effective treatment of postpericardiotomy syndrome after cardiac operations. A randomized placebo-controlled trial. J Thorac Cardiovasc Surg. 1990;100(2):292–6.
26. Imazio M, Bobbio M, Cecchi E, Demarie D, Demichelis B, Pomari F, et al. Colchicine in addition to conventional therapy for acute pericarditis. Results of the COlchicine for acute PEricarditis (COPE) trial. Circulation. 2005;112(13):2012–6.
27. Imazio M, Bobbio M, Cecchi E, et al. Colchicine as first-choice therapy for recurrent pericarditis: results of the core (colchicine for recurrent pericarditis) trial. Arch Intern Med. 2005;165(17):1987–91.
28. Imazio M, Brucato A, Cemin R, Ferrua S, Maggiolini S, Beqaraj F, et al. A randomized trial of colchicine for acute pericarditis. N Engl J Med. 2013;369(16):1522–8.
29. Verma S, Eikelboom JW, Nidorf SM, Al-Omran M, Gupta N, Teoh H, et al. Colchicine in cardiac disease: a systematic review and meta-analysis of randomized controlled trials. BMC Cardiovasc Disord. 2015;15(1):96.
30. Adler Y, Charron P, Imazio M, Badano L, Baron-Esquivias G, Bogaert J, et al. ESC guidelines for the diagnosis and management of pericardial diseases. Rev Esp Cardiol (Engl Ed). 2015;68(12):1126.
31. Leung YY, Yao Hui LL, Kraus VB. Colchicine-update on mechanisms of action and therapeutic uses. Semin Arthritis Rheum. 2015;45(3):341–50.
32. Imazio M, Brucato A, Cumetti D, Brambilla G, Demichelis B, Ferro S, et al. Corticosteroids for recurrent pericarditis. High versus low doses: a nonrandomized observation. Circulation. 2008;118(6):667–71.
33. Imazio M, Brucato A, Trinchero R, Shabetai R, Spodick D, Adler Y. Corticosteroid therapy for pericarditis: a double-edged sword. Nat Clin Pract Cardiovasc Med. 2008;5(3):118–9.

34. Vianello F, Cinetto F, Cavraro M, Battisti A, Castelli M, Imbergamo S, et al. Azathioprine in isolated recurrent pericarditis: a single centre experience. Int J Cardiol. 2011;147(3):477–8.
35. Lennard L. Implementation of TPMT testing. Br J Clin Pharmacol. 2014;77(4):704–14.
36. Imazio M, Lazaros G, Picardi E, Vasileiou P, Carraro M, Tousoulis D, et al. Intravenous human immunoglobulins for refractory recurrent pericarditis: a systematic review of all published cases. J Cardiovasc Med. 2016;17(4):263–9.
37. Brucato A, Imazio M, Gattorno M, et al. Effect of anakinra on recurrent pericarditis among patients with colchicine resistance and corticosteroid dependence: the airtrip randomized clinical trial. JAMA. 2016;316(18):1906–12.
38. Lazaros G, Antonatou K, Vassilopoulos D. The therapeutic role of Interleukin-1 inhibition in idiopathic recurrent pericarditis: current evidence and future challenges. Front Med. 2017;4:78.

Chapter 21
Adamantiades-Behçet's Disease

Petros P. Sfikakis

Introduction

Adamantiades-Behçet disease (ABD) is a distinct, chronic, relapsing systemic inflammatory disorder which affects small and large veins and arteries and is characterized by oral and genital ulcers, skin lesions, uveitis, arthritis and vascular and central nervous system manifestations. ABD is currently classified among the primary systemic vasculitides [41]. The name of the disease derives from the physicians who described the first patients. In 1937 the Turkish dermatologist Hulusi Behçet described three patients with the tri-symptom complex of oral and genital ulcerations and hypopyon uveitis. Seven years before, during the 1930 annual meeting of the Medical Association of Athens, the Greek ophthalmologist Venediktos Adamantiades had presented the first patient with ABD, a 20-year-old male patient with relapsing iritis, genital ulcers and arthritis [44].

Although ABD exists worldwide, it is more prevalent across the ancient trading route known as the "Silk Road", i.e. in countries of the Mediterranean Basin, the Middle East and the Far East. The highest rate (4 in 1000 adults) is found in Turkey, followed by Israel, Northern China, Iran, Korea, Japan, Saudi Arabia, Iraq, Morocco and Egypt. The disease is rare in Northern Europe and the Americas. In Western Europe ABD is a more common disease than previously thought, perhaps as a result of underdiagnosis, exceeding even the prevalence of polyarteritis nodosa [43].

ABD is rarely seen in children or in the elderly. Men are more commonly affected in Mediterranean and Middle Eastern countries, but a female preponderance is seen in the Far East. Familial cases have been reported [19]. The disease typically starts

P. P. Sfikakis
First Department of Propedeutic & Internal Medicine, National & Kapodistrian University of Athens, Medical School, Athens, Greece
e-mail: psfikakis@med.uoa.gr

P. Efthimiou (ed.), *Auto-Inflammatory Syndromes*,
https://doi.org/10.1007/978-3-319-96929-9_21

in the third or fourth decade of life; however, recurrent oral ulcers, which are most often the first symptom, may appear years before the diagnosis is established. ABD runs a remitting and relapsing course and may abate in the many patients after 20 years [41].

Aetiopathogenesis

ABD is not the typical autoinflammatory disease and should be viewed as a condition linking autoinflammation and autoimmunity [25, 26]. Even though ABD is considered a primary systemic vasculitis, no specific immune cell type can be recognised in vasculitic lesions. Moreover, vasculitis is absent in the pathergy skin reaction, in acne lesions and in synovitis, whereas it is always present in ocular lesions, veins, pulmonary arteries and epididymitis, being sometimes present in oral and genital ulcers, erythema nodosum, gut lesions and central nervous system lesions. Immune complex deposition is rarely seen [41]. Although both innate and adaptive immune responses are increased, autoantibodies are usually absent, unless the patient is under treatment with anti-TNF antibodies [10].

In addition to the distinct epidemiological features, a genetic contribution to the disease is supported by the high familial aggregation [12] and the strong association with HLA-B51, which, however, accounts for less than 20% of the genetic risk [13]. The HLA-B51 association was confirmed in two large genome-wide association studies and a second, independent association within the MHC class I region was found. Moreover, interleukin-10, interleukin-23 receptor and interleukin-12 receptor β2 were identified as susceptibility loci, whereas diminished IL-10 mRNA expression and low-protein production was associated with the disease-associated interleukin-10 variant [27, 30]. Moreover, in a recent meta-analysis, mutations M694 V and M6801 in familial Mediterranean fever (FMF) gene were identified as a probable susceptibility gene for ABD [40]. However, immune and inflammatory gene expressions seem to be variable in both the innate (CD14+) and adaptive (CD4+) immune responses in ABD and FMF patients compared to those in controls suggesting differences in immune regulation between the two [28]. Notably, using next-generation sequencing, it was recently found an influence in the pathogenesis of ABD of rare variants in the genes MVK, NOD2 and PSTPIP, which are commonly linked with autoinflammatory diseases [4].

Among the various proinflammatory cytokine-mediated interactions in ABD, an important role of TNF has been suggested by several ex vivo studies [6, 7, 9, 11, 20, 38]. The pathogenic role of TNF in the perpetuation of inflammation is also supported by the impressive clinical responses after therapy with anti-TNF antibodies in many patients with severe forms of ABD [2, 34, 36, 37].

Clinical Spectrum

The clinical spectrum of ABD is quite diverse (Table 21.1), whereas there are significant differences in the prevalence of clinical manifestations between various ethnic groups [41]. For example, there are fewer cases of intestinal disease in the Mediterranean Basin and less severe eye disease and less frequent skin pathergy among patients from the Northern Europe or America. Along this line, whether distinct clinical clusters exist in ABD remains to be clarified. For example, acneiform skin lesions (papules and pustules) seem to be more frequent in Turkish ABD patients with arthritis. This suggests that the arthritis seen in ABD may possibly be related to acne-associated arthritis [8]. Also, the increased presence of enthesopathy among Turkish ABD patients who had acne and arthritis compared with that among patients without arthritis supports the hypothesis that patients who also have arthritis and acne form a distinct cluster [14]. In contrast, the presence of such a cluster was not confirmed in other ethnic groups [1].

Prevalence of clinical manifestations in paediatric ABD may differ compared to adults (Table). In a recent study from 12 countries, boys more often than girls showed cutaneous, ocular and vascular symptoms and girls more often genital aphthosis. Age at disease onset and skin and vascular involvement were lower for European than non-European children. Oral aphthosis was the presenting sign for 81% of patients. The mean delay to the second symptom was almost 3 years [18].

Almost all patients with ABD develop mucocutaneous symptoms and signs. Recurrent oral ulcers which heal within 1 week without scarring constitute the cardinal disease feature. Ulcers may appear either as single or multiple lesions in the tongue, pharynx, buccal and/or labial mucosal membranes and usually are painful. Genital ulcers are usually larger and deeper than oral ulcers and may appear on the

Table 21.1 Frequency of clinical manifestations of ABD disease in adults and children

	Adults	Children
Oral ulcers	90–100%	90–100%
Genital ulcers	75–85%	<60%
Papulopustular lesions	55%	<40%
Erythema nodosum	45%	<35%
Arthritis	35–60%	30-
Fever episodes	25%	50%)
Uveitis	35–70%	35–70%
Superficial thrombophlebitis	25%	10%
Deep vein thrombosis	5–10%	5%
Aneurysms	3–8%	rare
Epididymitis	5–15% of men	rare
GI involvement	5–25%	5–35%
CNS involvement	10–20%	5–15%

scrotum, less frequently on the penis, or on the vulva and vagina in women. Skin lesions include erythema nodosum-like lesions, as well as pseudofolliculitis and acneiform nodules which can appear all over the body, and they are not always hair follicle-associated. Joint involvement is usually a non-erosive monoarthritis affecting the knee or the ankle or oligoarthritis. Recurrent epididymitis in men is manifested by testicular pain and is mostly self-limited. Gastrointestinal involvement is expressed by single or multiple deep penetrating ulcers which develop mostly in the terminal ileum, the ileocecal region and the colon. Ocular involvement may lead to blindness, and any part of the eye can be affected. Relapsing anterior uveitis with or without hypopyon, vitritis and sight-threatening inflammation of the posterior pole with vasculitis, retinitis, optic disc swelling and cystoid macular oedema may occur.

Thrombosis may occur in many different sites including deep veins (iliofemoral, superior or inferior vena cavae, axillary, brachial and hepatic) and superficial veins; superficial thrombophlebitis is transient and can be misdiagnosed as erythema nodosum. Thrombosis may also occur in the chambers of the heart and dural sinus. Arterial aneurysms may develop at the abdominal aorta, iliac, femoral, popliteal, carotid and renal arteries and can rupture suddenly. Central nervous system involvement includes parenchymal in 80% of cases and non-parenchymal. Parenchymal involvement is an inflammatory meningoencephalitis, with progressive (relapsing remitting) or monophasic pattern which is either diffuse (brainstem-plus) or affects only the brainstem, spinal cord and cerebellum. Non-parenchymal (cerebral venous thrombosis, intracranial hypertension, intracranial aneurysm or extracranial aneurysm/dissection) is secondary to vascular involvement and usually monophasic [17]. Very rare manifestations in less than 2% of patients include amyloidosis, nephritis, serositis, cardiomyopathy and pulmonary fibrosis.

Diagnosis

With no specific histologic, laboratory or imaging features, the diagnosis of ABD remains entirely clinical and requires the exclusion of other diagnoses based on clinical presentation. Due to the relapsing-remitting course of the disease, a careful past medical history is mandatory. There is no pathognomonic laboratory test, and HLA-B51 testing is not recommended for diagnostic purposes. The differential diagnosis may include almost all immune-mediated diseases and many infections and depends on the given constellation of clinical manifestations. For example, inflammatory bowel disease should be ruled out in a patient with intestinal involvement and arthritis, multiple scleroses in a patient with central nervous involvement and uveitis, or Takayasu's arteritis in a patient with arterial lesions.

The International Study Group Criteria set is the most widely used with a sensitivity of 85% and specificity of 96% [5]. This set of criteria has some limitations, especially in differentially diagnose Crohn's disease from ABD. According to these criteria, a patient can be diagnosed with ABD if, in the absence of other explanations, the patient has recurring oral ulcerations (aphthous or herpetiform) observed by the physician or the patient at least three times in a 12-month period, plus at least any two of the following:

(a) Recurrent genital aphthous ulceration or scarring
(b) Eye lesions: anterior uveitis, posterior uveitis, cells in the vitreous by slit lamp examination or retinal vasculitis observed by an ophthalmologist
(c) Skin lesions: erythema nodosum, pseudofolliculitis, papulopustular lesions or acneiform nodules in postadolescent patients not on corticosteroids
(d) A positive pathergy test (non-specific skin hyperreactivity in response to minor trauma) read by a physician at 24–48 h

The International Study Group Criteria do not perform well in paediatric ABD. The recently proposed paediatric classification criteria include the following six-item categories: (a) recurrent oral aphtosis with at least three attacks/year; (b) genital ulceration, typically with scar; (c) skin involvement (necrotic folliculitis, acneiform lesions, erythema nodosum); (d) ocular involvement (anterior or posterior uveitis, retinal vasculitis); (e) neurological signs (with the exception of isolated headaches); and (f) vascular signs (venous or arterial thrombosis, arterial aneurysms). A minimum of three of them is required to classify a child as having paediatric ABD [18].

Management

Morbidity and mortality are significant in ABD. Ocular involvement is the leading cause of morbidity and, if left untreated, may result in blindness in more than 70% of those affected. Young males have the worst prognosis, and major vessel and neurological involvement, both of which may occur even 10 years after diagnosis, are the main causes of death [31]. In general, ocular, vascular, gastrointestinal and CNS involvement may be associated with a poor prognosis. On the other hand, we should not forget that disease manifestations may ameliorate over time in many patients [41].

Treatment should be individualized according to age, gender, type and severity of organ involvement and patient's preferences, balancing the risks of therapy with the putative efficacy of a given approach. Adequately powered, randomized, controlled clinical trials are few. A multidisciplinary approach is necessary for optimal care. The aims of treatment are (a) to maintain the quality of life; (b) prevent irreversible damage, which usually occurs early in the course of disease, especially in the high-risk group of young men; and (c) prevent exacerbations of orogenital, cutaneous and joint manifestations. HLA-51 status has not been associated with severe disease or with a worst prognosis [15].

For oral ulcers, genital ulcers, papulopustular lesions, erythema nodosum, arthritis, epididymitis and superficial thrombophlebitis, which are all self-limited manifestations, the therapeutic aim is to control symptoms. Topical measures such as local steroids should be used for the treatment of oral and genital ulcers. Colchicine should be tried first for the prevention of recurrent mucocutaneous lesions especially when the dominant lesion is erythema nodosum or genital ulcer. Papulopustular or acne-like lesions are treated with topical or systemic measures as used in acne vulgaris. Leg ulcers might be caused by venous stasis or obliterative vasculitis. Treatment should be planned with the help of a dermatologist and vascular surgeon. Drugs such as azathioprine [42], thalidomide, interferon-a, anti-TNF or apremilast, which was efficacious in treating oral ulcers in a recent randomized controlled trial [16], should be considered in selected cases with refractory to the above mucocutaneous manifestations. Colchicine should be the initial treatment in acute arthritis. Acute monoarticular disease can be treated with intra-articular glucocorticoids. Non-steroidal anti-inflammatory agents and corticosteroids are used for epididymitis. Azathioprine, interferon-a or anti-TNF should be considered in recurrent and chronic cases. In general, for such manifestations that are not associated with serious organ involvement, chronic glucocorticoid use should be avoided because it may adversely affect arterial function [29].

On the other hand, for serious organ involvement, such as major vessel disease, gastrointestinal involvement, ocular involvement, and central nervous system, the use of immunosuppressive agents is mandatory [15]. The introduction of anti-TNF monoclonal antibodies [32, 33] represents a significant advancement in the management of patients with severe, refractory manifestations and especially in relapsing sight-threatening involvement of the posterior eye segment [35, 36]. Non-anti-TNF biologic agents, such as anti-IL-1 and anti-IL-6 agents, have been also used with variable beneficial results [3].

For the management of acute DVT, glucocorticoids and immunosuppressants such as azathioprine, cyclophosphamide or cyclosporine A, are recommended. For refractory venous thrombosis, anti-TNF mAbs could be considered. Anticoagulants may be added with caution, provided that the risk of bleeding in general is low and coexistent pulmonary artery aneurysms are ruled out. For the management of pulmonary artery aneurysms, high dose glucocorticoids and cyclophosphamide are recommended. Anti-TNF mAbs should be considered in refractory cases. For patients who have or who are at high risk of major bleeding, embolization should be preferred to open surgery. For both aortic and peripheral artery aneurysms, medical treatment with cyclophosphamide and corticosteroids is necessary before intervention to repair. Surgery or stenting should not be delayed if the patient is symptomatic [15].

For gastrointestinal involvement, glucocorticoids should be considered during acute exacerbations together with disease-modifying agents such as 5-ASA or azathioprine. For severe and/or refractory patients, anti-TNF mAbs and/or thalidomide should be considered. Anti-TNF mAbs have been officially approved in Japan in 2014 for intestinal ABD. Urgent surgical consultation is necessary in cases of perforation, major bleeding and intestinal obstruction [39].

Management of uveitis requires close collaboration with ophthalmologists with the ultimate aim of inducing and maintaining remission. Any patient with ABD and inflammatory eye disease affecting the posterior segment should be on a treatment regime such as azathioprine, cyclosporine A, interferon-a or anti-TNF mAbs infliximab and adalimumab. Infliximab has been shown to be efficacious in various ocular complications such as cystoids macular oedema or retinal neovascularization. Adalimumab has been officially approved for the treatment of noninfectious uveitis in 2016. Systemic glucocorticoids should be used only in combination with azathioprine or other systemic immunosupressants. Patients presenting with an initial or recurrent episode of acute sight-threatening uveitis should be treated with high-dose glucocorticoids, intravenous infliximab or interferon-a. Infliximab, however, has the fastest mode of action [22] and is efficacious for severe ocular complications such as cystoid macular oedema [21] and retinal neovascularization [24]. Intravitreal glucocorticoid injection and infliximab injection are also options in patients with unilateral exacerbation as an adjunct to systemic treatment [23].

Regarding CNS involvement, acute attacks of parenchymal involvement should be treated with high dose glucocorticoids followed by slow tapering, together with immunosuppressants such as azathioprine. Cyclosporine A should be avoided. Anti-TNF mAbs should be considered in severe disease as first line or in refractory patients. The first episode of cerebral venous thrombosis should be treated with high-dose glucocorticoids followed by tapering. Anticoagulants may be added for a short duration, but screening is needed for vascular disease at an extracranial site.

Finally, drug-free, long-term remission after withdrawal of successful anti-TNF treatment given for 2 years is feasible in some patients with severe ABD [37]. Because an anti-TNF agent-induced "cure" cannot be differentiated from a spontaneous remission by natural history, prospective studies should examine whether anti-TNF agents should be used as first-line treatment for the induction of emission in every patient with vital organ involvement.

References

1. Arida A, Vaiopoulos G, Markomichelakis N, Kaklamanis P, Sfikakis PP. Are clusters of patients with distinct clinical expression present in Behçet's disease? Clin Exp Rheumatol. 2009;27(2 Suppl 53):S48–51.
2. Arida A, Fragiadaki K, Giavri E, Sfikakis PP. Anti-TNF agents for Behçet disease: analysis of published data on 369 patients. Semin Arthritis Rheum. 2011;41:61–70.
3. Arida A, Sfikakis PP. Anti-cytokine biologic treatment beyond anti-TNF in Behçet's disease. Clin Exp Rheumatol. 2014;32(4 Suppl 84):S149–55.
4. Burillo-Sanz S, Montes-Cano MA, García-Lozano JR, Ortiz-Fernández L, Ortego-Centeno N, García-Hernández FJ, Espinosa G, Graña-Gil G, Sánchez-Bursón J, Rosa Juliá M, Solans R, Blanco R, Barnosi-Marín AC, Gómez De la Torre R, Fanlo P, Rodríguez-Carballeira M, Rodríguez-Rodríguez L, Camps T, Castañeda S, Alegre-Sancho JJ, Martín J, González-Escribano MF. Mutational profile of rare variants in inflammasome-related genes in Behçet disease: a next generation sequencing approach. Sci Rep. 2017;7(1):8453.
5. Criteria for diagnosis of Behcet's disease: international study group for Behcet's disease. Lancet. 1990;335:1078–80.
6. Curnow SJ, Pryce K, Modi N, Knight B, Graham EM, Stewart JE, Fortune F, Stanford MR, Murray PI, Wallace GR. Serum cytokine profiles in Behçet's disease: is there a role for IL-15 in pathogenesis? Immunol Lett. 2008;121(1):7–12.
7. Dalghous AM, Freysdottir J. Fortune F Expression of cytokines, chemokines, and chemokine receptors in oral ulcers of patients with Behcet's disease (BD) and recurrent aphthous stomatitis

is Th1-associated, although Th2-association is also observed in patients with BD. Scand J Rheumatol. 2006;35(6):472–5.
8. Diri E, Mat C, Hamuryudan V, Yurdakul S, Hizli N, Yazici H. Papulopustular skin lesions are seen more frequently in patients with Behçet's syndrome who have arthritis: a controlled and masked study. Ann Rheum Dis. 2001;60(11):1074–6.
9. Elezoglou AV, Sfikakis PP, Vaiopoulos G, Kapsimali V, Kaklamanis PG. Serum levels of soluble TNF-alpha receptor-II (P75), circulating gamma delta T-cells and Adamantiades-Behçet's disease activity. Adv Exp Med Biol. 2003;528:261–5.
10. Elezoglou A, Kafasi N, Kaklamanis PH, Theodossiadis PG, Kapsimali V, Choremi E, Vaiopoulos G, Sfikakis PP. Infliximab treatment-induced formation of autoantibodies is common in Behçet's disease. Clin Exp Rheumatol. 2007;25(4 Suppl 45):S65–9.
11. Emmi G, Silvestri E, Bella CD, Grassi A, Benagiano M, Cianchi F, Squatrito D, Cantarini L, Emmi L, Selmi C, Prisco D, D'Elios MM. Cytotoxic Th1 and Th17 cells infiltrate the intestinal mucosa of Behcet patients and exhibit high levels of TNF-α in early phases of the disease. Medicine (Baltimore). 2016;95(49):e5516.
12. Gül A, Inanç M, Ocal L, Aral O, Koniçe M. Familial aggregation of Behçet's disease in Turkey. Ann Rheum Dis. 2000;59(8):622–5.
13. Gul A, Ohno S. HLA-B*51 and Behçet Disease. Ocul Immunol Inflamm. 2012;20:37–43.
14. Hatemi G, Fresko I, Tascilar K, Yazici H. Increased enthesopathy among Behçet's syndrome patients with acne and arthritis: an ultrasonography study. Arthritis Rheum. 2008;58(5):1539–45.
15. Hatemi G, Silman A, Bang D, Bodaghi B, Chamberlain AM, Gul A, Houman MH, Kotter I, Olivieri I, Salvarani C, Sfikakis PP, Siva A, Stanford MR, Stubiger N, Yurdakul S, Yazici H. EULAR recommendations for the management of Behcet disease. Ann Rheum Dis. 2008;67:1656–62.
16. Hatemi G, Melikoglu M, Tunc R, Korkmaz C, Turgut Ozturk B, Mat C, Merkel PA, Calamia KT, Liu Z, Pineda L, Stevens RM, Yazici H, Yazici Y. Apremilast for Behçet's syndrome–a phase 2, placebo-controlled study. N Engl J Med. 2015;372(16):1510–8.
17. Kalra S, Silman A, Akman-Demir G, Bohlega S, Borhani-Haghighi A, Constantinescu CS, Houman H, Mahr A, Salvarani C, Sfikakis PP, Siva A, Al-Araji A. Diagnosis and management of Neuro-Behçet's disease: international consensus recommendations. J Neurol. 2014;261(9):1662–76.
18. Koné-Paut I, Shahram F, Darce-Bello M, Cantarini L, Cimaz R, Gattorno M, Anton J, Hofer M, Chkirate B, Bouayed K, Tugal-Tutkun I, Kuemmerle-Deschner J, Agostini H, Federici S, Arnoux A, Piedvache C. Ozen S; PEDBD group. Consensus classification criteria for paediatric Behçet's disease from a prospective observational cohort: PEDBD. Ann Rheum Dis. 2016;75(6):958–64.
19. Kural-Seyahi E, Fresko I, Seyahi N, Ozyazgan Y, Mat C, Hamuryudan V, Yurdakul S, Hl Y. The long-term mortality and morbidity of Behçet syndrome: a 2-decade outcome survey of 387 patients followed at a dedicated center. Medicine (Baltimore). 2003;82:60–76.
20. Lopalco G, Lucherini OM, Lopalco A, Venerito V, Fabiani C, Frediani B, Galeazzi M, Lapadula G, Cantarini L. Iannone F Cytokine signatures in mucocutaneous and ocular Behçet's disease. Front Immunol. 2017;8:200. https://doi.org/10.3389/fimmu.2017.00200. eCollection 2017.
21. Markomichelakis NN, Theodossiadis PG, Pantelia E, Papaefthimiou S, Theodossiadis GP, Sfikakis PP. Infliximab for chronic cystoid macular edema associated with uveitis. Am J Ophthalmol. 2004;138(4):648–50.
22. Markomichelakis N, Delicha E, Masselos S, Fragiadaki K, Kaklamanis P, Sfikakis PP. A single infliximab infusion vs corticosteroids for acute panuveitis attacks in Behçet's disease: a comparative 4-week study. Rheumatology (Oxford). 2011;50(3):593–7.
23. Markomichelakis N, Delicha E, Masselos S, Sfikakis PP. Intravitreal infliximab for sight-threatening relapsing uveitis in Behçet disease: a pilot study in 15 patients. Am J Ophthalmol. 2012;154(3):534–41.

24. Markomichelakis NN, Aissopou EK, Maselos S, Tugal-Tutkun I, Sfikakis PP. Biologic treatment options for retinal neovascularization in Behçet's disease. Ocul Immunol Inflamm. 2017;12:1–7. https://doi.org/10.1080/09273948.2017.1332228. [Epub ahead of print].
25. McGonagle D, McDermott MF. A proposed classification of the immunological diseases. PLoS Med. 2006;3(8):e297.
26. Mendoza-Pinto C, García-Carrasco M, Jiménez-Hernández M, Jiménez Hernández C, Riebeling-Navarro C, Nava Zavala A, Vera Recabarren M, Espinosa G, Jara Quezada J, Cervera R. Etiopathogenesis of Behcet's disease. Autoimmun Rev. 2010;9:241–5.
27. Mizuki N, Meguro A, Ota M, Ohno S, Shiota T, Kawagoe T, Ito N, Kera J, Okada E, Yatsu K, Song YW, Lee EB, Kitaichi N, Namba K, Horie Y, Takeno M, Sugita S, Mochizuki M, Bahram S, Ishigatsubo Y, Inoko H. Genome-wide association studies identify IL23R-IL12RB2 and IL10 as Behçet's disease susceptibility loci. Nat Genet. 2010;42:703–6.
28. Özdemir FT, Demiralp EE, Aydın SZ, Atagündüz P, Ergun T, Direskeneli H. Immune and inflammatory gene expressions are different in Behçet's disease compared to those in Familial Mediterranean Fever. Eur J Rheumatol. 2016;3(4):146–52.
29. Protogerou AD, Sfikakis PP, Stamatelopoulos KS, Papamichael C, Aznaouridis K, Karatzis E, Papaioannou TG, Ikonomidis I, Kaklamanis P, Mavrikakis M, Lekakis J. Interrelated modulation of endothelial function in Behcet's disease by clinical activity and corticosteroid treatment. Arthritis Res Ther. 2007;9(5):R90.
30. Remmers EF, Cosan F, Kirino Y, Ombrello MJ, Abaci N, Satorius C, et al. Genome-wide association study identifies variants in the MHC class I, IL10, and IL23R-IL12RB2 regions associated with Behçet' disease. Nat Genet. 2010;42:698–702.
31. Saadoun D, Wechsler B, Desseaux K, Le Thi HD, Amoura Z, Resche-Rigon M, Cacoub P. Mortality in Behcet's disease. Arthritis Rheum. 2010;62:2806–12.
32. Sfikakis PP. The first decade of biologic TNF antagonists in clinical practice: lessons learned, unresolved issues and future directions. Curr Dir Autoimmun. 2010;11:180–210.
33. Sfikakis PP, Theodossiadis PG, Katsiari CG, Kaklamanis P, Markomichelakis NN. Effect of infliximab on sight-threatening panuveitis in Behçet's disease. Lancet. 2001;358:295–6.
34. Sfikakis PP. Behçet's disease: a new target for anti-tumour necrosis factor treatment. Ann Rheum Dis. 2002;61(Suppl 2):ii51–3.
35. Sfikakis PP, Kaklamanis PH, Elezoglou A, Katsilambros N, Theodossiadis PG, Papaefthimiou S, Markomichelakis N. Infliximab for recurrent, sight-threatening ocular inflammation in Adamantiades-Behçet disease. Ann Intern Med. 2004;140(5):404–6.
36. Sfikakis PP, Markomichelakis N, Alpsoy E, Assaad-Khalil S, Bodaghi B, Gul A, et al. Anti-TNF therapy in the management of Behcet's disease: review and basis for recommendations. Rheumatology (Oxford). 2007;46:736–41.
37. Sfikakis PP, Arida A, Panopoulos S, Fragiadaki K, Pentazos G, Laskari K, Tektonidou M, Markomichelakis N. Drug-free long-term remission in severe Behcet's disease following withdrawal of successful anti-TNF treatment. Arthritis Rheumatol. 2017; https://doi.org/10.1002/art.40235. [Epub ahead of print].
38. Sugita S, Kawazoe Y, Imai A, Kawaguchi T, Horie S, Keino H, Takahashi M, Mochizuki M. Role of IL-22- and TNF-α-producing Th22 cells in uveitis patients with Behcet's disease. J Immunol. 2013;190(11):5799–808.
39. Vaiopoulos AG, Sfikakis PP, Kanakis MA, Vaiopoulos G, Kaklamanis PG. Gastrointestinal manifestations of Behçet's disease: advances in evaluation and management. Clin Exp Rheumatol. 2014;32(4 Suppl 84):S140–8.
40. Wu Z, Zhang S, Li J, Chen S, Li P, Sun F, Wen X, Zheng W, Zhang F, Li Y. Association between MEFV mutations M694V and M680I and Behçet's disease: a meta-analysis. PLoS One. 2015;10(7):e0132704. https://doi.org/10.1371/journal.pone.0132704. eCollection 2015.
41. Yazici H, Fresko I, Yurdakul S. Behcet's syndrome: disease manifestations, management, and advances in treatment. Nat Clin Pract Rheumatol. 2007;3:148–55.

42. Yazici H, Pazarli H, Barnes CG, Tuzun Y, Ozyazgan Y, Silman A, Serdaroglu S, Oguz V, Yurdakul S, Lovatt GE, et al. A controlled trial of azathioprine in Behcet's syndrome. N Engl J Med. 1990;322:281–5.
43. Yazici H, Seyahi E, Yurdakul S. Behcet's syndrome is not so rare: why do we need to know? Arthritis Rheum. 2008;58:3640–3.
44. Zouboulis CC, Keitel W. A historical review of early descriptions of Adamantiades- Behcet's disease. J Invest Dermatol. 2002;119:201–5.

Chapter 22
Amyloidosis

Michael Voulgarelis, Ioannis Mitroulis, and Athanasios G. Tzioufas

Introduction

The term amyloidosis refers to a family of heterogeneous diseases characterized by extracellular deposition of an abnormal protein-based material, called amyloid. Amyloidosis is caused by the production of misfolded insoluble proteins in increased amounts [1]. The proteins undergo partial proteolytic cleavage resulting in the formation of peptides, in an abnormal β-pleated sheet non-branching fibrillary conformation, which are resistant to further proteolysis and form linear, rigid, and 7.5–10 mm wide amyloid fibrils. Peptide P, apolipoprotein E, basement membrane components, as well as glycosaminoglycans, proteoglycans, and protease inhibitors are added to the fibrils, resulting to stabilization and deposition of amyloid [2] (Fig. 22.1). At least 30 different amyloidogenic proteins have been identified in humans, and they can be differentiated by mass spectroscopy after laser capture microdissection and genetic testing [3]. The physicochemical characteristics of amyloid will determine in which organs the amyloid will be deposited and therefore what lesions will occur. Although the amyloid composition changes according to the amyloidogenic protein, it has some common features: (i) It consists of protein fibrils, (ii) it is insoluble and resistant to proteolysis, and (iii) after Congo red staining, it gives an apple-green birefringence under cross-polarized light microscopy.

M. Voulgarelis · A. G. Tzioufas (✉)
Department of Pathophysiology, Medical School, National University of Athens, Athens, Greece
e-mail: agtzi@med.uoa.gr

I. Mitroulis
Institute of Clinical Chemistry and Laboratory Medicine, Technische Universität Dresden, Dresden, Germany

P. Efthimiou (ed.), *Auto-Inflammatory Syndromes*,
https://doi.org/10.1007/978-3-319-96929-9_22

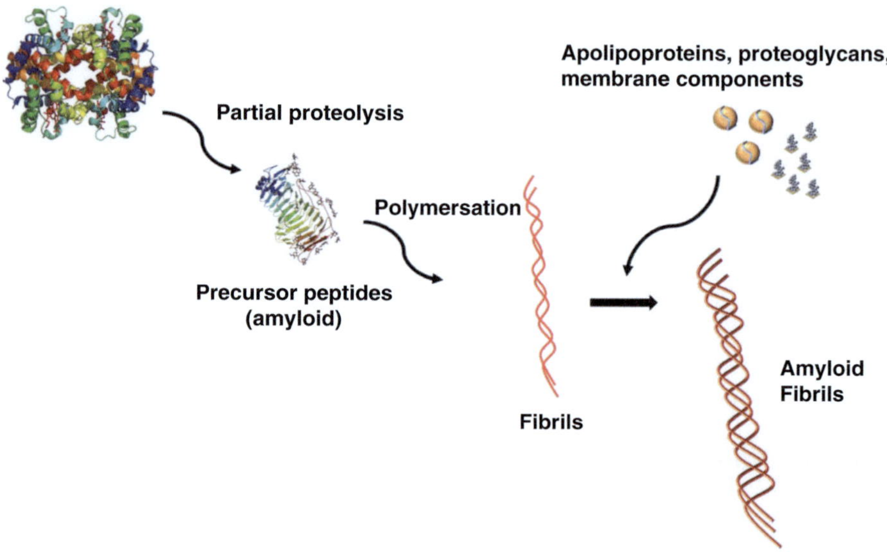

Fig. 22.1 Formation of amyloid fibrils. Proteins are partially cleaved forming precursor β-pleated sheet peptides (amyloids), which polymerize into fibrils. These fibrils interact with other components such as apolipoproteins, glycans, and membrane components to form proteolytically resistant and rigid amyloid fibrils

Classes of Amyloidosis

Amyloidosis is a rare disease. Systemic amyloidosis continues to be fatal and is responsible for about one in 1500 deaths per year in the UK. As mentioned, the amyloidosis classes are determined by the origin of the protein fibrils. Some amyloidoses are acquired, while others are inherited [4]. It is very important to define the amyloid type immediately when the diagnosis is made as treatment may be different. The most frequent types of amyloidogenic proteins are the light chain (AL) derived from monoclonal B-cell disorders producing amyloidogenic immunoglobulin light chains, serum amyloid A (SAA), and the mutant and wild-type transthyretin (TTR) (Table 22.1).

The responsible protein in AL amyloidosis (primary amyloidosis) is a light chain of immunoglobulins (part of the variable part of lambda chains in 75%) [5]. In AL amyloidosis, the abnormal folding is the result of either a proteolytic event or an amino acid sequence that causes a light chain thermodynamically instable and prone to self-aggregation [1]. Overproduction of the chains may be primary or accompany paraproteinemias (multiple myeloma, Waldenstrom macroglobulinemia). AL amyloidosis is the most common and most serious form of amyloidosis with incidence similar to that of Hodgkin's lymphoma or chronic myelogenous leukemia [5]. It is estimated to affect 5 to 12 people per million per year. In primary AL amyloidosis, the plasmacytic clone burden is low typically 5–10%; however in 10–15% of

Table 22.1 Classes of amyloidosis

Precursor protein	Human disease	Major causative association
Immunoglobulin light chain	Primary (AL) amyloidosis	Plasma cell disorders
Immunoglobulin heavy chain	Primary (AH) amyloidosis	Plasma cell disorders
Serum amyloid A	Secondary (AA) amyloidosis	Inflammation
Transthyretin (TTR)	Familial amyloidosis	Mutant ATTR
	Systemic senile amyloidosis	Wild-type ATTR
Beta2-microglobulin	Hemodialysis-related amyloidosis	Chronic hemodialysis patients

patients, AL amyloidosis occurs in association with multiple myeloma [6]. Evidence suggests that there is a correlation between immunoglobulin VL germline gene usage that are expressed by AL clones and amyloid-related organ involvement indicating that this tropism may be related to the antigenic affinities of the clonal light chains [7].

Extracellular deposition of amyloid protein A, which derives after processing of the acute-phase reactant serum amyloid AA (SAA), in several organs is the hallmark of AA amyloidosis. The accumulation of amyloid protein A results in tissue damage and progression toward organ dysfunction and failure, having a detrimental effect on morbidity and mortality in patients with inflammatory disorders [8]. Several inflammatory diseases, including rheumatoid arthritis (RA), systemic-onset juvenile idiopathic arthritis (SoJIA), Crohn's disease, ulcerative colitis, osteomyelitis, bronchiectasis, familial Mediterranean fever (FMF), tuberculosis, leprosy, sarcoidosis, Castleman's disease, injection-drug abuse, cystic fibrosis, and certain malignancies (kidney, cervix, Hodgkin's lymphoma), are characterized by an increased SAA production and hence increased chance of causing AA amyloidosis [9]. The underlying disorder, however, cannot be identified in a small number of patients (5–10%) at the initial diagnosis. In patients with idiopathic amyloidosis, the causing disorder can be identified later in the course of the disease [10]. Cytokines produced in these conditions, such as TNF and interleukins 1 and 6, are responsible for the increased production of SAA. The incidence of AA amyloidosis has declined in recent years due to effective treatment of chronic infections, such as tuberculosis, which were the main cause. In recent years the majority of cases in developed countries are due to rheumatoid arthritis. AA amyloidosis also complicates FMF, an inherited autosomal recessive condition due to a mutation of the pyrin gene, which has an aberrant effect on the inflammatory response to various stimuli. The condition is manifested by acute episodes of fever with serositis (that can mimic acute abdomen). Due to frequent inflammatory episodes, overproduction of SAA and AA amyloid deposition is induced.

TTR-related amyloidosis (ATTR) – also named "familial amyloid polyneuropathy" – was initially reported by the neurologist Corino da Costa Andrade in two villages of Portugal in 1950 [11]. The responsible protein (transthyretin or prealbumin) in ATTR is a normal serum transport protein (transfers thyroxine and vitamin A) mainly synthesized by the liver. The presence of mutation in TTR destabilizes the tetramer and leads to the release of monomers, which are believed to be amyloidogenic. ATTR can be caused by >100 mutations of TTR. The most commonly found mutation is the replacement of valine by methionine at position 50 (Val50Met), first described in the Portuguese population. TTR also accumulates with age, resulting in systemic senile amyloidosis (also called wild-type ATTR) in elderly, which results in the deposition of native TTR mainly in the heart. The prevalence of cardiac native TTR amyloid deposits is estimated at around 10% in people aged >80 years and 50% in those aged >90 years [12, 13].

Hemodialysis-related amyloidosis is a form of systemic amyloidosis; beta2-microglobulin (B2M) has been identified as the major constituent protein. The responsible protein β2-microglobulin is a protein found as a component of class I HLA antigens in the membrane of all nucleated cells. Because of its molecular weight (11.8 kd), it is not eliminated by conventional dialysis filters, which gradually accumulates in chronic hemodialysis patients. Finally, Alzheimer's disease is due to β-protein amyloidosis, while Creutzfeldt-Jakob disease is due to amyloidosis by prion proteins. In both cases, amyloid accumulates in the brain only. This amyloidosis is the only intracellular form of the disease.

Clinical Manifestations

Systemic amyloidosis is characterized by the accumulation of amyloid in various tissue and organs that produce specific clinical manifestations depending on the organ involvement (Table 22.2). Despite the fact that amyloid deposition can disturb the tissue architecture and lead to organ dysfunction, increasing evidence exists that amyloidogenic proteins have direct cytotoxic effects that also contribute to disease manifestations [14].

AL Amyloidosis

It is the most frequent and serious form of systemic amyloidosis and usually occurs after 50 years [15]. It affects more often the kidneys, heart, gastrointestinal tract, and nervous system [5, 16]. Rarely it affects the lungs, skin, and musculoskeletal

Table 22.2 Patterns of organ involvement

Amyloid type-class of amyloidosis	Heart	Kidney	Liver	Peripheral nervous system	Autonomic nervous system	Soft tissue
AL	++	++	+	+	+	+
Wild-type ATTR	++	–	–	–	–	–
Hereditary ATTR	++	++	–	++	+	–
AA	+	++	+	–	+	–

system. The main clinical manifestation of AL amyloidosis is nephrotic syndrome (10–15% of patients with nephrotic syndrome after 60 years old have AL amyloidosis). Rarely it occurs as asymptomatic albuminuria. The absence of hypertension (there may be orthostatic hypotension) and an increased kidney size are typical. Histologically, amyloid deposits give the specific apple-green birefringence under cross-polarized light microscopy. Amyloid deposits in vessels may be present alongside with or without glomerular lesions. Rarely, amyloid deposits are found in the interstitial space and the membrane of the collecting tubules [17]. The transmembrane injury may be manifested by renal tubular acidosis (usually type I and rarely type II) or nephrogenic diabetes insipidus. Cardiac AL amyloid deposition is accompanied by a restrictive cardiomyopathy characterized by progressive diastolic and subsequently systolic biventricular dysfunction and arrhythmia [16]. Infiltration of the myocardium causes concentrically thickened ventricular walls with reduced cavity size with subsequent impaired ventricular diastolic filling and both left and right ventricular insufficiency. Low QRS voltage on the electrocardiogram is found in a high proportion of patients and often is associated with a pseudoinfarct pattern, whereas a conduction tissue involvement (atrioventricular or sinoatrial nodes) is often complicated to ventricular arrhythmia and syncope. It has been indicated that certain circulating monoclonal LC may directly impair cardiac function, in addition to any mechanical effects of amyloid fibril deposition [14]. It has been published that AL cardiomyopathy seems to be associated with highest frequency of hemodynamic derangement and aggressive clinical course compared to that of TTR-related cardiomyopathies [18].

Peripheral nervous system involvement manifests as painful, bilateral, symmetric, distal sensory neuropathy that progresses to motor neuropathy. Autonomic nervous system in AL amyloidosis can lead to orthostatic hypotension, erectile dysfunction, and bowel motility dysfunction. Hepatomegaly is common, while splenomegaly is rarely observed [19]. Hepatomegaly can occur as a result of either congestion from right heart failure or amyloid infiltration of the liver. Profound elevation of alkaline phosphatase with only mild elevation of transaminases is characteristic. Soft tissue involvement is characterized by the presence of macroglossia, carpal tunnel syndrome, skin nodules, arthropathy, alopecia, nail dystrophy, submandibular gland enlargement, periorbital purpura, and hoarseness of voice due to larynx amyloid deposition.

AA Amyloidosis

The kidney is the most common affected organ, and renal manifestations are the more common feature of AA amyloidosis. Renal involvement is usually characterized by glomerular deposition of amyloid, leading to the development of nephrotic syndrome and subsequent renal insufficiency. Cardiac involvement, presented as systolic and diastolic dysfunction, and conduction disorders, including arrhythmia and heart block, and autonomic neuropathy are rare in patients with AA amyloidosis, compared to ATRR and AL amyloidosis, and therefore the prognosis is better than that of AL amyloidosis. Thyroid and adrenal glands can be also affected, whereas hepatomegaly is not uncommon. Gastrointestinal or urinary tract bleeding are also complications of AA amyloidosis due to vascular deposition of amyloid that results to increased vessel fragility [8, 10].

Dialysis-Related Amyloidosis

It is characterized by β2-microglobulin deposits in the joints and bones. The most common clinical manifestation is the carpal tunnel syndrome, which occurs at a significant rate after 10 years of long-term dialysis. Rarely it occurs with bone pain, fractures (bony cysts), and arthralgias (especially in the shoulder joint).

TTR-Related Amyloidosis

Mutations in several genes, such as transthyretin, fibrinogen, apolipoprotein A1, and apolipoprotein A2, can be responsible for hereditary amyloidosis, but by far the most common cause is variant ATTR amyloidosis (variant ATTR) caused by mutations in the transthyretin gene causing neuropathy and, often, cardiac involvement.

Systemic Amyloidosis in Autoinflammatory Syndromes

Reactive AA amyloidosis, with renal involvement leading to end-stage renal deficiency, is a severe complication of autoinflammatory syndromes, having a detrimental effect on morbidity and mortality. Amyloidosis is the most important complication of FMF, with an incidence of approximately 60% in untreated Turkish, Armenian, Arab, and non-Ashkenazi Jewish populations [20, 21]. Early-onset renal amyloidosis was the main cause of death in Jewish FMF patients, resulting in increased mortality compared to the general population [21]. Due to the increased risk of renal amyloidosis in patients with FMF, measurement of SAA and urinalysis every 6 months is recommended, even in low-risk patients [20]. *SAA* genotype, M694 V homozygosity, and environmental factors have a major role in the progression toward amyloidosis. The country of residence, rather than the country of origin, has been shown to be a major risk factor in the development of amyloidosis [22, 23]. The use of colchicine significantly diminishes the frequency of amyloidosis. Development of proteinuria, which is the first sign of renal amyloidosis, has been shown to decrease in a frequency of 1.7% of FMF patients under colchicine compared to 49% in non-compliant patients in a 10-year follow-up period [24]. Amyloidosis has been reported as the initial manifestation in asymptomatic patients with M694 V homozygosity in countries with increased frequency of amyloidosis. For this reason, colchicine could be considered for asymptomatic carriers with family members with amyloidosis [25]. Based on the efficacy of colchicine in the prevention of amyloidosis, colchicine should not be discontinued in non-responding patients treated with biologic agents [25, 26].

Reactive amyloidosis is also a severe complication in patients with cryopyrin-associated periodic syndrome (CAPS). It is uncommon in patients with familial cold autoinflammatory syndrome (FCAS), but it affects up to 25% of patients with Muckle-Wells syndrome. Blocking of IL-1 has been shown to be effective, not only in suppressing disease activity and normalizing SAA levels but also in improving renal function in patients with already established renal amyloidosis [27]. AA amyloidosis is also a complication in tumor necrosis factor receptor-associated periodic fever syndrome (TRAPS) and mevalonate kinase deficiency (MKD) [27, 28]. In a series of 158 cases, the frequency of amyloidosis was 10%. The median age of diagnosis of amyloidosis in patients with TRAPS was around 40 years [29]. Anti-cytokine treatment has been shown to be effective in inducing stabilization and even regression of the amyloid load in these patients, suggesting that early diagnosis and initiation of therapy to achieve regression of disease activity can inhibit the development of amyloidosis and preserve renal function [28].

Diagnosis of Amyloidosis

The suspicion of diagnosis of amyloidosis should be considered in every patient with a combination of several organ involvements. Especially the presence of nephrotic syndrome with increased kidney size, cardiomyopathy, autonomic nervous system involvement, the presence of macroglossia, and identification of monoclonal light chains in urine or serum by immunofixation are characteristic manifestations of AL amyloidosis. A medical history of chronic inflammatory disease in patients with nephrotic syndrome and hepatosplenomegaly suggests AA amyloidosis. Carpal tunnel syndrome in patients with chronic hemodialysis may be due to β-2 microglobulin deposition.

Confirmation of the diagnosis of amyloidosis is based on the histological examination of the affected organs where amyloid deposits are found after staining with Congo red, to have the specific apple-green birefringence under cross-polarized light microscopy [30]. The site of the screening biopsy does not involve in most cases the organ that is responsible for the clinical manifestation of amyloidosis, in order to avoid complication due to the surgical procedure. Rectal biopsy was commonly used in the past; however, this method was replaced by abdominal adipose tissue or labial salivary gland biopsy, which provides enough material for the diagnosis with practically no complications. In case of a negative abdominal adipose tissue biopsy and a strong clinical suspicion, a rectal biopsy should be performed [10, 30]. Immunohistochemical staining can then be used to determine the type of pathological protein and the type of amyloidosis. Significant diagnostic and prognostic assistance is provided by the scintigraphy with iodine-radiolabeled P peptide [31]. As this peptide is deposited in all cases of amyloidosis, the extent and location of its deposition gives information on the type and extent of organ involvement. It also serves to monitor the response of amyloidosis to treatment (change in the extent of deposition in sequential examinations). Interestingly, the combined findings of grade 2 or 3 myocardial radiotracer uptake on bone scintigraphy and absence of a monoclonal protein in serum or urine had a specificity and positive predictive value for cardiac ATTR amyloidosis of 100% [32].

Once the diagnosis of amyloidosis is established by the pathologist, confirmation of AL amyloidosis requires demonstration of a clonal plasma cell dyscrasia by a bone marrow biopsy or by the presence of a monoclonal light chain in the serum or urine. In this regard the serum free-light-chain (FLC) assay has a high sensitivity for circulating free light chains that is tenfold higher than that of immunofixation [33]. Thickening of the myocardial wall in combination with low potentials in ECG may also suggest cardiac amyloidosis. Cardiac ultrasound remains the first and most commonly used method to evaluate the patient with amyloidosis [16]. Echocardiographical findings typical to cardiac amyloidosis include the increased LV wall thickness ≥12 mm with "brilliant" speckled appearance of the myocardium, normal or small LV cavity, preserved LV ejection fraction, abnormal mitral filling pattern, due to LV diastolic dysfunction, right atrial enlargement, as well as dilated vena cave reflecting right ventricular (RV) filling pressure. Early experience suggests that magnetic resonance imaging (MRI) may provide an additional method for evaluation of cardiac involvement in amyloidosis and may be particularly useful in distinguishing ventricular wall thickening as a result of amyloid infiltration from ventricular hypertrophy caused by hypertension [34].

Mass spectrometry of amyloid deposits obtained after laser microdissection is the gold standard for the typing of amyloid fibrils but is available in very few laboratories. Genetic tests for the diagnosis of hereditary amyloidosis should be considered, especially if no paraprotein is found and in patients with a family history of the disease and in the presence of peripheral nervous system involvement as well as cardiac involvement. The presence of a serum monoclonal immunoglobulin does not necessarily mean AL amyloidosis since monoclonal gammopathy of undetermined significance (MGUS) is common in individuals over 65 years and wild-type ATTR amyloidosis of the heart. More specific more than 10% of patients with hereditary amyloidosis as well as 21% of wild-type ATTR in elderly have MGUS.

Pathogenesis of AA Amyloidosis

The deposition of extracellular amyloid fibrils in the affected organs is the hallmark of systemic amyloidosis. The insoluble fibrils are deposited at the extracellular space of the affected tissue and derive from precursor proteins that undergo changes in protein folding [3]. The precursor protein of the amyloid deposits in AA amyloidosis is the acute-phase reactant serum amyloid AA (SAA), a family of apolipoproteins produced mainly in the liver and associated with high-density lipoprotein (HDL) in plasma. SAA levels are low in healthy subjects and increase up to 1000-folds during inflammation. A sustained increase in SAA concentration in serum of patients with inflammatory disorders, suggestive of increased disease activity, is a prerequisite for the development of amyloidosis [10] (Fig. 22.2).

The genes that encode the SAA family members in humans are *SAA1*, *SAA2*, and *SAA4*. SAA1 and SAA2 are acute-phase proteins, whereas SAA4 is constitutively produced in the liver. In most cases, SAA1 is the precursor protein in reactive amyloidosis [10, 35, 36]. SAA1 and SAA2 production in the liver is regulated by pro-inflammatory cytokines like TNF, IL-1, and especially IL-6. In vitro stimulation studies have shown that IL-6 has the principal role in the transcriptional regulation of SAA through the transcription factors STAT3 and NFκB, whereas TNF and IL-1 mainly act as additional factors that increase the effect of IL-6 [37]. The important role of sustained inflammation, and especially of IL-6, in the progression of amyloidosis is also shown in experimental murine models. Transgenic mice expressing human IL-6 develop early-onset amyloidosis, sharing common features with human disease, which include high levels of SAA and amyloid depositions in the kidney, liver, and spleen [38]. To this direction, several clinical studies and case series suggest that the administration of tocilizumab, a humanized monoclonal antibody against the IL-6 receptor, normalizes the serum levels of SAA and stabilizes or even ameliorates amyloidosis in a wide range of disorders, including RA, SoJIA, FMF,

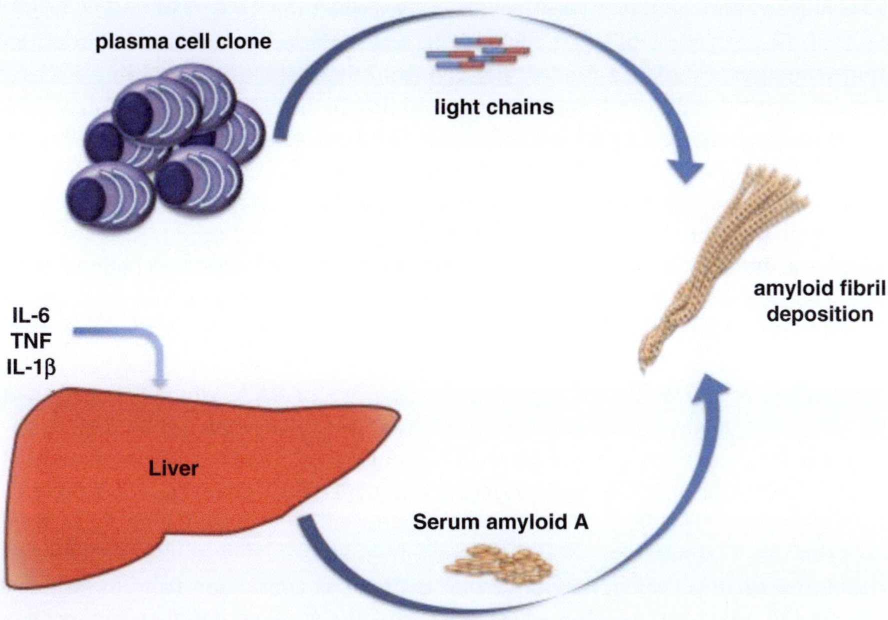

Fig. 22.2 Pathogenesis of AA amyloidosis. Pro-inflammatory cytokines in chronic inflammatory diseases induce the sustained production of serum amyloid A by hepatocytes. Serum amyloid A is processed and deposited as amyloid fibrils in the extracellular space of affected organs

and Castleman's disease [39–41]. Anti-TNF treatment has been also shown to decrease SAA levels and disease progression [10]. The role of IL-1 in the production of SAA and the subsequent progression toward amyloidosis has been shown in patients with autoinflammatory syndromes. Administration of anti-IL-1 agents results in the normalization of SAA levels and had a beneficial effect in the progression of amyloidosis [28].

These findings suggest that inhibition of pro-inflammatory cytokines decreases the SAA levels and can subsequently affect the progression of the disease. The correlation between SAA levels, amyloid load, and progression of amyloidosis has been also studied. In patients with AA amyloidosis, effective treatment of the underlying inflammatory disease and maintenance of SAA levels within the normal range (<10 mg/L) resulted in the regression or stabilization of amyloid load. Additionally, normalization of SAA levels was correlated with a stabilization or improvement of renal function, as assessed by the serum creatinine levels and proteinuria. However, relapses of the inflammatory disease resulted in a rapid increase of the amyloid load [42]. Taken together, amyloid deposits in patients with inflammatory disorders are in a dynamic balance, and tight disease control and achievement of remission prevent the further accumulation of amyloid or even result in the regression of amyloid deposits, revealing the critical role of early diagnosis and initiation of effective treatment strategies in patients with inflammatory disorders.

Except from the increased production of the precursor protein in the circulation, specific polymorphic variants of *SAA1* act as predisposing factors for amyloidosis. Five polymorphic coding alleles have been described for SAA1 (*SAA1.1*, *SAA1.2*, *SAA1.3*, *SAA1.4*, and *SAA1.5*). Even though there are minor differences in the amino acid sequence of the gene product derived from these alleles, several lines of evidence suggest that they influence the susceptibility in the development of amyloidosis. Homozygosity in *SAA1.1* is a risk factor for the development of amyloidosis in Caucasian patients, whereas Japanese patients with RA, homozygous for the *SAA1.3* allele, are in increased risk. Single cell polymorphisms (SNP) in the *SAA1* gene have been also linked to amyloidosis. For example, a C/T switch at position −13 of *SAA1.3* is associated with increased susceptibility to amyloidosis in patients with RA. The presence of these polymorphic variants and SNP can at least in part explain the fact that not all patients with increased SAA levels develop amyloidosis [10, 35, 43].

Amyloid A derives from the proteolytic cleavage of SAA, which is constituted by 104 amino acids, which results in the removal of C-terminus of the native protein. The most commonly found amyloid A protein associated with glomerular infiltrates is a 76-amino-acid-long N-terminal fragment of the precursor SAA protein. However, other deposits are formed by a mixture of short (approximately 44 residues) and long (approximately 100 residues) fragments. The lack of the C-terminus region results in a protein derivative that is prone to conversion from the α-helix structure to a β-sheet, which is characteristic of the amyloid deposits and enables the formation of typical cross β-structures of amyloidosis. There is evidence that macrophages play a role in the proteolytic cleavage of SAA. It has been shown that phagocytosis of SAA results in its dissociation from HDL. C-terminus truncation, misfolding, and accumulation in lysosomes then take place. Cathepsin B has been identified as a protease involved in lysosomal cleavage of SAA, whereas the metalloproteinases MMP1, MMP2, and MMP3 are identified in extracellular amyloid deposits [10, 43–45].

Except from amyloid A, which is the main fibril protein in reactive amyloidosis, several other components are present in fibril deposits, which are present in all different types of amyloidosis. The most important are heparan sulfate proteoglycan (HSPG) and serum amyloid P component (SAP). These components play a major role in the pathogenesis of amyloidosis. HSPG has been shown to mediate the dissociation of SAA from HDL and to contribute in the formation of the β-sheet structure of the amyloid fibrils [46]. SAP is a glycoprotein belonging in the pentraxin family and a component of extracellular matrix. Its relative concentration can reach up to approximately 15% in amyloid deposits [47]. In vivo data from mice deficient in SAP show that this protein is not necessary for the formation of amyloid deposits [48]. However, due to its resistance to proteolysis, SAP prevents amyloid fibril degradation.

Prognosis

The prognosis of patients with AL amyloidosis is related to the involvement of the heart [49]. From laboratory testing of patients with cardiac AL amyloidosis, elevated myocardial necrosis indexes such as troponin I and T can be observed. In patients with increased troponin, the mean survival is significantly lower compared to that of normal troponin patients (6–8 months versus 21–22 months) [50]. Determination of the circulating free light chain (FLC) levels as well as NT-pro BNP values represents two valuable modalities which can assess patient prognosis as well as treatment efficacy [33, 51, 52]. There are no approved therapies for AL amyloidosis. Plasma cell-directed therapies, such as high-dose chemotherapy in combination with autologous stem cell transplantation, alkylating agents, steroids, proteasome inhibitors, and/or immunomodulatory drugs, reduce production of the immunoglobulin LC. Overall, such therapies can induce a reduction in the concentration of the toxic LC by ~50% in 60% of patients, and this translates into cardiac or renal response, or both, in 20–35% of patients [53].

AA amyloidosis is a severe complication of inflammatory disorders, which if left uncontrolled leads to increased mortality. End-stage renal disease, heart failure, and gastrointestinal bleeding or perforation are the main causes of death in these patients. In a study involving 374 patients with AA amyloidosis, there was a significant correlation between amyloid prognosis, renal function and mortality, and SAA levels during follow-up period. A significant regression in amyloid deposits, assessed by SAP scintigraphy, was observed in patients with SAA levels within the normal range (10 mg/L), which had a major effect in survival of these patients.

The direct correlation between the levels of SAA and survival in patients with AA amyloidosis underlines the fact that the best treatment option is the early identification of affected patients and induction of remission of the underlying inflammatory disorder. Treatment with biologic agents targeting cytokines, and especially TNF and IL-6, has been shown to decrease the incidence of amyloidosis in patients with chronic inflammatory disorders, making reactive amyloidosis a rare disorder in Western countries [10, 39, 54]. These agents do not target the amyloid deposits per se, but decrease the liver production of SAA, leading to normalization of its levels in the circulation. In patients with FMF, despite the effectiveness of IL-1 targeting therapies, colchicine administration remains the gold standard in the prevention of amyloidosis [25, 26].

Concluding Remarks

Systemic amyloidosis is a life-threatening disorder, characterized by the deposition of misfolded proteins in the extracellular space, leading to the disorganization of the tissue architecture and finally to organ damage and failure. The timely identification and the initiation of effective treatment in patients with inflammatory disorders prevent the development of this fatal complication. This underlines the critical importance of the awareness of the medical community for the early diagnosis of patients under increased risk for amyloidosis.

References

1. Merlini G, Bellotti V. Molecular mechanisms of amyloidosis. N Engl J Med. 2003 Aug 7;349(6):583–96.
2. Kisilevsky R. The relation of proteoglycans, serum amyloid P and apo E to amyloidosis current status, 2000. Amyloid Int J Exp Clin Investig Off J Int Soc Amyloidosis. 2000;7(1):23–5.
3. Sipe JD, Benson MD, Buxbaum JN, Ikeda S, Merlini G, Saraiva MJM, et al. Amyloid fibril protein nomenclature: 2012 recommendations from the Nomenclature Committee of the International Society of Amyloidosis. Amyloid Int J Exp Clin Investig Off J Int Soc Amyloidosis. 2012 Dec;19(4):167–70.
4. Hazenberg BPC. Amyloidosis: a clinical overview. Rheum Dis Clin N Am. 2013 May;39(2):323–45.
5. Kyle RA, Gertz MA. Primary systemic amyloidosis: clinical and laboratory features in 474 cases. Semin Hematol. 1995 Jan;32(1):45–59.
6. Kyle RA, Linos A, Beard CM, Linke RP, Gertz MA, O'Fallon WM, et al. Incidence and natural history of primary systemic amyloidosis in Olmsted County, Minnesota, 1950 through 1989. Blood. 1992;79(7):1817–22.
7. Comenzo RL, Zhang Y, Martinez C, Osman K, Herrera GA. The tropism of organ involvement in primary systemic amyloidosis: contributions of Ig V(L) germ line gene use and clonal plasma cell burden. Blood. 2001;98(3):714–20.
8. Lachmann HJ, Goodman HJB, Gilbertson JA, Gallimore JR, Sabin CA, Gillmore JD, et al. Natural history and outcome in systemic AA amyloidosis. N Engl J Med. 2007;356(23):2361–71.
9. Bunker D, Gorevic P. AA amyloidosis: Mount Sinai experience, 1997–2012. Mt Sinai J Med N Y. 2012;79(6):749–56.

10. Westermark GT, Fändrich M, Westermark P. AA amyloidosis: pathogenesis and targeted therapy. Annu Rev Pathol. 2015;10:321–44.
11. Andrade C. A peculiar form of peripheral neuropathy; familiar atypical generalized amyloidosis with special involvement of the peripheral nerves. Brain J Neurol. 1952 Sep;75(3):408–27.
12. Pomerance A. Senile cardiac amyloidosis. Br Heart J. 1965;27(5):711–8.
13. Tanskanen M, Peuralinna T, Polvikoski T, Notkola I-L, Sulkava R, Hardy J, et al. Senile systemic amyloidosis affects 25% of the very aged and associates with genetic variation in alpha2-macroglobulin and tau: a population-based autopsy study. Ann Med. 2008;40(3):232–9.
14. Liao R, Jain M, Teller P, Connors LH, Ngoy S, Skinner M, et al. Infusion of light chains from patients with cardiac amyloidosis causes diastolic dysfunction in isolated mouse hearts. Circulation. 2001;104(14):1594–7.
15. Wechalekar AD, Gillmore JD, Hawkins PN. Systemic amyloidosis. Lancet Lond Engl. 2016;387(10038):2641–54.
16. Falk RH. Diagnosis and management of the cardiac amyloidoses. Circulation. 2005;112(13):2047–60.
17. Dember LM. Emerging treatment approaches for the systemic amyloidoses. Kidney Int. 2005;68(3):1377–90.
18. Rapezzi C, Lorenzini M, Longhi S, Milandri A, Gagliardi C, Bartolomei I, et al. Cardiac amyloidosis: the great pretender. Heart Fail Rev. 2015;20(2):117–24.
19. Park MA, Mueller PS, Kyle RA, Larson DR, Plevak MF, Gertz MA. Primary (AL) hepatic amyloidosis: clinical features and natural history in 98 patients. Medicine (Baltimore). 2003;82(5):291–8.
20. Giancane G, Haar NMT, Wulffraat N, Vastert SJ, Barron K, Hentgen V, et al. Evidence-based recommendations for genetic diagnosis of familial Mediterranean fever. Ann Rheum Dis. 2015;74(4):635–41.
21. Twig G, Livneh A, Vivante A, Afek A, Shamiss A, Derazne E, et al. Mortality risk factors associated with familial Mediterranean fever among a cohort of 1.25 million adolescents. Ann Rheum Dis. 2014;73(4):704–9.
22. Touitou I, Sarkisian T, Medlej-Hashim M, Tunca M, Livneh A, Cattan D, et al. Country as the primary risk factor for renal amyloidosis in familial Mediterranean fever. Arthritis Rheum. 2007;56(5):1706–12.
23. Akpolat T, Özkaya O, Özen S. Homozygous M694V as a risk factor for amyloidosis in Turkish FMF patients. Gene. 2012;492(1):285–9.
24. Zemer D, Pras M, Sohar E, Modan M, Cabili S, Gafni J. Colchicine in the prevention and treatment of the amyloidosis of familial Mediterranean fever. N Engl J Med. 1986;314(16):1001–5.
25. Ozen S, Demirkaya E, Erer B, Livneh A, Ben-Chetrit E, Giancane G, et al. EULAR recommendations for the management of familial Mediterranean fever. Ann Rheum Dis. 2016;75(4):644–51.
26. Hentgen V, Grateau G, Kone-Paut I, Livneh A, Padeh S, Rozenbaum M, et al. Evidence-based recommendations for the practical management of familial Mediterranean fever. Semin Arthritis Rheum. 2013;43(3):387–91.
27. ter Haar NM, Oswald M, Jeyaratnam J, Anton J, Barron KS, Brogan PA, et al. Recommendations for the management of autoinflammatory diseases. Ann Rheum Dis. 2015;74(9):1636–44.
28. Lane T, Loeffler JM, Rowczenio DM, Gilbertson JA, Bybee A, Russell TL, et al. AA amyloidosis complicating the hereditary periodic fever syndromes. Arthritis Rheum. 2013;65(4):1116–21.
29. Lachmann HJ, Papa R, Gerhold K, Obici L, Touitou I, Cantarini L, et al. The phenotype of TNF receptor-associated autoinflammatory syndrome (TRAPS) at presentation: a series of 158 cases from the Eurofever/EUROTRAPS international registry. Ann Rheum Dis. 2014;73(12):2160–7.
30. Libbey CA, Skinner M, Cohen AS. Use of abdominal fat tissue aspirate in the diagnosis of systemic amyloidosis. Arch Intern Med. 1983;143(8):1549–52.
31. Rapezzi C, Quarta CC, Guidalotti PL, Pettinato C, Fanti S, Leone O, et al. Role of (99m) Tc-DPD scintigraphy in diagnosis and prognosis of hereditary transthyretin-related cardiac amyloidosis. JACC Cardiovasc Imaging. 2011;4(6):659–70.

32. Gillmore JD, Maurer MS, Falk RH, Merlini G, Damy T, Dispenzieri A, et al. Nonbiopsy diagnosis of cardiac transthyretin amyloidosis. Circulation. 2016;133(24):2404–12.
33. Abraham RS, Katzmann JA, Clark RJ, Bradwell AR, Kyle RA, Gertz MA. Quantitative analysis of serum free light chains. A new marker for the diagnostic evaluation of primary systemic amyloidosis. Am J Clin Pathol. 2003;119(2):274–8.
34. Perugini E, Rapezzi C, Piva T, Leone O, Bacchi-Reggiani L, Riva L, et al. Non-invasive evaluation of the myocardial substrate of cardiac amyloidosis by gadolinium cardiac magnetic resonance. Heart. 2006;92(3):343–9.
35. Booth DR, Booth SE, Gillmore JD, Hawkins PN, Pepys MB. SAA1 alleles as risk factors in reactive systemic AA amyloidosis. Amyloid. 1998;5(4):262–5.
36. Kisilevsky R, Manley PN. Acute-phase serum amyloid a: perspectives on its physiological and pathological roles. Amyloid Int J Exp Clin Investig Off J Int Soc Amyloidosis. 2012;19(1):5–14.
37. Yoshizaki K. Pathogenic role of IL-6 combined with TNF-α or IL-1 in the induction of acute phase proteins SAA and CRP in chronic inflammatory diseases. Adv Exp Med Biol. 2011;691:141–50.
38. Solomon A, Weiss DT, Schell M, Hrncic R, Murphy CL, Wall J, et al. Transgenic mouse model of AA amyloidosis. Am J Pathol. 1999;154(4):1267–72.
39. Courties A, Grateau G, Philippe P, Flipo R-M, Astudillo L, Aubry-Rozier B, et al. AA amyloidosis treated with tocilizumab: case series and updated literature review. Amyloid Int J Exp Clin Investig Off J Int Soc Amyloidosis. 2015;22(2):84–92.
40. Okuda Y, Takasugi K. Successful use of a humanized anti-interleukin-6 receptor antibody, tocilizumab, to treat amyloid A amyloidosis complicating juvenile idiopathic arthritis. Arthritis Rheum. 2006 Sep;54(9):2997–3000.
41. Ugurlu S, Hacioglu A, Adibnia Y, Hamuryudan V, Ozdogan H. Tocilizumab in the treatment of twelve cases with aa amyloidosis secondary to familial mediterranean fever. Orphanet J Rare Dis. 2017;12(1):105.
42. Gillmore JD, Lovat LB, Persey MR, Pepys MB, Hawkins PN. Amyloid load and clinical outcome in AA amyloidosis in relation to circulating concentration of serum amyloid A protein. Lancet. 2001;358(9275):24–9.
43. Sun L, Ye RD. Serum amyloid A1: structure, function and gene polymorphism. Gene. 2016;583(1):48–57.
44. Stix B, Kähne T, Sletten K, Raynes J, Roessner A, Röcken C. Proteolysis of AA amyloid fibril proteins by matrix metalloproteinases-1, −2, and −3. Am J Pathol. 2001;159(2):561–70.
45. Chronopoulos S, Laird DW, Ali-Khan Z. Immunolocalization of serum amyloid A and AA amyloid in lysosomes in murine monocytoid cells: confocal and immunogold electron microscopic studies. J Pathol. 1994;173(4):361–9.
46. Noborn F, O'Callaghan P, Hermansson E, Zhang X, Ancsin JB, Damas AM, et al. Heparan sulfate/heparin promotes transthyretin fibrillization through selective binding to a basic motif in the protein. Proc Natl Acad Sci U S A. 2011;108(14):5584–9.
47. Bodin K, Ellmerich S, Kahan MC, Tennent GA, Loesch A, Gilbertson JA, et al. Antibodies to human serum amyloid P component eliminate visceral amyloid deposits. Nature. 2010;468(7320):93–7.
48. Inoue S, Kawano H, Ishihara T, Maeda S, Ohno S. Formation of experimental murine AA amyloid fibrils in SAP-deficient mice: high resolution ultrastructural study. Amyloid Int J Exp Clin Investig Off J Int Soc Amyloidosis. 2005;12(3):157–63.
49. Merlini G, Seldin DC, Gertz MA. Amyloidosis: pathogenesis and new therapeutic options. J Clin Oncol Off J Am Soc Clin Oncol. 2011;29(14):1924–33.
50. Dispenzieri A, Kyle RA, Gertz MA, Therneau TM, Miller WL, Chandrasekaran K, et al. Survival in patients with primary systemic amyloidosis and raised serum cardiac troponins. Lancet Lond Engl. 2003;361(9371):1787–9.
51. Kumar S, Dispenzieri A, Katzmann JA, Larson DR, Colby CL, Lacy MQ, et al. Serum immunoglobulin free light-chain measurement in primary amyloidosis: prognostic value and correlations with clinical features. Blood. 2010;116(24):5126–9.

52. Palladini G, Campana C, Klersy C, Balduini A, Vadacca G, Perfetti V, et al. Serum N-terminal pro-brain natriuretic peptide is a sensitive marker of myocardial dysfunction in AL amyloidosis. Circulation. 2003;107(19):2440–5.
53. Wechalekar AD, Gillmore JD, Bird J, Cavenagh J, Hawkins S, Kazmi M, et al. Guidelines on the management of AL amyloidosis. Br J Haematol. 2015;168(2):186–206.
54. Esatoglu SN, Hatemi G, Ugurlu S, Gokturk A, Tascilar K, Ozdogan H. Long-term follow-up of secondary amyloidosis patients treated with tumor necrosis factor inhibitor therapy: a STROBE-compliant observational study. Medicine (Baltimore). 2017 Aug;96(34):e7859.

Index

P. Efthimiou (ed.), *Auto-Inflammatory Syndromes*,
https://doi.org/10.1007/978-3-319-96929-9

D

R

S

MIX
Papier aus verantwortungsvollen Quellen
Paper from responsible sources
FSC® C105338

If you have any concerns about our products,
you can contact us on
ProductSafety@springernature.com

In case Publisher is established outside the EU,
the EU authorized representative is:
Springer Nature Customer Service Center GmbH
Europaplatz 3, 69115 Heidelberg, Germany

Printed by Libri Plureos GmbH
in Hamburg, Germany